La Mettrie

Medicine, Philosophy,

and Enlightenment

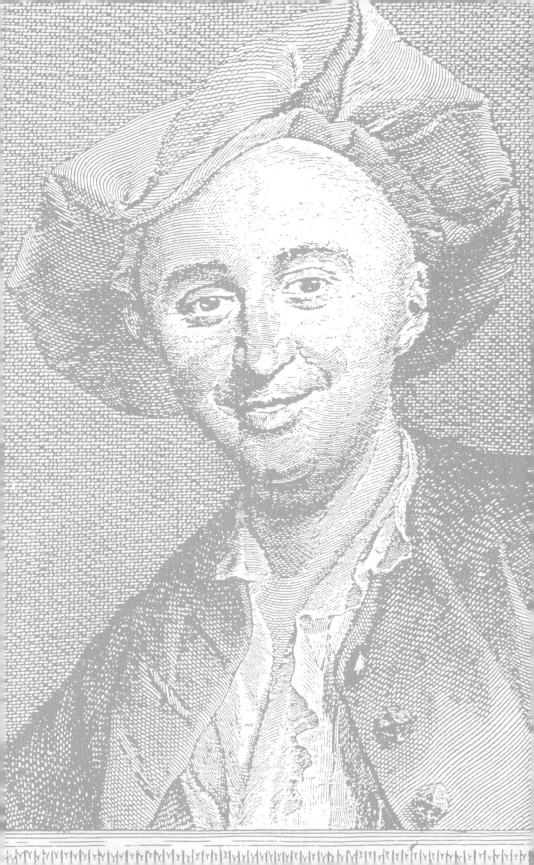

La Mettrie

Medicine, Philosophy, and Enlightenment

Kathleen Wellman

Duke University Press

Durham and London

1992

Chapter 5 is a revised version of a previously published article,
"La Mettrie's *Institutions de Médecine*: A Reinterpretation of the
Boerhaavian Legacy," *Janus* 72, no. 4 (1985): 283–304.

Library of Congress Cataloging-in-Publication Data
Wellman, Kathleen Anne, 1951–
La Mettrie : medicine, philosophy, and enlightenment / Kathleen Wellman.
p. cm.
Includes bibliographical references and index.
ISBN 0-8223-1204-2 (acid-free paper)
1. La Mettrie, Julien Offray de, 1709–1751.
2. Physicians—France—Biography.
3. Philosophers—France—Biography. I. Title.
R507.L193W46   1992
610'.92—dc20
[B] 91-23992
CIP

*Frontispiece illustration: Engraving of Julien Offray de La Mettrie.
Courtesy of the National Library of Medicine, Bethesda, Maryland.*

for Dennis

Contents

Preface

This project began as an attempt to reassess the role of La Mettrie in the Enlightenment by studying his medicine as well as his philosophy. I was and remain convinced both that the medical tradition is the most convincing way to understand La Mettrie's philosophy and that it defines a prominent strain in the thought of French materialists which distinguishes their contribution to the French Enlightenment. Construed narrowly, then, this study argues that medicine makes sense of La Mettrie and to a significant degree of the other French materialists as well. But I also want to suggest that an integration of medicine and philosophy adds a crucial component to the Enlightenment as a whole. Medicine, understood in its broadest dimensions as encompassing physiology, philosophical discussions of nature, and the pragmatic and therapeutic concerns of the practitioner, is a significant feature of Enlightenment criticism of traditional metaphysics and absolutist institutions and of arguments for the utility of science. Eighteenth-century medicine, as an amalgam of theory and practice wedded to a broad philosophical base, played a fundamental role in the evolution of the Enlightenment, a movement with a new sense of the nature and purpose of philosophy, with new tools and agendas for reform and new roles and definitions for intellectuals. Specifically, medicine suggested an integration of the abstract and the utilitarian, afforded empirical evidence for a critique of metaphysics, allowed the development of a naturalist understanding of human nature, and impelled an examination of existing institutions and their effects on human beings in light of a new understanding of human nature. La Mettrie is a crucial figure in the articulation and evolution of this medical concern.

Because the compartmentalization of disciplines and the divisions which we have constructed between the humanities and the sciences was foreign to the eighteenth century, an integration of medicine and philosophy not only affords a clearer view of the mental landscape of the eighteenth century but also allows one to integrate the historiographic treatment of the Enlightenment and the history of science. These two traditions have followed the same general evolution in the past thirty years: from a discussion of great figures, to the involvement of those figures in political and scientific institutions, to institutional histories, to the impact of eighteenth-century medicine on popular culture. All of these approaches have broadened our understanding of the eighteenth century, and they must affect the way in which history is subsequently written. We must understand great figures within their context and be aware of the political dimensions of intellectual change; the effects of institutional evolution on individuals and events must be taken into account. In general, recent approaches to the Enlightenment have impelled a heightened responsiveness to the context of ideas, individuals, and events. But as we learn more about the past, we must also reexamine what we take for granted about its intellectual dimensions. Does the traditionally acknowledged muddle of Newtonianism and Lockeanism accurately reflect the intellectual inheritance which the philosophes used as a foundation for social reform? This study argues that this picture needs to be amplified and emended. Consider, for example, Enlightenment studies written fifty years ago, before the Enlightenment could be used to foreshadow totalitarianism, before the "discovery" of Diderot and the *Encyclopédie*, and long before the acknowledgment of anything but an elite culture. These studies assert a more positivistic Enlightenment, a movement with clear and direct connections to American democracy, concerned almost solely with political reform. More recent pictures are more diverse but less conclusive. Did the real Enlightenment take place among the philosophes in salons or the literary hacks on grub street? The philosophes, no longer gifted with political omniscience, are allowed a degree of political insight, albeit marred by a fundamental conservatism and disdain for the common man. But they have also been cast as diabolical initiators of schemes which produced totalitarianism. And the once obvious ties between the Enlightenment and the French Revolution have all but dissipated, leaving the connection between ideas and events in a netherworld and the question of the decisive cause of the political events of the Revolution, as distinct from centuries of bread riots, indeterminate. These are just a few of the issues which were not commonly raised when earlier truisms about the intellectual roots of the Enlightenment came into vogue. Just as our understanding of the Enlightenment has been broadened, so too must assessments of its important intellectual forebears and the roles of certain individuals in the movement be reexamined in light of evolving perceptions and new information about the Enlightenment and its ramifications. To this end I offer this study of La Mettrie and his role in the medicalization of the Enlightenment.

In carrying out this study I have made certain assumptions and followed certain directions which allow me to avoid some of the questions which have structured and, I would suggest, plagued La Mettrie scholarship. First, I have not tried to follow out literary references to determine influences on La Mettrie. There are significant seventeenth-century literary influences on his work, some of which have been well discussed elsewhere.[1] But instead of following out these sometimes illuminating, sometimes tantalizingly inconclusive comparisons, I have chosen to take La Mettrie's literary, philosophical, and scientific heritage as he explicitly used them. Second, I have been concerned to present La Mettrie as the author of a fundamentally coherent body of writings on medical and philosophical issues. This is a change of emphasis from most of the recent scholarship on La Mettrie, which has produced annotated editions of specific texts with monographic introductions. These editions assert the importance of a particular work by presenting it as a distinctive evolution or break in La Mettrie's thinking. While shifts of emphasis do occur,[2] La Mettrie's philosophical and medical works present a striking consistency, a consistency explained in part by the short span of the author's writings, 1735–1750, and borne out by internal references and allusions to the development of themes across La Mettrie's writings. Finally, I have chosen to consider only in the final section the problematic question of La Mettrie's personality and the reception of his works, because such discussions usually degenerate into apologies or denunciations. I am attempting an apology in that I mean to argue that medicine ties together his whole corpus and that his medical interpretation of

Enlightenment issues gave him an important role to play in the Enlightenment. While other philosophes have had new reputations rescued from previous disrepute and neglect (consider, for example, the striking resurgence in interest in Diderot), La Mettrie is apparently in an almost unsalvageable position because he had no contemporary defenders. Recent scholarship has cast him into a new kind of disrepute, as insane or as an early source of totalitarian thought, or has caused him to suffer a new kind of neglect, considered important for only one idea, *l'homme machine*. My purpose is to present the whole of La Mettrie's medical and philosophical work, to claim that the whole is structured and informed by the concerns of eighteenth-century medical practice and theory, and to chronicle his application of medical concerns to the fundamental issues of the French Enlightenment.

Acknowledgments

The completion of a first book is the result of such a long history of influence that the debts incurred are too numerous to fully acknowledge. Friends and colleagues at the University of Chicago, in Paris, at Stanford, the University of Dallas, the University of Wisconsin-Milwaukee, and Southern Methodist University all form part of this project. They have provided the support and stimulation of intellectual communities and made scholarship both rewarding and part of a common endeavor.

This project owes a great deal to the Georges Lurcy Foundation, which funded my research in Paris and gave me a year to devote my entire attention to La Mettrie. In Paris, Jacques Roger made me welcome in his seminar, which helped me to define certain issues in the natural sciences of the eighteenth century. To Marjorie Grene and the members of the National Endowment for the Humanities seminar she directed, I owe a greater understanding of Descartes. My earliest interest in the philosophy of this period was awakened and nurtured by Norton Nelkin.

I am particularly indebted to members of my dissertation committee at the University of Chicago. Allen G. Debus developed my interest in the history of science, and I appreciate his continued enthusiasm for this project. Keith M. Baker has been an inspiring model of excellence in eighteenth-century studies, and I am grateful to him for his always perspicacious reading of my material.

I would like to thank Larry Malley and Pam Morrison of Duke University Press for their expeditious handling of the manuscript.

My children, Elizabeth and Matthew, have understood with

good cheer the demands of my book their entire lives. My husband, Dennis Sepper, has also lived with this book a long time. I am grateful to him not only for his sustaining love and support but also for his editing skills. This book is dedicated to him.

La Mettrie

Medicine, Philosophy,
and Enlightenment

Introduction

The first half of the eighteenth century was a period of intense intellectual germination which flowered in the movement commonly called the Enlightenment. This movement reappraised the institutions and conventions of the eighteenth century with daring and verve. One of the most appealing things about the Enlightenment is its tremendous intellectual energy. With no compartmentalization of disciplines, it was the last era when all of human knowledge was assumed to be accessible to the well-educated individual. As a result, the philosophes, as the standard-bearers of the new movement called themselves, felt free to explicate Newtonian physics or popularize the metaphysics of John Locke. They assumed that the past could be recast in terms which would allow them to address not only the intellectual issues of the day but also the social and political concerns. Modest souls they were not. The story of the reinterpretations of the past has been admirably told in works of the intellectual history of the movement. The evolution from the classical literature of the seventeenth century to the polemical, philosophical literature of the eighteenth, from the metaphysics of the seventeenth-century rationalist to the social sciences of the eighteenth-century philosophe has come to form part of the conventional understanding of the Enlightenment. But this evolution is perhaps less straightforward and less consistent than a historiographical overview suggests. An examination of the careers and writings of such diverse eighteenth-century intellectuals as Montesquieu, Voltaire, Rousseau, and Diderot suggest that there were many distinct routes to Enlightenment. Julien Offray de La Mettrie chose a particularly unconventional but fruitful approach to both the traditions of the past and the emerging new intellectual movement. Both his criticisms of the old and his involvement in the new were determined by his understanding of medicine. In essence, he medicalized the Enlightenment.

Medicalization has been cast by historians like Michel Foucault as a modern villain, an authoritarian imposition by the medical profession of its authority at the expense of rival but less powerful popular practitioners. Whether or not these charges can be empirically substantiated, this diabolical intention does not seem relevant to the kind of authority La Mettrie intended for the reform-minded physician or surgeon. In fact, La Mettrie also campaigned for public health, or a control by the public of their own health which would have challenged all medical authorities.

La Mettrie's medicalization must also be understood in large part as an attempt to interpret the concerns of the Enlightenment in medical terms. His entire body of work, both medical and philosophical, is clearly the product of the medical concerns, issues, and theories of the late seventeenth and early eighteenth centuries. But he took those medical concerns and cast them in Enlightenment terms, deliberately identifying himself with the new intellectual movement and arguing the concerns of public health and public knowledge against corporate privilege. His medicalization reinterpreted the past and commented on the social, scientific, and intellectual issues which produced the Enlightenment. For example, he attacked conventional metaphysics and addressed the notion of nature and human nature, and the nature and purpose of the philosophes, by the standards of good medical theory and practice. In the hands of La Mettrie, the Enlightenment was to be understood as a movement informed by the principles of medical practice and theory, a movement in which the concerns of the theologian had to yield to the reform-minded physician, discussions of nature had to be sustained by empirical observation, and discussions of human nature had to take into consideration the aberrant and the deviant; that is, primacy was to be given to the evidence of direct observations of both sick and well individuals. The philosophe was to judge by the standards of medicine. The issues of contemporary medicine gave La Mettrie a critical perspective and a reformist stance. His analysis and criticism of the established medical order made him an able polemicist well equipped to use those stylistic tools and the evidence of contemporary science in the cause of Enlightenment.

Although some recent studies of the history of science and philosophy in the eighteenth century take serious enough note of La Mettrie to dedicate a few pages to him, general studies in the Enlightenment rarely accord him more than a few perfunctory remarks, which serve either to perpetuate simplistic notions of his philosophy or to repeat the defamatory remarks of his critics. For example, Paul Hazard mentions La Mettrie only to turn *L'Homme machine* into a joke at La Mettrie's expense. "There was more matter in him than in the general run of men . . . his machine broke down, indigestion was the trouble." Ernst Cassirer treats La Mettrie, Helvétius, and d'Holbach as a collective unit, denigrating the writings of the materialists as "having no characteristic significance" and as a "retrogression into the dogmatic mode of thinking which the leading scientific minds of the eighteenth century oppose and endeavor to eliminate." Because they rejected the certainty of the mathematical sciences and chose instead to orient their thought around biological and physiological considerations, Cassirer demotes the materialists to the rank of scientific dilettantes. Although Peter Gay readily concedes that La Mettrie influenced d'Holbach, Helvétius, and Diderot and mentions him in connection with eighteenth-century science and the fight against excessive rationalism, he is primarily concerned with his "little flock," which does not include La Mettrie.[1]

In part, the neglect of La Mettrie in general discussions of the Enlightenment is due to his problematic chronological relationship to it. He wrote during the 1740s and was dead by 1751. On the eve of the encyclopedic movement, he produced works of materialist philosophy, a philosophy more characteristic of the 1770s than of the early Enlightenment. Though he identified with them, La Mettrie was a liability to the philosophes in the 1750s, especially since their enemies singled him out as representative of the excesses and the dangers posed to society by philosophy. Defamed in the 1750s and 1760s by philosophe and antiphilosophe alike and tarred with a thoroughly unsavory reputation, La Mettrie was an unlikely candidate for rehabilitation by the philosophes in the 1770s. Indeed, few subsequent historians have looked beyond defamatory remarks about La Mettrie or his own outrageous statements to investigate the content of his philosophical work.

More problematic than the expedient disavowal of La Mettrie by the philosophes or his neglect in general works on the Enlightenment are the uses to which his most outrageous remarks have been put by some modern historians. The materialists as a group have been much abused. Historians such as Jacob L. Talmon have decried their political theories as responsible for the rise of the totalitarian state.[2] Marxist historians have distorted them into early, if not particularly perceptive, forerunners of Marx.[3] La Mettrie in particular has been resurrected from relative obscurity to be held responsible for the ills of the twentieth century. Lester Crocker considers de Sade to be the founder of nihilism and the only possible culmination of Enlightenment efforts for political and social reform. Crocker explains de Sade by turning to La Mettrie as the author of a philosophy which denied man a special place in the universe and created the "absurd." The moderate Enlightenment is cast as a doomed battle against the nihilist implications of La Mettrie's ethics. Without God and the Christian world order, the progression from La Mettrie to de Sade to twentieth-century totalitarianism and nihilism is, for Crocker, inevitable.[4]

Recent studies have accorded La Mettrie some measure of importance and influence in eighteenth-century philosophy by studying specific texts. Aram Vartanian's edition of *L'Homme machine* with his monographic introduction has been most influential in provoking interest in La Mettrie. Vartanian considers La Mettrie to be significant in the evolution of the concept of *bête machine* to *homme machine*, which he traced in his work *Diderot and Descartes*, and his critical edition of *L'Homme machine* thoroughly discusses the evolution of that notion. By virtue of his extensive footnotes to La Mettrie's text, Vartanian is able to demonstrate the connection between La Mettrie's text and biological, physiological, and philosophical issues of the seventeenth and eighteenth centuries. John Falvey's critical edition of the *Discours sur le bonheur* draws connections between La Mettrie and seventeenth-century moralists. Ann Thomson's introduction to her critical edition of the *Discours préliminaire* discusses the structure and themes of the text and influences on it. And Theo Verbeek's recent edition of the *Traité de l'âme* has discussed the sources, especially in the clandestine literature, of this fundamental work.[5] All of these studies have been important in adding depth to our understanding of La Mettrie, a depth which has taken him beyond the simplistic clichés and disparaging remarks which are the basis of his critical reputation.

However, these critical editions have been most concerned with establishing the antecedents of La Mettrie's work. As a result, they invariably place him in the context of the seventeenth century rather than treat his contemporary impact.

All of these uses and abuses of La Mettrie's philosophy have failed to treat it as a whole. But what seems particularly striking in La Mettrie's work is its seamless quality.[6] His entire philosophy applies his scientific knowledge to philosophical questions such as the nature of matter and human beings and the relationship of human beings to nature and society. La Mettrie investigated with an eye to humanitarian reform, especially to the alleviation of human suffering, specifically of those unfortunates whose physiological constitutions inclined them to nonconformism. Reforming zeal, rather than nihilism, motivated some of his most shocking remarks.

La Mettrie's philosophic works are clearly interrelated in terms of the issues they discuss and the examples they use, and they quite clearly follow one from another. In his earliest works he defined an epistemology, then provided empirical evidence for it, and finally addressed its implications for our understanding of nature and man in society. Through his philosophy, he expanded his humanitarian quest for medical reform and public health to address broader issues of Enlightenment. He intended to destroy metaphysical notions of human beings and to enforce a naturalistic understanding of man so that social institutions could better serve human needs. His most vehement crusade was for tolerance and understanding of the con- stitutionally maladjusted, the individual who is "socially ill."

The outlines of La Mettrie's biography are well known because he was such a scandalous figure. But beyond the general outline there is such a dearth of documentary evidence that the main source of information remains the *éloge* delivered by Frederick the Great.[7] Some details of that *éloge* have been corrected or questioned by the painstaking research of Pierre Lemée and Ann Thomson.[8]

La Mettrie was born in Saint-Malo in Brittany on December 19, 1709. Thus he was approximately the age of the second generation of philosophes (Diderot, b. 1713, and Buffon, b. 1707), those whose philosophic works began to appear at mid-century. La Mettrie was the son of a well-to-do textile merchant, who was able to give him a good education. He attended the provincial colleges of Coutance and Caen and then the Collège du Plessis in Paris, where he was very much influenced by Jansenism, so much so that, at least according to Frederick's *éloge*, he produced a Jansenist tract, which unfortunately has never been found. In 1725 he enrolled in the Collège d'Harcourt to study philosophy and natural science. (The college was the first academic institution to permit the introduction of Cartesianism into the curriculum.) After he received his degree, he spent five years at the Faculty of Paris studying medicine. In order to evade the high cost of completing a medical degree in Paris, La Mettrie went to the University of Reims for three months and at the end of that period received his medical degree. Finding his medical education an insufficient preparation for medical practice, he went to Leyden to study with Hermann Boerhaave for two years before returning home to practice in Saint-Malo. He subsequently served as a personal physician to the Duke de Grammont and as physician to a battalion of the *gardes françaises*. During this period he began to publish the works that made him a pariah to both the Faculty of Paris and to the orthodox—that is, his medical satires and his materialist philosophy. Because of the outrage provoked by the satires and his first philosophical work, *L'Histoire naturelle de l'âme*, he was exiled to Holland. When *L'Homme machine* (1747) proved to be too radical even for the tolerant Dutch, La Mettrie sought refuge at the court of Frederick the Great, where he died in 1751 after eating contaminated pâté.[9]

The facts of this sketch are common knowledge, but a more detailed account of La Mettrie's life has proven frustratingly elusive. Few letters have been found, and no personal papers exist to illuminate the man behind the notoriety. Historians have been tempted to flesh out the persona of La Mettrie on the basis of his published writings. This has been a popular technique for both those who seek grist for a defamatory mill and those who seek greater recognition for a misunderstood thinker. The stylistic complexities and obscurities of his texts have led some to conclude that he was insane or drunk.[10] Others have reveled in his concern with sexuality as an aspect of human health, hailing him as a prescient source of modern attitudes.[11] Intriguing as some of these speculations are, they cannot be conclusively supported and do not provide enough material to add appreciably to the basic biographical sketch. As a subject of study La Mettrie poses certain difficulties not only because of the lack of biographical material but also because of the nature of his specific context. Intellectual historians, responding to the legitimate criticisms of social historians, have sought to ground intellectual figures in concrete contexts of their class, profession, career, and so forth. However, La Mettrie is also frustrating in this respect; his specific context is the world of elite medicine, which places him squarely within the *intellectual* context of the contemporary issues of physiology and philosophy. In this study I therefore have sought to contextualize La Mettrie's philosophy in the world of medicine, both theoretical and practical.

La Mettrie was made acutely aware of the issues of the profession and the practice of medicine while he was a medical student in Paris. The primary issue of that period was the conflict between the doctors and the surgeons. It was a quarrel not only about the issues of professionalism—that is, who would control education, who would have preeminence among medical practitioners, and how membership in the profession would be controlled—but also about such crucial questions as the proper education for the practitioner and the correct method and theory of practice.

La Mettrie aroused the indignation of his fellow physicians by espousing the cause of the surgeons in their pamphlet war with the doctors. He was the only doctor to do so. He accepted the surgeons' arguments that they, not the doctors, represented the hope for the progress of medicine and incorporated Enlightenment ideals. He also apparently found the surgeons closer to his ideal medical practitioner than the doctors, whose foibles he used as rich material for satire. Within the context of the issues raised in the pamphlet war, he came to develop a conception of the ideal physician.

Hermann Boerhaave was his model of both medical theory and practice. Boerhaave's classes revealed to him the poverty of his own medical education and led him to expose the failings of members of the Parisian medical community. Boerhaave's medical theory provided the foundation for his own discussion of the philosophy of nature. In fact, La Mettrie's critical assessment of Boerhaave's medicine enabled him to develop fundamental perspectives from which he later investigated philosophical questions.

La Mettrie's involvement in issues of medical practice and theory must be thoroughly discussed because medicine was the determining factor in the formation of his entire philosophy. It was the basis of his conception of nature, especially human nature, and was the cutting edge against which any metaphysical notions were to be examined. Medicine thus epitomized the true method of scientific investigation and experimentation, and its empirical rigor could vanquish metaphysics.

Though disillusioned with the practice of medicine in France, La Mettrie considered the competent medical practitioner to be the quintessential man of humanity and social responsibility. Where medicine offered a hope for a more naturalistic understanding of nature, the *médecin-philosophe* might be able to reform social institutions in accord with that understanding. This book will examine the development of La Mettrie's medical philosophy and his deliberate and explicit redefinition of crucial Enlightenment issues according to the concerns of medicine.

1

A Source of Medical Enlightenment

The Conflict between the Doctors
and the Surgeons

Medicine was particularly important to the philosophes because of their concern with the social utility of the sciences. As one historian has neatly summarized this interest, "Nothing could be plainer than this: Medicine was philosophy at work; philosophy was medicine for the individual and society."[1] This interest in science, particularly in medicine, proclaimed by Enlightenment thinkers themselves, should provoke us to seek an understanding of the practice and theory of science and medicine in the eighteenth century and its influence on Enlightenment philosophy. La Mettrie provides a particularly illuminating perspective from which to examine the intriguing relationship between science, medicine, and philosophy.

But despite the concern of the philosophes with medicine, concrete and explicit connections between medicine and the Enlightenment have not received a great deal of attention. Histories of eighteenth-century medicine quite frequently purport to treat the entire century but then rush eagerly from the chaos of eighteenth-century theory and practice to the more appealing saga of the medical reforms of the Revolution and the professionalization of medicine in the nineteenth century. Perhaps this neglect is the result of the fact that in some respects eighteenth-century medicine does not lend support to a Whiggish story of medical progress, since it confronts one at every turn with the arcane. The descriptions of diseases found in eighteenth-century medical texts are only sometimes recognizable to modern physicians. Even discussions of the treatment of diseases found in the works of the best-educated medical practitioners are much more likely to horrify than to edify. Poor education (or at least what seems an impractical education for the physician), dishearteningly ineffective methods of treatment (reflected in high patient mortality rates), bizarre and arcane discussions of diseases and treatments, and vested self-interest, venality, and chaos in medical practice are factors that might discourage one from investigating this unsavory scene in detail. In sum, eighteenth-century medicine is both baffling in its diverse manifestations and somewhat unedifying in its lack of efficacy.[2]

In fact, the actual practice of medicine in eighteenth-century France might lead one to think that the nature of the relationship between Enlightenment and medicine was simply one of vain and unreasonably optimistic hopes on the part of the philosophes. But while the actual practices and professional standards of eighteenth-century medicine are not edifying, the records left by physicians in medical texts and case studies produce a more positive assessment thereof. In other words, removed from the considerations of whether the practices of physicians actually produced decisive improvements in health, medical texts treat issues in ways which can be correlated to Enlightenment concerns, especially to its crucial quest to ameliorate the human condition. The pamphlet war between the doctors and the surgeons, which was waged with particular intensity between 1724 and 1750, offers a possible source for reform which the philosophes recognized as implicit in the application of medicine to the ills of society. That is not to suggest that the philosophes were directly inspired by the intense vituperative and sometimes even violent demonstrations of professional rancor involved in this pamphlet war. (Indeed, the concerns of philosophes with the destructive tenor of the pamphlet war are explicitly demonstrated in Diderot's "Lettre d'un citoyen zélé.")[3] Nonetheless, the issues developed during this polemic might well have suggested to the philosophes reasons to be hopeful about what medicine offered and might be able to accomplish.

The pamphlet war itself was the crucial professional issue for the doctors and surgeons of Paris in the formative years of the Enlightenment. In the narrowest sense it dealt with issues of professionalization and provided a particularly useful vehicle for gauging professional issues. While the heat of polemic invited charges and countercharges and promoted inflammatory rhetoric exaggerating the merits of one's case and the deficiencies of one's opponents, a pamphlet war also provided the opportunity for developing a clear and cogent set of arguments about good medicine and the social advantages good medicine would produce. And this particular pamphlet war advocated a new criterion by which medical practice and education should be judged. Some pamphlets were addressed to the king, the traditional adjudicator in disputes between doctors and surgeons, but as the arguments came to focus less on questions of precedent and more on the issue of public good, the surgeons in particular sought to present their case before a new body, one remote from royal strictures and a corporate hierarchy that deemed them subservient to the doctors; they made their arguments in the interest of the public and sought to bring those arguments before the undefined and unspecified authority of public opinion. Thus they sought to shift authority from the king and the medical corporation to public opinion and to redefine the nature of the profession as independent from traditional privilege, sustained instead by public service.

Although the pamphlet war suggests that the surgeons succeeded in defining and implementing the agenda for medical reform in France, it is a limited source for the complicated social history of medical practice.[4] Participants did not address the specific issues of medical education and practice outside of Paris, nor did the advocates on either side see their positions as rectifying medical deficiencies in rural areas. It was instead a controversy between the two most elite medical groups in France. And while they had influence outside of Paris and were certainly interested in extending it, they did not actually practice except among the wealthiest members of Parisian society. (The practice of elite surgeons would have been somewhat more extensive in both social and geographical terms.) Thus their contentious disputes over medical practice and theory would have had very little immediate impact beyond their narrow circle. However, this debate set the agenda and defined the shape of medical reforms that were more widely extended and imposed in the nineteenth century. Although the pamphlet war does not provide a detailed picture of the diversity of French medical practice, it effectively underscores the affinities between the positions taken by the surgeons of Saint-Côme[5] and the optimistic expectations for medicine held by the philosophes.

The barrage of invective, charges, and countercharges produced suggest that the pamphlet war, which raged in Paris between 1724 and 1750, appears to be simply a particularly vociferous professional squabble. However, the professional issues and medical concerns which divided the doctors and surgeons had important ramifications. Within the context of this war, both doctors and surgeons came to articulate positions on medical practice and theory. From those positions emerged attacks on privilege and arguments for medical reform, criticisms of existing institutions and systems of education, and the beginnings of a campaign for public health. While the initial point of contention was whether the surgeons would be allowed to throw off their subservience to the doctors, especially insofar as the education of the surgeons was concerned, the debate had far broader implications.

The surgeons of Saint-Côme used every legislative gain to work toward the establishment of a university-educated surgical elite, a goal which set them definitively apart from the uneducated empirics. They also argued for reforms in medical education and practice, emphasizing, even as early as the 1720s and 1730s, the empirical and the clinical as the proper foundation of medicine. They asserted the necessity of practical education and the incorporation of chemistry and anatomy into medical education and practice. Offering an education based on both theory and practice, and identifying themselves with the promulgation of the fruits of the scientific revolution, the surgeons also defined the medical reforms that were decisive in the revolutionary period in France.[6] Those reforms united the doctors and the surgeons under the surgeons' standards of medical practice and education rather than those of the physicians. In distinct contrast to the physicians, the surgeons argued for a new kind of medical education, one which was to be both empirical and theoretical. Their practice made extensive use of the clinics and the hospitals. Moreover, the surgeons of the eighteenth century proposed to set themselves up as men educated in the liberal arts and well studied in the practical application of their art and craft; the surgeon was to be a model of the Enlightenment man of science and a foreshadowing of the nineteenth-century physician. Thus the history of the surgeons may well be a key to bridging both the differences in medical practice of the eighteenth and nineteenth centuries and the epistemic differences between these periods as defined by Foucault.

Finally, the surgeons seemed to formulate and embrace Enlightenment hopes for medicine better than the doctors. The surgeons espoused the empirical, pragmatic perspective of the philosophes and adopted empirical modesty as a philosophical stance more readily than the more conservative physicians. They adopted a loosely Lockean epistemology, a stance characteristic of the Enlightenment, because it corresponded to the way they perceived disease. (No doubt this connection exists in part because Locke's *Essay* is so thoroughly colored by his close contact with the English empirical physician, Thomas Sydenham.)[7] Furthermore, the surgeons were able to serve as a model of Enlightenment hopes for the integration of the mechanical and liberal arts; for example, the *Encyclopédie* used plates of surgical instruments as outstanding examples of the benefits derived from the craft tradition.[8] Surgery rather than medicine also served as a model of the utilitarian benefits of medicine for two reasons. The surgeons were more successful in tying their goals to the broader issues of the Enlightenment. And the Faculty of Medicine, representing privilege, monopoly, and ignorance, and thus epitomizing some of the ills of the ancien régime, was too resistant to innovation.

The Historical Roots of the Conflict

The surgeons' specific concerns and projects for reform grew in part out of the long history of their problematic position within the medical community, particularly their relationship to the powerful Faculty of Medicine.[9] A guild of surgeons, whose members came to be called "surgeons of the long robe," had been established in the fourteenth century. Although some of these early surgeons may have been university educated, they did not constitute an academic body until 1533, when the surgical College of Saint-Côme was established. In 1544 Francis I granted them the right to wear the cap and gown and to give public courses in anatomy and surgical operations, concessions which meant higher status and financial privileges for the small academic surgical community. The barber-surgeons, or "surgeons of the short robe," who had also established a guild at about the same time as the surgeons of the long robe, were a larger group who trimmed hair and performed minor operations.[10]

In 1505 the barber-surgeons signed the first of many agreements with the doctors, agreeing to deal only with the manual operations of surgery and to treat patients only after the doctors-regent of the Faculty of Paris had given their approval. This document in effect conceded the doctors' superiority and control and provided them with the basis for their arguments from legal precedent in the pamphlet war. In 1655 the situation was further complicated by the formal union of the barber-surgeons and the surgeons of the long robe.[11] For the eighteenth-century surgical polemicists, the most famous of whom was the influential physiocrat, François Quesnay, this union was the product of a conspiracy by the doctors to gain control over all the surgeons and produced the decline of French surgery. He described the relationship this way: "On the one side, one sees the barbers, pushed by ambition, revolting against their masters, usurping the rights of our Art. In league with the Faculty of Medicine to support their charges, they became the instruments of the hate of all doctors against the surgeons. On the other side, one finds the surgeons completely tied to their profession, enemies of trouble, regretfully obligated to refute injustice and jealousy, and always disposed to sacrifice a portion of their interests for the love of country."[12] As a corrective to this obviously biased account, Toby Gelfand has pointed to the economic factors that inclined the surgeons of the long robe to work with the barber-surgeons. For example, the state of the surgical art in the sixteenth century could not support an academic surgical guild whose principal medical function was to perform major operations. Given the pain, expense, and very low success rate of major operations, it is not surprising that there was little demand for them.[13]

But even if the surgeons and the barber-surgeons had reasons to unite, their expectations of the union were strikingly different from its actual results. The barber-surgeons wished to unite with the surgeons to escape the chafing confines of medical subjugation. The surgeons wished both to share some of the more lucrative practices of the barbers' craft and ultimately to establish a faculty of surgery to rival the medical faculty. But the doctors quickly precluded these possibilities and used the move toward union for their own ends. By appealing to the king they gained the letters-patent of 1655, which granted them the right to order and supervise all "médicaux se-cours," including surgical operations; the surgeons were to be considered merely instruments of physicians.[14] Instead of gaining a surgical faculty equivalent to the medical faculty, or at least independent of the doctors, the surgeons lost all control over the education of surgeons. And the barber-surgeons did not evade medical control but instead found it more consistently applied.

Whether or not it was a misapprehension of their past, the theory that the union of 1655 was a conspiracy on the part of the doctors allowed surgical polemicists of the eighteenth century to portray the pre-1655 company of surgeons of the long robe as a Utopian picture of the proper role and status of surgeons. More realistically, it gave them a historical precedent for an academic company of surgeons which they would attempt to reestablish throughout the course of the eighteenth century.

Moreover, the doctors, not content with the subjugation of the entire surgical profession, continued to lobby for and to gain legislative strictures against the surgeons late in the seventeenth century. For example, in 1660 the Parlement of Paris decreed that this new community had to submit itself to the Faculty on the same basis as the barber-surgeons. This meant that all signs of academic status were prohibited, and public teaching and the defense of academic theses by surgical students was forbidden. In 1670 further legislation required that the surgical community of Saint-Côme render financial and honorific signs of deference to the medical community.[15]

Although these strictures were considered insufferable by eighteenth-century surgeons, they in fact separated the entire surgical community from the Faculty of Medicine and provided an opportunity for the surgical company to develop on its own. Although the legal status of the surgeons did not change from 1650 to 1699, this period witnessed a strengthening of the surgical company and a separation, in practice though not in legislation, of the surgeons from the barber-surgeons.[16] The dictates of fashion had heightened the demand for barbers, and thus those barber-surgeons who were primarily barbers were quick to take advantage of the lucrative sideline of wigmaking. A royal ordinance of 1673 separated the wigmaker from the surgeon, forbidding the barber-wigmakers to perform any act of surgery and the members of Saint-Côme to sell wigs.[17] The separation that had developed between the spheres of practice of the academic surgical community and other surgeons was recognized in the statutes of 1699, which explicitly enjoined that those surgeons who gave up barbers' work and limited themselves to "the art of surgery purely and simply will be considered to practice a liberal art and will enjoy all the privileges attributed to the liberal arts."[18] It should be noted that while these distinctions were clearly defined in law, they were not maintained in practice even in Paris, and in the provinces such distinctions tended to break down entirely.[19]

The surgeons of the long robe also offered an alternative to the doctors in terms of medical practice. Even though the surgeons were legally restricted to external symptoms, in fact they also treated medical problems with internal symptoms because of the great demand for medical services which the doctors could not meet. It was in part simply a question of numbers.[20] The case of Paris, where surgeons were the principal medical practitioners, provides a telling example. In the eighteenth century, the Faculty of Medicine of Paris consisted of about 100 physicians for a population of half a million. The Faculty of Medicine maintained that number to ensure their control over the profession and the ability of their members to support themselves and maintain their social position. At the same time in Paris there were approximately two hundred and fifty master surgeons and about the same number of "privileged surgeons,"[21] those who rented the privilege of working under a master surgeon. Since the ratio of surgeons to doctors was about 5 to 1, it is not surprising that they encroached on the physicians' practice of medicine and were in fact the principal licensed medical practitioners of Paris.

Social factors were also involved in the growing influence of surgeons. Doctors belonged to the high bourgeoisie and generally treated members of that class or the nobility, many of whom acted as their patrons. Doctors were also frequently members of eighteenth-century salon society. Several physicians, notably Helvétius, Chirac, and Sylva, were ennobled in the 1720s, indicating the rising social status of physicians.[22] Surgeons, on the other hand, treated most other social classes, with the very lowest seeking out the barber-surgeons. Surgeons rather than doctors thus served as the ordinary medical practitioners for the bulk of the population. As one surgeon noted in a charge against the doctors, "the faubourgs of Paris, refuges of poor citizenry, contain more people than a good many cities of the kingdom; yet no physicians live in the faubourgs"; he concluded, "surgeons will always be the physicians of the poor." And a doctor indignantly claimed that surgeons received 90 percent of medical revenues.[23] Surgeons in fact met a burgeoning demand for medical services. They staffed the hospitals and followed the king's army.[24] The advent of the standing army in the seventeenth century required a large medical staff, and these positions were usually filled by surgeons. Military service gave the surgeon not only an opportunity to extend his activity to the treatment of wounds, which would have been outside his normal experience,[25] but also a legitimate way for him to treat a whole range of medical problems despite the traditional division of medical practice into internal and external symptoms.

Most importantly, the surgeons were in a position to profit from and participate in the renewed interest in anatomy and physiology awakened by Harvey's discovery of the circulation of the blood and by attempts to apply Cartesian mechanism to medicine. This progress in anatomy and its direct application to surgery gave the College of Saint-Côme greater prestige, and in the late seventeenth century several Parisian surgeons were admitted into the Academy of Sciences.[26] In general, the association of surgeons with new developments in the sciences gave surgery greater credibility, undermining the notion that surgery was simply a manual operation and acknowledging the surgeons as standard-bearers of the new science in France.

The surgeons were also able to capitalize on the great popularity in the seventeenth century of all things scientific. As part of the course at the Faculty of Paris, a doctor lectured while a surgeon demonstrated anatomy and surgical technique. Certain surgeons became so renowned for their abilities as demonstrators that surgeons could reasonably argue that the doctor was superfluous to the procedure. Because of the popularity of the surgical courses, young surgeons also were able to offer private courses to supplement their income, and surgeons of great repute offered courses in public institutions. For example, the public courses in surgery and anatomy given by the surgeon Pierre Dionis at the Jardin du Roi strikingly overshadowed those of the *premier médecin* in terms of attendance, and his lectures were gathered together in a popular textbook.[27] As a result of the popularity of these surgical demonstrations, the College of Saint-Côme was authorized to construct a public amphitheater, and a royal edict of 1699 specifically ordered the surgeons to continue their public demonstrations despite the opposition of the Faculty of Medicine.[28]

The surgical community was also able to carve out an important educational niche. The separation of the doctors and the surgeons left a void in surgical education, since the Faculty of Medicine ceased to train barber-surgeons after they merged with the surgeons of the long robe and did not reinstitute a course for surgeons until 1720. The surgeons themselves attempted to fill this void. They had always had an education by apprenticeship, and from their union with the barbers in 1660 until the royal edict of 1724, they introduced a series of increasingly rigorous examinations.[29] These examinations effectively separated the surgeons from the barbers, raised the overall educational level of the surgeons, and created an educational elite within the surgical profession. The surgeons thus had grounds to claim that they alone were capable of educating surgeons, since only their system offered a practical education that not only was grounded in empirical investigation but also implemented the most recent developments in medical theory and practice. Pride in the strengths of that education also gave the surgeons zeal in the fight to control their own education and the fervor of the righteous in pressing the claim that they offered the soundest medical education.

In contrast to the surgical emphasis on empirical investigation and practical experience, medical education in France in the eighteenth century remained staunchly oriented around the exegesis of ancient texts and rigidly resistant to innovation.[30] Medical students were taught by professors who were generalists. With rare exceptions, there was no notion of medical specialization within the Faculty of Paris and very little sense that research was worthwhile. Instead, the faculty was dominated by the conviction that everything to be known about medicine was to be found in the texts of Hippocrates, Galen, and Aristotle. Consequently the requirement for success as a medical student was a good grasp of those texts and a defense of a thesis. The medical thesis of four pages in quarto was based on the work of the candidate's major professor and designed to show the candidate's skill in the use of syllogism. One historian who has studied these theses concluded that "it would be in vain that one would hope to find in these works originality, a taste for research, or intellectual independence."[31] The education offered by the Faculty completely neglected midwifery, chemistry, and anatomy; in addition, it offered no bedside instruction and only four dissection classes annually. Acknowledging the decline of standards of French medical education, a royal edict of 1767 condemned "the relaxation which has taken place in some of the faculties of medicine, both in regard to the duration and quality of studies and in regard to the number and nature of exams leading to a degree."[32]

The decline of French medicine was also reflected in the growing influence of the king's first surgeon at the expense of the first physician. Traditionally, the king of France had a first physician and a first barber-surgeon. But when the barber-surgeons and the surgeons of the long robe merged, the king's council ordered the *premier barbier* to sell his "rights and privileges over the art of surgery to the *premier chirurgien*, François Félix."[33]

The surgeons were particularly fortunate in the abilities of the first few holders of that office. Their skills enabled them to effect cures of members of the royal family which increased their professional standing and their influence with the king. For example, in 1686, Félix successfully operated on Louis XIV for an anal fistula. Georges Maréchal, the next first surgeon, also advanced the cause of the surgeons by correctly diagnosing Louis XIV's last illness and recommending treatment. The first physician, Guy-Crescent Fagon, had insisted that the king's health was good; he prevailed, only to be dismissed upon the king's demise. Maréchal was also in good standing with the new regent, Philip, Duke of Orléans, for he had successfully treated him for a dislocated shoulder in 1710; more significantly, in 1711 Maréchal defended the Duke against charges of poisoning the heirs to the throne. Predisposed to favor the cause of the surgeons, Philip supported Maréchal when he defied the doctors by ordering the surgeons not to pay the deferential fees to the medical faculty.[34] These influential first surgeons defined for themselves a role as advocate for the surgeons, and they lobbied to upgrade the educational level and social status of the surgeons.[35]

The history of the conflict between the doctors and the surgeons not only provides a background to a discussion of the pamphlet war but also indicates critical differences in the evolution of the two bodies, particularly the advances made by elite surgeons at the expense of the Faculty of Medicine.[36] The history also demonstrates the surgeons' willingness to contest and challenge the doctors in their areas of professional exclusivity such as university education and training. Perhaps the most interesting conclusion to be drawn from the history of the conflict is that the new discoveries and approaches to science of the seventeenth century, for example, anatomical discoveries and arguments for empiricism, worked in favor of the surgeons and put them in a position to manipulate these innovations in their own interests. In the course of the pamphlet war this implicit possibility was explicitly argued and developed by the surgeons. They did not simply claim that the new sciences enhanced their professional status and reenforced their notions of practice, but rather that their understanding of the new sciences was the way to progress. These tactics allowed the surgical community in the course of the pamphlet war to espouse the new, to take command of it, and to claim that their commitment to the new sciences legitimated them and authorized their control of medicine.

The most concrete and immediately influential result of the increase in surgical visibility, in the domain of surgical practice, in educational level, and in proximity to the crown was the ordinance of 1724, which began a long process of returning surgical education to the surgeons and enabled the surgeons to claim that they rather than the doctors set the standards for medical practice. The pamphlet war which ensued in the wake of the ordinance was not simply a renewal of the centuries-old professional dispute. Although issues of professional preeminence and control remained significant, the debate also provided a forum within which the surgeons presented ideas for educational reform, claimed to embody the new sciences and philosophy, and portrayed the doctors as reactionaries who clung to outmoded and ineffectual practices. The ordinance of 1724 thereby ushered in a new stage in the dispute, in which issues of medical education and practice were featured more prominently and the academic community of the surgeons asserted a new model for the profession.

The Battle to Define Medical Practice and Epistemology, 1724–1743

The royal ordinance of 1724 violently reopened the traditional battle between the doctors and the surgeons by granting the College of Saint-Côme the right to appoint five surgeon demonstrators to give public courses in anatomy and surgery. This ordinance in effect sanctioned the establishment of a surgical academic elite and abrogated the monopoly which the Faculty of Medicine claimed over medical education, including surgical education. It denied the authority of the doctors to teach the surgeons their craft and thus challenged their hegemony over the entire medical profession by questioning their expertise in surgery. The conflict became one between the authority of the doctors and the innovative practices of the surgeons, between the traditional, textually based education of the doctors and the empirical, clinical practice of the surgeons. The doctors could not tolerate such a challenge to their authority and expertise, and they vented their indignation in a pamphlet war which raged from 1724 to 1750.

In the first salvo, the doctors protested the encroachments by the surgeons on their traditional preserves and cited specific grievances. For example, the doctors addressed a *mémoire* to the king to remind him of their rights and to argue for the repeal of the hated ordinance; it was, they claimed, totally unnecessary because they were more than able to educate the surgeons. They pointed out that the Faculty had recently granted the enormous concession of teaching its surgical course in French because the surgeons were not well versed in Latin. Furthermore, if the surgeons gave demonstrations in their own college, they would have to contend with overcrowded quarters and to fit their courses in between all their exercises, dissections, and operations. In other words, for all concerned the status quo was a better and more convenient arrangement.[37]

In another pamphlet a doctor contended that the right of the first surgeon to appoint the five demonstrators gave him too much power, making him not only the leader of the surgeons but also placing him in charge of all instruction in the art of surgery. The doctors were voicing their concern over the very real change in power that had occurred within the medical profession[38] and indicating the threat that a centralized surgical profession could pose to the authority of the Faculty of Paris. As head of the entire surgical profession, the first surgeon was able to effect greater centralization and exercise greater control over surgery than any medical figure could wield in medicine. Although the first physician had the prestigious position of serving the king, he had no influence within the Faculty of Paris. The dean of the Faculty of Paris had extensive control over medical practice in Paris but virtually none outside it, and he could not become a real force within the profession because he was elected by lot for a term of only two years.[39] In contrast to this divided authority in medicine, the first surgeon was able to further consolidate and extend his authority. The edict of 1724 revived the offices of lieutenant to the first surgeon in regional surgical communities. The sale of these offices both guaranteed the economic health of the first surgeon and the College of Saint-Côme and considerably extended the first surgeon's control through his personal appointment of four hundred local lieutenants who reported directly to him.[40] This particular pamphlet expressed concern about the first surgeon's power vis-à-vis the first physician but also noted that the organization of the surgical profession allowed far more centralization, and that the edict, by reviving the office of lieutenant, fostered not only centralization but also more effective continuing control from Paris over provincial surgeons. The doctors were incensed enough to claim in one pamphlet that the rights granted to the first surgeon in effect authorized a conspiracy against the prerogatives of the first physician.[41]

The doctors vehemently contested the surgeons' newly acquired right to teach on the grounds that they had neither the authority nor the ability. Doctors, they argued, could both teach and operate, although they ordinarily chose to operate only when a surgeon was unavailable. (They did concede that it was occasionally useful to have a surgeon who knew theory and could therefore consult with the physician.) But regardless of the ability of the individual surgeon, the profession of the surgeon, the doctors claimed, was to operate, and he was therefore "sans qualité et sans titre"[42] to teach. Furthermore, they argued, there was no need to alter the present system of surgical education. They cited the merits of the public courses offered at the Jardin du Roi. There, they claimed, La Peyronnie, one of the most noted of contemporary surgeons, admirably fulfilled the proper role of the surgeon by acting simply as a demonstrator for the doctor who lectured. The fundamental issue for the doctors was to maintain their position of preeminence over the surgeons. Therefore, they insisted that doctors without training must be allowed to operate, that surgeons, whether trained or not, must not be allowed to teach, and that the subordinate position of the surgeons in the medical hierarchy must be reinforced by law. Most important to these outraged physicians, this ordinance "would overturn the subordination which should exist between the doctors and the surgeons."[43]

Though the doctors conceded that there were those rare surgeons like Maréchal and La Peyronnie "who know more than their trade," they charged that the education of the surgeons did not prepare them to teach. They found the surgeons' education deficient in two specific respects: their knowledge of theory was inevitably limited and outmoded because they did not know Latin, and, more important, their education did not teach them to reason. They were therefore unable to "penetrate the true reasons for the operations of nature; the uniform and universal and first reasons which are, however, the source of all the varieties which are found in the mechanism of our bodies."[44] These sorts of claims for clear and certain knowledge gleaned through their conservative, classical mode of education shows the way in which the Faculty was out of step with the empirical basis and the epistemological modesty which characterized the claims to knowledge of the natural scientist, the philosophe, and the surgeon.

The doctors also found fault with the education of the surgeons because it neglected chemistry. As a result, the surgeons "have no knowledge of elements or compounds, or moving forces and their effects, or of liquids and their differing proportions. Nor do they know anything about the formation, growth, or causes of destruction of minerals, vegetables, or animals."[45] This charge seems especially ironic since the Parisian medical community had so violently opposed the introduction of chemistry, especially chemical remedies, into French medicine. For example, Pierre Le Paulmier was formally censured by the Faculty in 1566 simply for consulting the iatrochemist Joseph de Chesne.[46] And the Faculty of Paris did not even offer courses in chemistry until 1770.[47]

The surgeons defended their system of education against these charges, claiming that the advances made in surgical practice and the high degree of prestige enjoyed by French surgeons was not the result of their education by the Faculty of Medicine but was instead due completely to the ways the surgeons had circumvented the education offered by the Faculty.[48] Furthermore, according to the surgeons, it was essential that control of surgical education be placed completely in their hands. Only then could the educational level of the surgeons continue to rise and the public health continue to benefit from surgical advances. In other words, they explicitly connected their educational innovations with the improvement of public health. True, they acknowledged, this right or control (as they preferred to call it) had traditionally belonged to the doctors, but they had not put it to good use; in fact, the control which the doctors so proudly proclaimed "had been gained only by intrigue, and had become a shameful yoke around the surgeons which the ordinance had removed, restoring them to their natural liberty."[49] The surgeons challenged that right because the doctors had proven themselves to be incapable of fulfilling the responsibilities it entailed. A doctor's bonnet, after all, did not necessarily make one a good teacher. One particularly bold surgeon proclaimed that only four doctors in a hundred could teach, a particularly acute problem because those doctors who did teach had not been selected for their pedagogical skill. The surgeons, he maintained, would unfailingly cultivate good surgical teaching because of their consistent emphasis on empiricism and demonstration.[50]

Ultimately, according to the surgeons, the ordinance of 1724 only legitimated the situation which already existed; that is to say, the surgeons educated themselves in fact. They challenged the doctors to produce one surgeon they had trained. Perhaps facetiously, one surgeon suggested that the doctors must recognize this was true since they claimed that the surgeons did not know Latin, yet the doctors had condescended to teach in French for only the past five years! "Who then has really educated the surgeons in the centuries that the doctors were in charge, if not the surgeons themselves?" asked a surgeon. Furthermore, the surgeons contended, it took an entire lifetime to "apply oneself to the cultivation and practice of this art"; however, the course of surgery offered by the doctors was merely eight days long. The surgeons also claimed that since the doctors themselves so scorned the practice of surgery they must also have neglected the theoretical aspects of the art. But despite neglect by the doctors, the surgeons proudly proclaimed that the art of surgery had made great strides as a result of its cultivation by the College of Saint-Côme. Because they had fostered and improved the art of surgery while the doctors neglected it, the surgeons claimed to have merited the right to teach surgery. Or, they asked, "has the great diligence with which the surgeons have applied themselves to their art made them deserving of the servitude in which the doctors leave them languishing?"[51]

The surgeons attempted to refute the arguments of the doctors that their education could not teach them the essence of the operation of nature by staunchly adopting a position of epistemological modesty and arguing for the value of the practical over the theoretical. And, the surgeons noted, knowledge of first causes was no more likely to be accorded to doctors than to surgeons. "I wonder whether it is sufficient to be a surgeon to be ignorant of this knowledge, or if it is enough to be a doctor to be knowledgeable?"[52] queried a surgeon. More importantly, according to the surgeons, the very fact that the doctors presumed to plumb the depths of nature made it much less likely that they would learn anything significant. They considered it unsurprising that the doctors had made so little progress in surgery since they "lost themselves in their systems." The surgeons pointed out to the doctors that "by abandoning experience, you have nothing which can fix your reason when it wanders. Thus is it at all astonishing that the product of all your efforts can be reduced to a useless mass of abstract ideas?"[53] Surgery, on the other hand, the surgeons claimed, made great progress because the surgeons never ceased to be guided by experience and they did not maintain the artificial and counterproductive distinction between theory and practice. If the doctors succeeded in their quest to reestablish their control over surgical education, the surgeons warned that the level of surgical practice would inevitably decline. These surgeons were not simply arguing that their practice of medicine was as good as or better than that of the doctors but also that their understanding of medical theory and epistemology was much more likely to be productive.

In formulating their arguments the surgeons took positions which were later espoused by the philosophes and have come to be identified as crucial characteristics of the Enlightenment. For example, they adopted epistemological modesty as the appropriate philosophical position for the scientist. Just as virtually every philosophe later did, the surgeons acknowledged that one can have no knowledge of first causes. They also shared with Enlightenment thinkers a firm belief in the efficacy of empirical investigation. But beyond these philosophical affinities, surgeons shared with the philosophes an explicitly reformist concern. As practitioners of experimental philosophy, they held out hope of immediate benefit to mankind from their practice. In other words, the surgeons, like the philosophes, saw medicine as the most obvious and concrete source of the benefits science could provide for mankind. And the surgeons, like the philosophes, claimed to work for the amelioration of social conditions by reforming institutions. The surgeons directed their reforming zeal specifically to challenging the control the Faculty of Medicine exercised over them.

The surgeons pointed with pride to their reputation throughout Europe for excellence in both surgical education and practice, noting the "crowd of foreigners who never set foot in the Schools of the Faculty, who came to Paris to follow the exercises of the school of Saint-Côme."[54] This boast is legitimated by the fact that French surgery had attained a great reputation in the late seventeenth century, built on successful techniques in major operations and extensive anatomical work, which brought surgeons and physicians from all over Europe to study surgery in Paris. An eighteenth-century proverb that recognized this preeminence advised one to go to England to study medicine, to Germany to study pharmacy, but to France to study surgery.[55]

To gain a wider audience and a more sympathetic hearing for their arguments, the surgeons sought to make their dispute with the doctors a public issue by directly addressing the reader of their pamphlets and by haranguing crowds on the street corners of Paris. They claimed that surgical education ought to be of paramount interest to every citizen of the realm because the surgeons were, in fact, the primary medical practitioners in France. As the surgeons noted: "Doctors practice in the cities, surgeons practice in the rest of the country, follow the army, and accompany the fleet."[56] They consistently argued that it was they and not the doctors who best served the public well-being. They pointed out to their readers that the doctors, in formulating their arguments, never claimed to serve the public interest. Instead they raised issues of power and prestige.[57] The surgeons, on the other hand, appealed to public opinion as a control on privilege because public opinion represented a rational and disinterested consensus which would make reform possible and because it would invariably address the public good.[58]

While the surgeons were certainly right that the doctors' pamphlets rarely addressed the issue of the public good, nonetheless their arguments tended to neglect, as polemics generally and sometimes deliberately do, certain important issues. The doctors might have failed to argue for the public well-being either because they saw it as peripheral to the issue raised by the ordinance, because they considered an appeal to the public an inappropriate forum for the discussion of professional issues, because they took it as axiomatic that they, at the pinnacle of the medical hierarchy, would best serve the public well-being, or perhaps, as the surgeons insinuated, because they recognized that this was not where the strength of their position lay. The surgeons, honing their own polemical skills, also failed to acknowledge that the doctors were legitimately concerned about the attack made on their profession by the surgeons and that the surgeons themselves were not disinterested partisans of the public good but were also seeking professional gains.

Although the doctors generally concentrated their efforts on defending the traditional system of education, they occasionally tried to encroach further on surgical practices, challenging several domains traditionally held by the surgeons. In general, the division of medical practice between the doctors and the surgeons was based on a distinction between diseases with external symptoms and those with internal symptoms, a division of practice dating from the incorporation of the barber-surgeons under the control of the doctors in 1505. The basis for the division seems to have been the notion that a surgeon would be able to resolve external problems completely evident to the eye by means of pragmatic, somewhat mechanical skills. The doctors, with their theoretical approach to education and practice, would be better able to diagnose hidden symptoms. One of the bones of contention in the pamphlet war was the treatment of venereal disease, which, according to this distinction, fell within the province of the surgeons.[59] Because venereal disease reached epidemic proportions during the sixteenth and seventeenth centuries, it was a significant segment of the surgeon's practice and perhaps his chief source of income.[60] The doctors certainly recognized the lucrative nature of this practice. Perhaps they also realized that the surgeons' control over such a prevalent disease had carved for themselves an important niche in medical practice and so constituted another encroachment on the authority and practice of the doctors. Thus they argued vehemently that the nature of the disease required treatment by a physician.

The doctors challenged the surgeons' right to treat venereal disease on two grounds. First, regardless of the external symptoms, venereal disease was simply too complicated for surgeons to be able to treat it competently. The symptoms were both terrible and equivocal, and so, the doctors contended, its treatment "unquestionably merits the most serious attention of the most enlightened physician." Secondly, the doctors claimed that even according to the traditional distinction between external and internal symptoms they ought to treat venereal disease, for the external symptoms were only minor reflections of a great internal disturbance of humors, complications which cried out for the enlightened judgment of a physician.[61] Once again, according to the doctors, the deficiencies of surgical education made surgeons incapable of treating venereal disease. Doctors supported this claim by calling into question the value of experience. "Without speaking of the most accomplished sort, experience is nothing but an uncertain, not to say murderous, routine when it is not directed by prudence and discernment. How many unfortunate victims are there of experiments conducted by these observers?"[62]

In contrast to the uneducated surgeons, the doctors presented themselves as well educated and especially well read in the belles lettres. One doctor acknowledged that this sort of education might be thought irrelevant to the practice of medicine, yet he contended that "belles lettres which adorn the spirit make it more susceptible to other learning." Furthermore, this familiarity with great literature could reasonably suggest to the patient that his physician had a certain quality of character. Thus the doctors *ought* to treat venereal disease because they are endowed with "the sentiments of honor and a proven probity," presumably by virtue of their classical education. (The empirical education of the surgeons evidently could not endow them with these attributes.) The superior quality of medical education ought to make venereal disease the preserve of the doctors. "For instructed in the nature of the mechanism of man and the help which medicine furnishes, they alone are capable of reestablishing this mechanism when it no longer functions in its whole or in some of its parts."[63]

One surgeon responded directly to these attacks on the character and ability of the surgeons. First of all, he argued that within the distinction between external and internal symptoms there could be no question but that venereal disease had external symptoms requiring treatment. Second, he wondered how these men, who had been depicted by the doctors as "grossiers et sans culture," could have gained the confidence of the public, often at the expense of their trust in doctors, who had, in contrast, been portrayed as men of culture and honor. He concluded that the eloquence of success spoke for the surgeons. Finally, the surgeons wrote the important treatises on venereal disease and taught their students how to treat it. The surgeons were staunch in the defense of their system of education, particularly its emphasis on experience and apprenticeship as a method of instruction, for "habilité" in the treatment of disease could be communicated only by the assiduous formation of students. Doctors who might be able orators or poets by virtue of their education would nonetheless be less adept in the treatment of disease than the empirically educated surgeon.[64]

Both the doctors and the surgeons claimed to exercise their skills on behalf of the public good, but they used different arguments. The doctors claimed to protect the public good by virtue of their education. The surgeons based their claim on their experience, particularly on the fact that because of the rigid control of medical faculties over the number of physicians they, the surgeons, were the primary medical practitioners in France.

During the most intense period of pamphlet warfare, from 1724 to 1743, the surgeons made crucial gains.[65] Though the doctors had hoped to effect a revocation of the ordinance of 1724 by this airing of their objections to the surgeons, the pamphlet war worked to the advantage of the surgeons. The surgeons were able to assert convincingly certain professional goals, such as their claim to educate their own and to treat venereal disease and their right to control the surgical profession independently of the Faculty of Medicine. The surgeons also raised the broader question of the nature of the most appropriate education for medical practitioners. These issues were not immediately resolved, but the surgeons continued to gain public and royal support and influence within the scientific community. They became more centrally organized and their educational standards became more stringent. In articulating their particular professional and educational goals, the surgeons allied themselves with the forces of progress such as the new science and the Enlightenment.

The subsequent royal ordinance of 1743 granted important concessions to the surgeons: they were given the right to confer university degrees and to approve degree candidates in surgery; they formed a lay faculty with the same stature as the other four within the university; and they gained the right to govern themselves without any supervision or control by the Faculty of Medicine.

The pamphlet war continued with unabated furor after the new edict, but the tenor of the debate changed. The doctors began to argue more defensively as their power eroded over the course of the dispute. They also tended to argue in support of privilege while the surgeons argued from concerns of practice. With every legislative victory the surgeons argued with greater confidence, a confidence based on the sense that the burden of proof in the pamphlet war now rested on the physicians. No doubt they felt that they, and not the physicians, epitomized the spirit of the age and the goals of Enlightenment. Before the ordinance of 1743 the surgeons simply argued the legitimacy of their systems of medical education and practice. After 1743, not content with the separate but equal status spelled out by the ordinance, they increased their demands for independence from the physicians and argued the primacy of the empirical tradition they represented. They based most of their claims on the superiority of their education in preparing them for practice and used that superiority, or that particular combination of the theoretical and practical, to argue that they ought to be considered the preeminent medical practitioners.

As the pamphlet war came to an end in the 1750s, the elite surgeons of France were in an enviable position. They had unequivocally gained the right to educate their own, and they were no longer required to proffer homage to the doctors. Their influence in the medical profession in France and abroad was officially sanctioned and solidified by new professional institutions and status. Their practice of medicine made them essentially general practitioners with a specialization in surgery. They had established a system of medical education which concentrated on both the theoretical and the practical aspects of medicine. In addition to their adherence to the empirical craft tradition, which connected them to the manual arts glorified by the encyclopedists, the surgeons also enjoyed the benefits attached to membership in a liberal profession. Their firm ties to hospitals and to the military placed them in the forefront of clinical practice. They alone in the medical profession incorporated disciplines such as pathology, anatomy, clinical pathology, and chemistry into their system of education and could thus claim to be the initiators of medical development through the cultivation of the new sciences. In 1750 the amphitheater of Saint-Côme was transformed into an official College of Surgery, independent of the Faculty of Medicine. Under continued royal patronage, the college emerged as the most vital center of medical instruction in the kingdom, and surgery, with its emphasis on hospital training and pathological anatomy, made a major contribution to the subsequent development of Parisian clinical medicine.[66]

The conflict was restricted to the members of two educated, elite bodies of Parisian medical practitioners. Thus it cannot be assumed that the innovations in practice and theory argued by the surgeons had an immediate or direct effect on the practice of medicine outside of Paris or that this debate set new standards of practice or defined new intellectual approaches to medicine for medical practitioners in general. Nonetheless, the pamphlet war itself played a crucial role in the development of French medicine. In particular, the pamphlet war was fought over the control and delimitation of certain essential professional concerns, especially the legal status and training of members and the standardization of practices. The pamphlet war was also crucial in changing the nature of the relationship between doctor and surgeon and between patient and medical practitioner.[67] The war both fostered increased competition between doctors and surgeons and served to develop a loose network among surgeons. Surgeons also enjoyed an enhanced relationship with patients at the expense of physicians: in this period patients chose surgeons not only for economic or social reasons but also because of surgical claims to technical competence, especially in one of the most crucial areas of eighteenth-century medical practice, bloodletting. The claims made by elite surgeons in the pamphlet war were crucial to professionalization in that they helped to winnow out the unqualified and uneducated from those with more developed standards of training and practice.

Although the surgeons in the pamphlet war made claims for standards of education and practice that were not immediately influential in the medical community at large, nonetheless those demands were ultimately critical to future professional medical development: they prefigured the reforms of medicine enacted during the Revolution. Medicine and surgery were united in the *école de santé* in 1794 in a way that shows the extensive influence of the surgical tradition. The new system of medical education incorporated surgical institutions such as bedside teaching, clinical apprenticeships, and practical schooling in anatomy and dissection, as well as surgical concepts such as the cultivation and development of pathology, and it placed surgical personnel in key positions in the new medical hierarchy. Thus the reformed medical profession had a profoundly surgical character.[68] The fact that the Revolution adopted some of the proposals launched by the surgeons does not argue for a direct influence of the surgeons on revolutionary reformers so much as suggest an analogy between their concerns. In the first half of the century, the surgeons had successfully attacked the Faculty as an entrenched privileged body; by the end of the century, the Revolution had abolished the physicians' professionally privileged status. But the importance of the pamphlet war is not restricted to the prescience of the surgeons on the issue of medical reform. In this period surgeons articulated a reformist view of medical practice and distinguished themselves, as the surgeons of Saint-Côme, both from less well educated and more unorthodox practitioners and from charlatans. The pamphlet war cannot be dismissed as simple wrangling based on professional jealousy, for it allowed the surgeons to articulate a medical philosophy and a program of education.

The debate also had an impact beyond the sphere of Parisian medical practice: the surgeons, by identifying corporate privilege as an impediment to reform, had launched a political challenge which could not be ignored by contemporaries interested in reform in other areas. Beyond the general philosophical affinities between the surgeons and the philosophes previously discussed, the surgeons understood the uses of science in the same way the philosophes would later define them. For example, for the surgeons as for the philosophes, science was practical and utilitarian rather than systematic or abstract. Science in general and specific positions taken in scientific debates were clearly seen by both surgeons and philosophes as having concrete social and political ramifications. The attacks made by surgeons on medical education were akin to philosophical attacks on metaphysicians and Scholastics. Both groups felt the need to argue their intellectual authority and professional credibility not on the grounds of tradition or privilege but rather because of their service to the public.

Important comparisons can also be drawn between the reformist concerns of surgeons and the philosophes. Both groups argued against the corporate structure of French society because it restricted the development of talent in order to enhance the privilege of elites. Surgical tracts and philosophical writings both demonstrate the moral indignation of new claimants to power. Both surgeons and philosophes sought the endorsement of their claims in the arena of public opinion, using polemics to their advantage and to the discomfiture of the privileged groups they challenged. These correlations between the goals of philosophes and surgeons caused them to use similar methods and similar strategies. It is unlikely that any Parisian would have been unaware of this hotly contested professional dispute, which sometimes erupted into street fighting. It thus seems improbable that the philosophes in particular could have failed to note the arguments and strategies of the surgeons. La Mettrie identified himself as a philosophe and, in a series of medical satires and pamphlets, took the revolutionary or philosophical potential inherent in the issues of the pamphlet war and elaborated it into an explicit campaign for Enlightenment reform. The implicit correlations between philosophes and surgeons thus become explicit and sharply defined in La Mettrie's satires.

2

La Mettrie's Medical Satires

The Formation of a Philosophe

The connection between the concerns, methods, and claims of the surgeons and those of the philosophes presents interesting parallels and suggests the surgeons as a positive medical model that might in part explain the enthusiasm of the philosophes for medicine. But although there are many statements in the writings of the philosophes about the great hope medicine offered and many doctors and surgeons participated in the growing philosophical movement, clear-cut discussions of the surgical position and its relationship to the Enlightenment are not easily found. However, the career of La Mettrie as a surgical polemicist and satirist suggests some connections; La Mettrie's personal involvement in the pamphlet war between the doctors and the surgeons led him to the cause of reform and to define himself as a philosophe.

La Mettrie was a medical student in Paris from 1727 to 1731, during the period of intense pamphlet warfare provoked by the ordinance of 1724. Finding his Parisian medical education wanting, La Mettrie went to Leyden to study with Hermann Boerhaave. When he returned to France La Mettrie attacked the physicians; he seems to have realized that the surgeons, not the doctors, were concerned with the progress and reform of medicine, and he took up the surgeons' cause in the pamphlet war. The pamphlet war gave him a forum for articulating his concern with medical reform and for arguing the integral relationship between public well-being and good medical practice. La Mettrie's involvement in the pamphlet war was a first step in his own evolution into a philosophe, and from the reformist concerns of the surgeons he was able to forge his own crusade for Enlightenment.

His espousal of the surgeons' cause was certainly grounds enough for his fellow physicians to condemn La Mettrie as a medical heretic. Although some physicians attempted to conciliate the surgeons or to mediate the dispute, they did not argue against their own or suggest that there were faults in either their system of education or their practice. They did not contend, as La Mettrie did, that the experience of the surgeons made them better qualified to deal with illnesses than the classically educated physicians. La Mettrie did not simply become involved in this dispute in the abstract, arguing the position of the surgeons from a purely theoretical point of view. Instead, he ridiculed the principal members of the Faculty of Medicine of Paris, who were also, not surprisingly, the chief advocates for the doctors against the surgeons. Nor was this interest in the contemporary medical situation merely a passing concern: La Mettrie wrote seven volumes of satiric comment on the medicine of his day from 1737 to 1750, and at the time of his death he was preparing a collected volume of his *Oeuvres polémiques* to stand with his *Oeuvres philosophiques* and his *Oeuvres de médecine*.[1]

In his years as a medical student, a period in which the pamphlet war between the doctors and the surgeons was *the* crucial professional issue, La Mettrie supported the cause of the doctors and shared the opinion of his fellow physicians that the surgeons were at best untrained empirics and at worst unscrupulous charlatans.[2] The first question which bears some investigation is why, a mere four years later, he wrote vituperative, satirical portraits of his medical confreres. These would have, at the very least, provided ammunition for the enemies of the doctors in the professional battle to retain their privileged status in the face of the incursions of the surgeons. But La Mettrie's satires did not simply provide ammunition for the surgeons' cause; rather, they were part of a concerted, deliberate campaign on behalf of the surgeons and their clinical education and empirical practice. As a result, La Mettrie was pilloried by the doctors as a traitor from within, a renegade.

There were several significant sources of La Mettrie's disaffection with the Parisian medical community. First, as a provincial medical student in Paris, he would have been a marginal member of the medical establishment and, as he never became a more central figure, perhaps his loyalty would not have been particularly strong. No doubt any alienation he may have felt would have increased when he found himself unable to pay the exorbitantly high cost of graduating from the University of Paris and was instead constrained to complete his degree requirements in three months at the University of Reims. A degree from Reims would also have considerably restricted the extent of his medical practice. For example, graduates of provincial faculties were required to pay large fees and take extensive examinations to practice in the jurisdiction of other regional medical corporations.[3] Furthermore, as did so many in this age of the new science, La Mettrie found his classical, text-oriented education wanting.[4] In addition to this general dissatisfaction with his education, he concluded that it had been particularly inappropriate for the actual application of medicine to the treatment of patients: he discovered to his chagrin that his doctor's bonnet did not confer on him the ability to diagnose and treat disease. His practice as an army doctor primarily in the company of surgeons demonstrated that the surgeons, much maligned by his fellow physicians, were better trained to be effective medical practitioners. La Mettrie's disaffection was expressed in his career as a medical satirist, which afforded him the opportunity to take vengeance on the medical establishment, to assert the superiority of his own subsequent education in Leyden, and to gain a certain notoriety that might well have advanced the career of an unknown provincial physician.

Because he challenged the Parisian physicians, La Mettrie's books were condemned to be burned by the hangman. In his last polemical work, the *Ouvrage de Pénélope*, La Mettrie reflected on his career as a satirist; he wrote this work realizing full well the outrage his satires would provoke and knowing that the medical community would be galvanized to frustrate his reform efforts and to persecute him. He proclaimed his involvement in the pamphlet war as an act of courage motivated primarily by concern for the public well-being at the expense of his own self-interest. Placing himself firmly within the context of the republic of letters, he asked, "But should one balance one's own gain against the public well-being?" His own satires were broad in order to provoke the public to recognize the need for medical reform. He recognized that the satires had given him a reputation as a cantankerous troublemaker but hoped that posterity would vindicate his efforts. And he vehemently claimed his right to satirize as "a liberty which is always permitted in the republic of letters." Furthermore, he insisted, his satires did no real harm, merely depriving certain physicians of "an ill-acquired esteem." In fact, he noted with irony, he and the doctors both suffered the same fate as a result of his satires, that is, "the loss of the profit which accrues from a good reputation."[5]

La Mettrie's self-proclaimed lofty motives have not been considered or acknowledged by scholars, who have instead usually dismissed the satires as either completely malicious pieces or as insignificant works. Raymond Boissier, the only biographer of La Mettrie who has discussed them in any detail, has argued that La Mettrie wanted the king to appoint Jean Senac as first physician and that these satires were an elaborate scheme to discredit all the other notable Parisian physicians.[6] To support this contention, he notes the extremely laudatory description of Senac in the last few pages of La Mettrie's *Ouvrage de Pénélope*.[7] Frederick the Great's *Éloge*, one of the few contemporary sources about La Mettrie's life (although it has been questioned by historians on many specific points), also suggests that influencing the appointment of Senac was La Mettrie's motive for writing the satires, but, in a spirit appropriate to an *éloge*, Frederick claims that La Mettrie was Senac's unwilling pawn.[8] But this argument is implausible: Senac was not the only physician spared La Mettrie's barbs, and it would not have been so worth his while to secure the appointment of a physician he favored that La Mettrie would have both risked incurring the wrath of all the other Parisian physicians and campaigned tirelessly for this end for thirteen years and over 1,500 pages. It is possible that La Mettrie praised Senac because he was one of the few Parisian physicians who were concerned about the deplorable quality of French medical education. Senac was also an outstanding anatomist, an area of competence La Mettrie considered absolutely essential for the physician.

The charge of malice is not so easily dismissed. Some of La Mettrie's attacks were undeniably malicious, and the satirical point of his pen was frequently used to jab his arguments home at the expense of his rivals, especially Jean Astruc.[9] La Mettrie also used his pen to redress personal wrongs and to cast doubt on the skills of doctors who questioned the merits of his own work or that of either of his mentors, Pierre Hunauld or Hermann Boerhaave. And it is certainly true that the notoriety of the satirist, gained by the effective use of polemical venom, would have enhanced, or at least highlighted, the career of an obscure provincial physician.

Although these personal and petty motives might undercut an attempt to canonize La Mettrie as a noble, disinterested crusader for the cause of public health, they are not sufficient to account for the wide range of his satiric portraits, particularly since La Mettrie did not know many of the physicians he satirized or have a personal grievance against them. Instead, the one principle of selection that La Mettrie consistently employed in choosing his satiric targets was the position a doctor took in the debate between the doctors and the surgeons. Without exception, all those La Mettrie satirized had written on behalf of the doctors or had taken a public stand against the surgeons.[10] Furthermore, La Mettrie's pen left unscathed those doctors who argued for conciliation between the doctors and the surgeons or advocated medical reforms. He clearly and deliberately used the arguments of the surgeons and understood that his satires would be construed as part of the pamphlet war.

Furthermore, the possible self-interest of the author should not allow one to entirely discount the content of La Mettrie's satires, which went well beyond personal or professional concerns. His efforts were not narrowly focused on the specific gains the surgeons sought, that is, they were not simply another salvo in the pamphlet war. Instead, his satires were an attack on the foibles of members of the medical community, an indictment of the corporate workings of the Faculty, and finally an exposé of the ways in which proper standards of medical education and practice had been completely undermined by the society physician. His satires rework in a more dramatic fashion the concerns of the surgeons, and through his reworking those concerns become a forceful expression of Enlightenment ideology. The target of his attack expands beyond personal slights and narrow professional disputes into a full-scale attack on the Faculty of Medicine, its corporate structure, its privileged status, and the system of education it fostered.

The Surgeons' Case

The scope of La Mettrie's satire gradually widened. His first polemical work, *Lettre à Monsieur Astruc* (1737),[11] was a straightforward academic challenge to the arguments of Astruc in *De orbis venereis* (1736)[12] on the nature, origin, and treatment of venereal disease. La Mettrie no doubt felt a need to defend himself and his mentor, Hermann Boerhaave. In 1735 he published a translation of Boerhaave's treatise on venereal disease, to which he added a hundred pages of his own observations.[13] Astruc attacked certain points made by both of them. La Mettrie's *Lettre* is both a stirring defense of Boerhaave's methods and an argument in a rather arid academic controversy. The focus of the polemic is narrowly defined, raising very specific areas of disagreement with Astruc about venereal disease. Both the style—heavy-handed sarcasm used as a bludgeon—and the narrow range of this initial polemical work are completely uncharacteristic of La Mettrie's other satires, which have a more biting style and address the broader issues of the practice of medicine, the nature of medical education, and the character of the physician.

Though his next work, *Saint Cosme vengé* (1737),[14] continued his controversy with Astruc, La Mettrie changed his tactics radically. He did not attempt to refute Astruc directly, but instead ridiculed him, a stylistic device which seems suited to La Mettrie's skills and an appropriate tactic to employ against Astruc's pretensions. Perhaps La Mettrie had realized that his direct attack on Astruc was ineffectual and that through satire he, the medical David, might be able to vanquish a Goliath of the Parisian medical faculty. For example, to ridicule Astruc's pedantic scholarship, La Mettrie chided him for not referring to every one of the writings of the church fathers; Astruc might thus have neglected the *one* conclusive reference. Furthermore, despite his claims to scholarly expertise, Astruc, according to La Mettrie, borrowed heavily from the work of Dom Calmet.[15] Here La Mettrie objected not only to pedantry and plagiarism but also to the use of theological sources as evidence in a scientific discussion. If La Mettrie had not swayed his readers by challenging Astruc on questions of medical diagnosis and treatment, he intended to cast aspersions on the methods Astruc used and thus discredit his conclusions. But *Saint Cosme vengé* is more than a recasting of La Mettrie's original dispute with Astruc. In this text, La Mettrie first raised a theme which persists throughout his career as a medical satirist: he questioned scholarship as an effective way to learn about diseases and cast doubt on the system of medical education which produced preeminent scholars who were untrained and uninterested in empirical medicine. More problematic than pedantry, as far as La Mettrie was concerned, was the fact that Astruc had no firsthand experience. Thus La Mettrie was able to call into question all of Astruc's conclusions. For example, he claimed that Astruc contributed nothing to the treatment of venereal disease because the surgeons treated it; Astruc had probably never even seen a case. This lack of experience led Astruc to misinterpret many other authors who had written about it.[16] La Mettrie's disagreements with Astruc on the origin and treatment of venereal disease led him to question the relevance of medical scholarship and medical education. In arguing that experience, not scholarship, made one competent to practice, he argued the cause of the surgeons, because they had practical experience in the treatment of venereal disease.

It was not just a question of their role in the treatment of venereal disease. The surgeons, according to La Mettrie, were the real physicians, because they alone were concerned with the treatment of disease. By contrast, the ranks of the medical profession were swollen with men who either did not practice medicine or practiced it poorly. La Mettrie noted with approval that in recent years some honors and a higher status had been accorded the surgeons because the public recognized the vital role they played in France's wars. However, he contended that the role of the surgeons must continue to be emphasized and honored so that the profession would attract highly qualified men. This had been difficult in the past because the doctors enjoyed such a high social status. Yet La Mettrie vehemently maintained that it was important to cultivate the surgeons because they were "citizens so necessary in these unhappy times of war and calamity, always so much more useful than those who let themselves be blinded by the false lures of physics, leaving experience behind, getting lost chasing vain theory."[17]

Thus, with the publication of *Saint Cosme vengé*, La Mettrie became a proponent of the surgical position in the pamphlet war. He supported their principal claims that by virtue of their experience they, and not the doctors, were the most competent medical practitioners, and that they best served the public good because they upheld practice over theory and experience over erudition.

That La Mettrie's satires were part of the pamphlet war has not been recognized for several reasons. Many scholars have scorned them as the least significant of La Mettrie's writings;[18] physician-historians were unwilling to acknowledge the treachery of a fellow physician;[19] and La Mettrie's own position on the surgeons evolved over the course of his medical practice. It is even possible to argue that his position vis-à-vis the surgeons was ambiguous, for La Mettrie was not so partial a defender that the surgeons were completely spared the venom of his pen. In his earlier medical works, he parroted the common opinions doctors held of the surgeons. For example, in his treatise on venereal disease, La Mettrie claimed that the surgeons had not contributed to the understanding of the disease because they could not read the other treatises on the subject—they were written in Latin. As the concluding point of a particularly scathing review, he asked, "Is it necessary to add that the author of this book is either a charlatan or a surgeon?"[20] However, these remarks were made before La Mettrie practiced medicine in Saint-Malo or in the army, two experiences which might well have changed his opinion of the surgeons.

As if to forestall just such a discussion of his position on this issue, La Mettrie assessed the merits of each side in the pamphlet war and his own involvement in the war in his last medical satire, the *Ouvrage de Pénélope* (1748–50).[21] Although La Mettrie was vehement in proclaiming the value of surgical experience and the empirically based education of the surgeons, he was not a blind partisan of their cause. He discussed in some detail his view of both the ideal and the actual relationship of surgery to medicine. For example, he noted that if a doctor wishes to practice surgery, he will find that he lacks a certain "adresse de la main" and the knowledge of certain practical details. However, if his failings are more significant and he is, for example, completely ignorant of anatomy, La Mettrie claims the fault is completely the doctor's own, because cadavers are readily available and there are many competent anatomists who can provide instruction. On the other hand, the surgeon who wishes to practice medicine has many more deficiencies in his education to overcome. For example, he might well discover that he knows only anatomy, and gross anatomy at that! His understanding of medicine will perhaps reflect the limits of his education, "a lack of literature and of penetration of spirit which is ordinarily so little cultivated. From which one sees what an enormous distance separates surgery from medicine." Thus the doctor has only one step to make to become a proficient surgeon; a course of operations on a cadaver will provide the foundation for knowledge which can be further amplified by practice, observation of surgeons, and work in hospitals. But the surgeons must undertake a much broader program of education and practice. Therefore, La Mettrie acknowledges that the position of the doctors ought to be above that of the surgeons "by virtue of the fact that they know medicine more profoundly, with all its accompaniments of physics and mechanics, too subtle to be seized by men who have not studied."[22]

However, La Mettrie also vigorously maintained that the proper relationship between doctors and surgeons cannot be implemented because the doctors in no way resemble the idealized characters he here portrays. The doctors of Paris, in fact, do not study anatomy, and according to La Mettrie, any physician who is ignorant of anatomy and surgery is not only unworthy to involve himself in surgical consultation but also "can only be a detestable doctor." Furthermore, although it is common knowledge that doctors know nothing of surgery, nonetheless they insist on teaching surgery, or rather, as La Mettrie describes it, on giving "très beaux discours." The audacity of the doctors astonishes La Mettrie as he exclaims, "Having never delivered a child into this world, don't they also presume to teach the art of delivering," inviting the midwives of Paris to these lectures, as if the midwives could possibly learn anything from them. He compares the doctors to "gens de cabinet," who are too delicate to deal with cadavers and so imagine that they can learn anatomy from books or chemistry from the proceedings of learned societies. Although La Mettrie was somewhat sympathetic to the doctors' claim that, because their education was much broader than that of the surgeons, they should control the practice of medicine, nonetheless he claimed that the doctors had forfeited that privileged status by their failure to cultivate the practice of medicine. And he blamed the doctors for the pamphlet war, noting that if the doctors in fact exemplified his ideal of medical practice and education, the surgeons would not have engaged in the battle but would instead have cooperated with the doctors to advance the cause of medicine. As La Mettrie put it, "If the doctors had not neglected anatomy, the surgeons would not have had such sport."[23]

Though he thought that the surgeons' case in the dispute was a good one, La Mettrie charged that both the surgeons and the doctors wasted time, made themselves the laughingstocks of Paris, and, most important, failed to serve the public good.[24] La Mettrie contended that the separation of medicine and surgery in France made both groups lose sight of their essential responsibility to care for the sick. Holland provided a useful counterexample; there surgery and medicine were essentially united, and the physicians had adopted the essentials of experimental medicine, clinical education and practice, and the study of anatomy and surgery.

Although not unaware of the surgeons' faults, La Mettrie evidently saw them as less ambitious and less avaricious than the doctors and as providing a real service to the public. The pamphlet war gave La Mettrie a forum for arguing the integral relationship between public well-being and good medical practice. The ever-widening gap between his sense of the proper physician and the spectacle of medical practice in Paris led him to espouse the methods of practice and the empirical education the surgeons advocated. Outraged, he exposed the failings of Parisian doctors in stinging satiric portraits.

Into the Fray

Satire as a literary genre, direct and relatively free of stylistic conventions, could be adapted readily and effectively to La Mettrie's concern with medical reform. The genre of satire, with its characteristic features of a topical subject and a quasi-realistic style designed to both shock and amuse,[25] was an appropriate tool for bringing an issue to public attention, using wit to attack a specific target. In the hands of Enlightenment pamphleteers,[26] satire emerged as a frequently employed instrument of social and ethical reform, for the satirist was "a moral agent, often a social scavenger, working on a storage of bile."[27] Even though philosophes like Voltaire apologized for using such an unsophisticated literary genre, satire was well suited to the cause of Enlightenment both because it sought to subvert and because its ultimate appeal was to reason and common sense.[28] While La Mettrie's medical satires may not be the best examples of the genre, nonetheless his satires served his purpose well, attracting a popular response and drawing attention to the issues of medical education and practice.

With the publication of *Politique du médecin de Machiavel, ou le chemin de la fortune ouverte aux médecins*, La Mettrie became a full-blown polemicist. He constructed an elaborate fable which thinly veiled his meaning and allowed him greater license in making his arguments. The text is supposedly a French translation of an ancient Chinese medical treatise handed down from generation to generation. Perhaps the use of this device was meant to afford La Mettrie some protection from the authorities, but since this pamphlet and his next one, *La Faculté vengée*, provoked enough outrage from the Faculty of Paris to have him expelled from Paris and his books burned, it was obviously not sufficient. It failed in part because La Mettrie was much more intent on making his criticisms than on maintaining the fiction.

He claimed to have translated this supposedly ancient text because, as he put it, "I was touched by the miserable condition of French letters today and I wanted to enrich my poor country with this excellent piece."[29] He deduced that the author was a judicious critic, and "an honest man, like Linacre himself, he was occupied only with distinguishing charlatanism from true medicine."[30] La Mettrie praised the author extravagantly for his lack of self-interest: "At the expense of his own fortune, which depends on the friendship of his colleagues, he has revealed their ruses and artifices, and as he himself said, he wished to be a true doctor, *only to be a better citizen*."[31] This phrase is telling for, despite the literary artifice, it is perfectly obvious that La Mettrie is the author of these defamatory portraits of his colleagues and that his defense of the author is a self-justification. Very much in keeping with the Enlightenment tradition, he argued that zeal for reform, even if, or perhaps especially if, it opposed self-interest, was the acid test of the good citizen.

La Mettrie dedicated his preface to Emperor Kein-long, a thinly disguised Louis XV,[32] reminding him that after his death he would be judged by posterity, which grants a good reputation only to those kings who have done good for their subjects. La Mettrie praised the king for having quashed the spirit of fanaticism, which he acknowledged was far more dangerous to a kingdom than "la liberté de penser des Philosophes de tous les siècles."[33] But La Mettrie pointed out that there was another monster to be slain by the king, more dangerous to his realm than fanaticism, "le brigandage de la médecine." This treatise was written to expose to the king those "alleged physicians" and to suggest simple means by which the king could remedy their "deadly abuses."[34]

La Mettrie thus proclaimed his sympathy with Enlightenment efforts to quash fanaticism, to effect a reform of philosophy, and to change the way men thought. But he was also intent on pointing out in all his medical and philosophical works that if one wished to ameliorate social and political conditions, the reform of medicine was a good place to begin. Though the abuses of medicine had garnered little attention from reformers, La Mettrie contended that such reforms were absolutely essential since the life and well-being of the citizens were directly in the hands of incompetent and badly educated practitioners. Thus, according to La Mettrie, kings, philosophes, and reformers of all kinds should first turn their attention to medical reform to correct the most flagrant abuses affecting the human condition.

Though the literary devices La Mettrie employed in this particular satire were transparent and not at all subtle, they did present certain opportunities for him. For example, he could claim that the points he made were not simply another piece in a propaganda war but rather an attempt to reform medicine by criticism. By pointing out the flaws in the character of certain physicians, he could work toward a redefinition of the ideal medical practitioner and raise questions about the nature of medicine and its role in society. Specifically, he allied the issue of medical reform to social reform and concern for public well-being.

The Parisian physicians must have been incensed by the absolute transparency of the portraits found in the *Politique*. They were so ingeniously presented that one medical historian has suggested that La Mettrie must have had spies within the Faculty reporting to him on the foibles of its members.[35] Each portrait of a physician begins with a description of his outstanding physical characteristics; the physician could be identified either by that characteristic or by a play on his name. For example, Sylva is de la Forêt, Mancot is Jaunisse because of his yellow complexion, and Astruc is called Savantasse for his intellectual pretensions. By the time the second edition was published in 1762, a key to the personages was listed on the frontispiece, the satirical guise virtually abandoned.

The essential part of each portrait was a description of the "politique" employed by each physician that explained the success of his practice. For example, Bouillac acquainted himself with the plots of the latest novels and therefore was thought by all of Paris to be well informed. One canny physician from Montpellier, Mancot, took care not to seem to infringe upon the practice of Parisian doctors and thus spent all his time in cafés, visiting his patients by stealth in the dark of night. Another spent all his time with the theater crowd and Freemasons to assure their patronage. Others catered to the vanity of women, acting more as cosmetologists than physicians. Another adopted the practice of visiting his patients frequently to ensure a good income. La Mettrie's harshest portrait claimed that Astruc assured his success by espousing Molinist theology to gain a Jesuit clientele and by criticizing the surgeons to raise his status in the medical community.[36]

Because these different practices governed medicine, the methods and treatments of these physicians were likely to be ineffective or even absurd. La Mettrie cited misdiagnoses of Mancot that had had fatal results. Sylva, La Mettrie claimed, saw medicine as "haute cuisine" for wealthy patients; therefore the medicines he prescribed were inevitably expensive and exotic. Helvétius, he charged, had no medical knowledge and was therefore an empiric of the worst kind and a "marchand d'ipécacuana" for the treatment of dysentery.[37] Other physicians violated medicine by failing to practice it, like Falconet, who gave up medicine for the life of "un homme savant," or, even worse, Procope, who abandoned it for the high life.

Two of La Mettrie's harshest descriptions were reserved for Ferein and Chirac, dead and venerated members of the medical community. The virulence of these portraits seems to stem from a feeling that if the medical establishment was to be effectively challenged the pillars of its society had to be assailed. Chirac, or, as La Mettrie called him, the Emperor Julian, had tried to establish the philosophical principles of medicine but failed because he had no experience on which to base his principles. Ferein had presumed to teach medical students even though he knew nothing of medical practice. His knowledge of anatomy was so limited, according to La Mettrie, that any knowledge his students derived from his classes was actually conveyed to them by the surgeon Ferein used as a demonstrator! These two venerable members of the medical community had violated the standards of medicine set forth by the surgeons and ultimately espoused by La Mettrie. They sought to base medicine on philosophical first principles rather than on experience and taught medicine without experience or knowledge of anatomy. Another probable motive behind La Mettrie's singling out of Chirac and

Ferien for his most devastating criticism was that both of them had attacked La Mettrie himself and his two mentors, Boerhaave and Hunauld.[38] Chirac had attacked Hunauld and failed to recognize the greatness of Boerhaave's contribution to medicine; Ferein had presumed to teach Boerhaave's physiology, though his knowledge of anatomy was nil, and to set himself up as an authority on Boerhaave. La Mettrie no doubt saw this as a blow both to the reputation of his teacher and to his own claim to be the sole French translator of Boerhaave's works. Ferein was also disparaging of one of La Mettrie's own works; it was reported that after reading several pages of La Mettrie's *Observations de médecine pratique* he said "to all the physicians he met that he could never give his approval to ideas of practice so despicable," which led La Mettrie to wonder "how a mediocre anatomist had become a judge of practitioners."[39] Chirac had also posed a particular threat to the Parisian surgeons; as first physician he had tried unsuccessfully in 1730 to centralize the power of the physicians by creating a medical academy whose members would have been allowed to practice in Paris.[40]

Though La Mettrie was clearly willing to use his pamphlets to redress personal grievances and to defend his mentors, the *Politique du médecin de Machiavel* reveals the complexity of La Mettrie's motives in writing these satires. It is no coincidence that his satiric portraits lampooned those who wrote against the surgeons; he had taken as his own their arguments for medicine based on experience and service to the public. Yet this attack is far too focused on specific members of the Faculty to be seen as simply another piece in the pamphlet war. Unlike the surgeons, La Mettrie did not mean merely to proclaim the merits of surgical education and practice. As a result, his satires do not address specific professional issues or argue for specific advances by the surgical community. Instead, they are broader, wittier, and, as a result, more effective and potentially more damaging to the doctors than the specific claims the surgeons made on their own behalf. La Mettrie meant to indict medical practice in Paris. He claimed that the doctors were self-seeking social climbers whose medical practice was based on ignorance. In essence, their medical practice catered to the whims of the wealthy and was dictated by popular trends. Because they scorned practical experience and anatomy, their practice of medicine could have no legitimate foundation. But while the failings of individual physi-

cians, so ably ridiculed in these early works, were indeed reprehensible, the dealings of the corporate body of the physicians, the Faculty
of Medicine, cried out even more stridently for exposure and reform. The Faculty should be ridiculed because, according to La
Mettrie, it perpetuated the low standards of medical practice in
France.

Taking on the Faculty

La Faculté vengée (1747)[41] is La Mettrie's most concerted attack on
the corporate entity of the medical profession, the Faculty of Medicine of Paris. This satire was popular enough to warrant republica-
tion in 1762 under the title *Les Charlatans démasqués* because, as
the editor put it, "the spectacle of a doctor writing to discredit his
colleagues is sure to amaze and interest Paris."[42] To add insult to
injury, this work was published by the printer used by the Faculty,
and in it La Mettrie claims to be a "docteur régent de la Faculté de
Paris."[43] It is written in a very light style, with far less of the
bludgeoning overkill of his earlier satires. Instead of launching a
virulent, polemical argument, this satire is a play in which the
characters speak for themselves, freely acknowledging all the character flaws and violations of medical standards which La Mettrie
attributed to them in the *Politique du médecin de Machiavel*.

The first act establishes La Mettrie's relationship to the Faculty.
He is disguised as Chat-Huant (the owl), "so called by comparison
to that animal, who preys on other birds and then sees them all
against him when he falls into a trap." He and several friends meet
the Porter and discuss the Faculty with him. The Porter, a laconic
old man, says of doctors, "I regard a physician, even one of the best,
as a machine which when tapped always resonates Hippocrates or
Galen and never makes another sound." He informs the disguised
La Mettrie and his friends that the Faculty is convening to decide
what to do about La Mettrie because "he has revealed all the secrets
of our synagogue so well that, to speak 'Christian,' our feasts are
greatly diminished and our patriarchs complain." The members of
the Faculty are so incensed over La Mettrie's satires that they have
prevailed upon their most illustrious members to return from hell to
take vengeance on him. La Mettrie's friends advise him to flee,

because with "les beaux esprits, les dévots, et les médecins" for enemies, he is safe nowhere.[44]

The next act of the play exposes the way the Faculty acts as a body. As they file in, they make much ado over their respective ranking within the Faculty, remarking that such questions are the primary considerations of a "facultatiste." They must address the problem of La Mettrie because his satires are endangering their sources of income by arousing their patients' suspicions. Since money is the balm of their profession, they conclude that La Mettrie's works should be banned and the author burned.[45]

Besides the venality, pettiness, and arrogance the doctors reveal when gathered together, their discussion of their patients in scene 5 brings their callousness to the fore. One physician recounts how he lost a patient; he was thinking of the card game *quinze*, so that when asked how many grams of medication should be given to the patient he unthinkingly replied "fifteen," and the patient died of an overdose.[46] Another physician proudly proclaims his ability to announce with perfect equanimity the death of a patient to his relatives. After all, he remarks, "What is man at bottom? Nature loses a thousand to make one."[47] The doctors conclude that they have no cause for concern about the demise of a patient because their role in society is population control.

The Faculty is then shown to operate as a mutual support system, sustaining and perpetuating the foibles of its membership. For example, Moulin makes light of his lack of anatomical knowledge and says that it is only important to know that the brain is not in the abdomen. Bordelin praises Astruc as a compiler and plagiarizer and says that he himself intends to defend a thesis proving that the "new theory" of the circulation was not contained in ancient works of medicine.[48] The members of the Faculty have thus proclaimed the barrenness of their notions of scholarship, discounted the concerns of their patients, and revealed their consuming interest in rank and privilege.

In the third act the devil arrives, summoned by his minions to more effectively impose judgment upon La Mettrie. As the estimable physicians of Paris gather before their ruler, they eagerly confess to all the sins La Mettrie had laid at their door. Moulin boasts of his complete ignorance of chemistry and botany and crows, "I have, to my great satisfaction, changed the Seine into a river of blood."[49]

Before the devil, Astruc glories in his pedantry. The devil, the patron of the physicians, is a common visitor at Faculty gatherings, because the deplorable practices of the physicians bring so many souls to hell. All the medical practices which La Mettrie has so heartily condemned are praiseworthy in the court of the devil.

The doctors then present to the devil a list of the grievances they would like him to redress. They entreat him to reestablish the authority of the doctors over the surgeons. Specifically, only doctors should have the right to authorize bloodletting by surgeons in exchange for a fee paid to the doctors. The doctors also request that the devil reaffirm the authority of the medical faculty by decreeing that only the faculties of Paris and Montpellier be allowed to *sell* degrees and that all the other, small, rival faculties be abolished. Finally, they ask the devil to address the problem of La Mettrie, who has done so much to warn the public of their malfeasance.[50]

The devil chides the doctors for their foolishness in taking La Mettrie's satires to heart. Because the public has no desire to be disabused of its illusions about doctors, it not only protects them despite their faults but turns those faults into virtues. "It is in this way that the vanity of the sick is in complicity with that of the doctors." The devil also points out to his disciples that reformers are ineffectual and satire has never corrected anyone. "Therefore," he advises, "be tranquil, laugh with the public to make it appear, if possible, that all in the satire is the opposite of what you actually are!" The doctors should also continue to behave as they always have, unconcerned with the cure of disease and preoccupied with financial and social success. The devil advises the doctors to "develop in your overheated imaginations and in the minds of the idiots who listen to you the most blatantly false ideas and the hollowest dreams. Do not waste time in the observation of nature. It is a tortuous path from which one never escapes. Above all, protect the fools, knaves, and rogues; wipe out merit and genius, and regard whoever has virtues and talent as a double enemy."[51] The advice of the devil, La Mettrie cleverly suggests, conforms to the actual standards of medical education and practice endorsed by the Faculty.

La Mettrie then pleads his case before the devil, claiming that he reported only what he himself saw or what was reported to him by unimpeachable sources. If, as the doctors claim, he is a scourge of society, La Mettrie asks what name can then be applied to the doctors? He characterizes them as "this vile troop of men whose union should reign as a blessing to the country, but where, in fact, union never reigns, where instead there are so many wolves in the forest trying to set traps for each other, to supplant each other, and to devour each other."[52]

La Mettrie apologizes for his satirical career, just as Voltaire deplored his satirical campaigns of the 1750s and 1760s.[53] Both of these writers seem to have recognized that although it was an effective style, it was undignified, a kind of literary brawling. Their apologies reflect a fear that a satiric treatment might garner the wrong kind of attention, perhaps compromising or trivializing a serious philosophical issue. But neither Voltaire nor La Mettrie could abandon such an attention-getting technique. Admitting that he was ashamed to have prostituted his pen in polemical writings and contending that "the role that I play, sire, is not at all in my character," La Mettrie proffers the following arguments in his defense. First, he notes, the history of medicine is full of examples of admirable physicians, such as Guy Patin and Phillippe Hecquet, who have written satires. In addition, although he admits that his satires have attacked both "l'intérêt et l'amour propre," he hopes that posterity will vindicate him so that the outrage he now provokes will turn to praise "when I will have no more enemies and my book will be widely enjoyed." Most importantly, he protests, "my excuse is the hope, very much in vain, no doubt, that the most perverse of doctors, those furthest removed from the right path, will perhaps one day correct their errors."[54]

The devil is torn in making his judgment. La Mettrie's indictment of the character of the doctors has been corroborated by their own testimony. Though he admires La Mettrie's courage in attacking a group more despicable than the devil himself, the devil must support and sustain his minions. Yet, as La Mettrie hoped, the devil shows himself to be more merciful than the doctors who wished to burn him; he merely exiles La Mettrie to Holland, where he can pose no threat to the Faculty.[55]

This is La Mettrie's most successful satire. It is not as serious in tone or as polemical in style as *Saint Cosme vengé*, and it does not resort to the convoluted twists of plot of the *Politique du médecin de Machiavel*. Unlike the writing in the *Politique*, where the satire is sometimes heavy-handed, the satire in *La Faculté vengée* is lighter because the doctors eagerly espouse the pictures La Mettrie drew of them. But this subtler satirical style does not blunt his effective attack on corporate privilege.

The Faculty became the focus of La Mettrie's reformist zeal because he held the corporate structure of the Faculty responsible, in large part, for the sorry state of medical education and practice in France and, perhaps more reasonably, for the lack of medical progress and innovation in France. His fundamental claim seems to have been that the very nature of the corporate privilege which the Faculty vehemently asserted in order to protect and further the interests of its membership could only work to the detriment of public health. La Mettrie argued that since the Faculty had taken as its primary goal the restriction of the number of physicians to ensure that they all could earn a good living, it had, in effect, directed the concern of the profession away from the care of the sick and toward an increase in social status. Unconcerned with the care of patients, the Faculty was instead vitally interested in increasing the wealth and social status of the physicians and with preserving the privileges of their corporate order.[56] But this privilege then was indefensible, because the physicians acted out of self-interest rather than from motives of public concern. Like many Enlightenment reformers, La Mettrie used privilege as a pejorative term for unwarranted and undeserved benefits. In this case, he intended to raise questions about the degree to which the exalted social status and protection conveyed by privilege were warranted by the caliber of the services the doctors provided. Thus his attack on the Faculty was designed to expose it as a corporate body which primarily fostered self-interest as opposed to public well-being.

According to La Mettrie, the demands of the doctors in the pamphlet war with the surgeons documented the overriding concern of the Faculty with questions of precedence. Like other entrenched, corrupt bastions of ancien régime privilege, the medical corporation focused its attention on the preservation of all sources and signs of status and position. Where this concern had no effect on public health, La Mettrie suggested that it was perhaps all to the good that the doctors were preoccupied with issues of prestige rather than issues of public health. After all, he noted, "a lazy fabricator of systems will not then present himself, to the risk of one and all, to try to remedy a malfunction of a machine that he knows only through speculation."[57] However, the dispute between the doctors and the surgeons, though perhaps from the doctors' point of view only a question of precedence, was far more disturbing to La Mettrie because of the possible deleterious effects on public health which would accrue if the doctors' claims to control surgical operations were reestablished. La Mettrie agreed with the surgeons that they should preside over surgical operations, since they, not the doctors, had practical experience in operating.

La Mettrie expanded the scope of his satires by moving beyond attacks on individuals to focus on the Parisian medical community and its corporate privilege. In *Ouvrage de Pénélope* (so called because the first two volumes weave a picture of the outrageous and despicable Parisian physician, a picture unraveled by the third volume, which seriously discusses the good physician) La Mettrie hones his attack by discussing the most detrimental result of corporate medical monopoly: the standards of medical education allowed by the Faculty and the code of professional conduct it endorsed.[58]

A Parisian Physician

In *Ouvrage de Pénélope*, La Mettrie made use of all the knowledge he had gleaned of the workings of the medical profession to give satirical counsel to his son on the steps he must take to ensure his acceptance by the profession and his rapid rise within it. The words of advice, he notes in the preface, are meant to cause revulsion, to cry to the reader, "Don't follow me or you will be dishonored!" Nonetheless, the work is dedicated to the doctors of Paris, who, La Mettrie claims, "have dictated every word."[59]

This satire shows a bitterness uncharacteristic of La Mettrie's earlier analyses of the medical community. Perhaps, at the end of his long campaign for medical reform, La Mettrie was daunted by the spectacle of such flagrant abuses of medical authority. While his pictures of specific physicians were harsh, it is less the vigor of his satire than his underlying purpose which separates La Mettrie from the long tradition of medical satire. Though his satires are frequently quite witty, the humor always gives way to the deadly earnest of his reforming zeal. Unlike Molière, whose famous physicians also reveal overwhelming ignorance, La Mettrie was not poking fun at the foibles of men, the conceit of doctors, and the complicity of the public in fostering it. He was engaged instead in a campaign for reform; the stance of the committed philosopher overshadows Moliéresque ridicule. Thus at times La Mettrie's wit flags, exposing his disgust with his fellow physicians and his despair of reforming deplorable medical practice.

La Mettrie's bitterness in this satire might also have been provoked by the failure of the Parisian medical community to correspond in any way to the ideal of medical practice and education he had experienced in Leyden under Boerhaave's tutelage. Perhaps the most succinct statement of the ideal medical practitioner is to be found in Boerhaave's text *De comparando certo in physicis*, in which he set forth the following three qualities as absolutely essential for the physician: "that he have a good mind, and be well instructed in the science of physic [medicine], that he have a readiness or promptitude to exercise his science, and that he exercise it for the benefit of the sick."[60]

La Mettrie found all these canons flagrantly violated by the physicians of Paris. Medical education in Paris certainly did not foster knowledge of the science of medicine. In fact, in the *Ouvrage de Pénélope*, La Mettrie advised the prospective physician to avoid entire fields of medical knowledge because they would not facilitate his quest to be a successful doctor. For example, anatomy is obviously useless to the aspiring physician because one can adopt a theory of the cause of all disease without actually having to deal with the parts of the body, and the study of anatomy will not earn for the doctor the respect of his colleagues; even William Harvey was not highly regarded by his contemporaries. Chemistry is positively detrimental to a medical career. Confined to a laboratory, the young physician will be covered with ashes. Since no physicians study chemistry, anyone who does will simply arouse envy or scorn. The manifest uselessness of surgery to medicine, La Mettrie claims, is shown by the large number of doctors who have made their fortunes without knowing anything of surgery. They gain preeminence even though their diagnoses are frequently proven wrong by the surgeons on the operating table.

Though scientific knowledge is useful only insofar as it contributes to the social status of the physician, La Mettrie notes that cultivation of the arts can be a most effective means to advancement in medicine. Literature, for example, is most helpful to the physician, for the "bon mot" is always appropriate and the study of literature enables him to construct "hypotheses which are as brilliant as they are intangible."[61] The very limited cultivation of some of these arts will give one the appearance of knowledge, and with the appearance of knowledge comes medical and social prestige. Thus, according to La Mettrie, the successful practice of medicine does not require that one be, as Boerhaave counseled, "well instructed in the science or knowledge of physic."[62]

The corporate control of the medical profession, according to La Mettrie, has worked to the detriment of medical education because the faculty determines which areas of scholarship are appropriate or essential for the successful physician. Hence La Mettrie contends that the study of physiology and the adoption of new discoveries have always been absolutely irrelevant to the Faculty, citing only the most notable case, the failure of the Faculty to accept the circulation of the blood more than one hundred years after Harvey. Because medicine is entirely theoretical, specific physiological study is to be abhorred, and as La Mettrie notes, "the lack of physiology will not prevent you from entering the Academy [of Science] provided that you know how to imagine a few surprising facts, if chance does not furnish you with any observations."[63] La Mettrie held that the reason medical education had become so bankrupt was that the Faculty of Medicine scorned the new sciences. As a result, university medical education continued to reject the empirical and the clinical in favor of textual disputation, and medical theories were held or abandoned solely on the basis of contemporary medical trends. Therefore, the best product of the Parisian medical system was a pedant who understood medicine as a scholarly pursuit, without practical application.[64] But the more typical graduate knew nothing of medical practice or theory, and his practice, or "politique," like that of the targets of La Mettrie's satires, reflected no more than the shifting sands of medical trends fostered by those who practiced society medicine.

Not only did the Faculty of Medicine support incompetent practitioners, it also reinforced the corporate cohesiveness of its membership, which, according to La Mettrie, worked to the detriment of public health. He cited loyalty to each other as the determining factor in all strictures of professional etiquette, a principle stringently invoked by the faculty in their battle with the surgeons. As Sylva put it, "I will act as an advocate for my greatest enemies rather than any friend among the surgeons."[65] Another general rule of medical conduct is that a physician, if he has a well-established reputation, treat his colleagues with scorn. Since a young physician cannot yet have attained such an enviable status, La Mettrie suggests that he cultivate the patronage of older physicians who can introduce him to their organizations.

Medical practice has also been corrupted by the Faculty, which has enforced unanimity and perpetuated conservative practices. La Mettrie used the medical consultation as an outstanding example. While the public is under the delusion that medical consultations exist to provide greater care for the patient, La Mettrie claims that they instead care for the physician by sharing his burden and effectively diluting his responsibility. When the doctors assemble to consult, no one takes charge, and only the most innocuous remedies are suggested so that everyone can concur in the treatment. Then the doctors can "let the patient go tranquilly into the next world without risking the reputation of a doctor." According to La Mettrie, the young physician must realize that unity of opinion is the most important factor in the medical consultation, for it provides protection for all involved. If a doctor should hold a contrary opinion about a case, he should advance it only if he has a hope of convincing the others. As a general rule, La Mettrie suggests to his son that he always espouse the views of the ancients on any issue, for the older physicians see any disparagement of modern innovations in medicine as flattery.[66] In general, the physician should eschew the novel or the innovative.

Certain professional practices also protect the physician in his dealings with patients. For example, the physician should affect a profound meditation while considering a case. If one has been fortunate enough to overhear the patient's self-diagnosis, one should solemnly repeat it. If not, La Mettrie advocates the following method of diagnosis. "I prefer one of the qualities of Matter, *impenetrability*. Medicine is a secret from the public. Why reveal what nature and art rarely reveal to the doctor?" In prescribing medicine, La Mettrie notes, one should never prescribe remedies which are uncommon or seem in any way to be mysterious to the patient, but only those medications which are in vogue and therefore beyond question. In the event of a patient's death, he should simply say that "nature is good and wise." Consigning the responsibility to nature, La Mettrie notes, is the most effective way for the physician to deal with death. Another valuable method is always to exaggerate the severity of the disease so that one will not be taken unawares by the death of a patient. After the fact, one can say, "I could have predicted it. I would not even have believed that he would have lasted so long."[67] In other words, the successful practice of medicine requires that the physician be most concerned with maintaining a reputation and with professional solidarity, rather than with "a readiness to exercise his science for the benefit of the sick," as Boerhaave had advised.

La Mettrie's critique of medicine as practiced in Paris focused on two fundamental issues: medical education and practice. He found contemporary medical education a bastion of ignorance because the physician refused to concern himself with the knowledge the new sciences could give him and instead persisted in the pursuit of erudition. This concern left the physician with a completely illusory basis for his practice, as he was uneducated in both the theory and the practice of medicine. In addition to being ignorant, the physician in Paris practiced society medicine. He used only popular remedies and acted to fulfill public expectations about the role of the doctor. Unconcerned with the care of patients, these physicians were vitally concerned with increasing their social status and preserving their privileges.

By participating in a public debate and by using the popular and effective medium of satire, La Mettrie meant to increase public involvement in medical issues. Specifically, he meant to goad the public to see that the proper physician ought to be the antithesis of the spectacle his satires presented. Because the true physician is concerned with issues of public health rather than social prestige, the public must demand that sort of physician. And since the physician can only be as good as the education he receives, the public must insist that the sort of medical education the surgeons supported be implemented.

La Mettrie's satires must also be placed within the context of the pamphlet literature and the periodical press that flourished in the 1740s and that was directed in part to weakening the jurisdiction of the established order, in this case the Faculty of Medicine.[68] His satires have particular significance within this context because they suggest four explicit bases of comparison between medicine and programs of Enlightenment reformers. First, La Mettrie satirized the Parisian medical community by contrasting their practice and education with the more enlightened standards of empirical and clinical medicine as he had seen it practiced in Leyden. Second, he indicted the corporate control exercised by the Faculty of Medicine as an unwarranted exercise of privilege, using the explicitly pejorative connotation of privilege common to Enlightenment rhetoric. Third, he contrasted the deficiencies characteristic of medical education and practice with the education and practice of the surgeons, who provided effective and therefore socially beneficial medical treatment. Finally, La Mettrie directed his campaign for medical reform to the public, charging that public with the mission of insisting that private or corporate control of medical knowledge by the Faculty be made public so that it could be reformed.

La Mettrie's satires also had significant ramifications for his later philosophical works. He demonstrated the same kind of iconoclasm in his philosophical works, subjecting philosophical authorities to ridicule; in philosophical matters he espoused with equal enthusiasm a concern with the standards of empiricism and utility; and he regarded the ultimate agent of both philosophical and medical reform to be the *médecin-philosophe*, as defined in his satires. The role of the *médecin-philosophe* in the philosophical sphere is an important theme of La Mettrie's philosophical works and will be discussed later. In the medical sphere, the *médecin-philosophe* was to be an amalgam of the zealous, reform-minded philosophe, the adept, empirical surgeon, and the well-educated, idealistic physician. La Mettrie's model for such a physician was Hermann Boerhaave. But La Mettrie also expanded the role of the physician to fit the context of Enlightenment France, for the *médecin-philosophe* must also, as La Mettrie himself had done, acknowledge the practice of the surgeons as more effective, attack medical privilege as corrupt and dangerous to public health, and conduct a campaign to inform the public on medical issues in the interest of public health. The reformist campaign of the satires had to be couched in such vehement terms because, as La Mettrie boldly asserted, "Medicine is, without question, the most useful and the most necessary of all the sciences. Physicians are even the only philosophers who are useful to the Republic and serve the State. All the others are lazy men who are content to admire nature, with arms crossed, without the power to bring to the state the least service."[69]

It is ironic that when La Mettrie's involvement in medical issues is noted, he is assumed, generally as a result of the above quotation, to be a staunch proponent of the medical profession.[70] No cognizance is taken of his career as a critic of the established medical order. However, despite his criticism, La Mettrie did not become antagonistic towards medicine. He did not, for example, advocate turning away from medicine in favor of less orthodox treatments or practice. Instead, he concentrated his efforts on a redefinition of the standards of medical education and practice.

At some levels, La Mettrie made his arguments for a new medical order on the same basis as the old arguments for privilege, that is, a specific kind of education and practice ought to entitle one to a position of preeminence. The difference, like the difference between the philosophes and traditional philosophers, is one of motive and reformist concern. For example, the old, privileged medical order is characterized, according to La Mettrie, by self-interest, passivity, concern with metaphysical and systematic knowledge, and deference toward the established order. The new medical practitioner, cloaked in the authority of the positions argued by the surgeons, is instead involved in issues of public health, concerned with providing essential public services, informed by concrete observation, and frankly irreverent in the face of established authority. The proponents of the new order do not appeal to tradition or attempt to keep knowledge secret within corporations. Rather, they appeal to public interest and attempt to educate the public.

Despite his excoriation of eighteenth-century practices and practitioners, medicine was still, for La Mettrie, the source of hope for the ills of society. And the ramifications of medical reform were not restricted to the medical profession or the practice of medicine: just as new standards of medical practice could be imposed as correctives to the old, so too, as La Mettrie was to suggest, medical theory could be used against metaphysics. In essence, La Mettrie wanted a reform of medical education and practice not only for the obvious utilitarian benefits reform would produce but also so that medicine could provide the foundation for a new understanding of human nature.

3

Boerhaave

The Medical Heritage

No doubt members of the Faculty of Medicine had some justification for the ire which provoked them to have La Mettrie's works
burned. After all, La Mettrie was a young French physician whose
French university experience was perhaps dissolute[1] and at best
undistinguished, whose medical experience was restricted to a
backwoods practice in Saint-Malo and a brief stint as an army
physician. These were hardly positions from which to assail the
authority of the Faculty of Medicine. La Mettrie, a physician without high standing in the profession, returned from abroad to set
himself up as the authority on Boerhaave, with exclusive rights to
translate his works into French. Those works themselves argued a
position on medical theory and practice greatly at odds with that
taken by the Faculty of Medicine of Paris. Furthermore, the authority of Boerhaave gave La Mettrie, a provincial upstart without even
the credentials to practice in Paris, the audacity not only to find
French medical education and practice defective but also to take up
the cause of the surgeons, the doctors' enemies, and to hone his
abilities as a satirist in his personal attacks on the doctors.
    While it might be wondered if La Mettrie was simply endowed
with an extraordinary quantity of chutzpah, the real source of his
confidence seems to have been his direct exposure to Boerhaave, the
preeminent medical teacher of the eighteenth century. Boerhaave
opened La Mettrie's eyes to the possibilities for medical practice and
reform that clinical experience, dissection, and the study of comparative anatomy offered. Boerhaave familiarized him with the leading
authorities, the prominent issues, and the latest theories of medical
practice. In return, La Mettrie translated Boerhaave's medical works

and wrote treatises on diseases in an attempt to apply Boerhaave's theory and practice of medicine. He also reappraised the synthesis of iatromechanism and iatrochemistry that was the foundation of Boerhaave's physiology. The new medicine, as defined and taught by Boerhaave, dramatically revealed the failings of La Mettrie's own education, and combined with his own experience as an army doctor, that knowledge gave him the confidence with which to assail the Faculty. Most importantly, La Mettrie used Boerhaave's physiology as the basis of his own philosophy.

Although Hermann Boerhaave (1668–1738) was a heroic figure of unquestioned importance in the eighteenth century, praised by his contemporaries for his innovations in the theory and practice of medicine, his merits have been more difficult for medical historians to appreciate. They have been able to salvage little of his system for use in modern medicine. So with varying degrees of opprobrium they have looked upon him as a rather interesting relic of the eighteenth century or, worse, as a misguided and blind mechanist. Sometimes they have attempted to preserve some of Boerhaave's former luster by associating him with the acknowledged heroes of the scientific revolution: it is a rather backhanded way of acknowledging that Boerhaave had some insight to say that he very early recognized the importance of Newton or that he in some way reflects the teachings of Francis Bacon.[2] Nonetheless, his medicine has been generally neglected by recent historians of science despite its unquestioned importance to his contemporaries.

Boerhaave was born at Voorhout in 1668, the son of a local pastor. Destined for a career in the ministry, he embarked on a program of studies in theology and philosophy at the University of Leyden. Unfortunately, the mere rumor that he had defended Spinoza was enough to prohibit a career in the church.[3] Boerhaave then turned to what had previously been an avocation, medicine. He cannot have had much respect for the medical education of his day, for instead of enrolling in a degree program he undertook an extensive, systematic, independent study of medical writers, attended public dissections, and dissected animals. He passed the exams necessary for a medical degree in 1693 at Harderwijk. He supported himself by giving private courses in medicine until 1701, when he was appointed lecturer in medicine at Leyden. In 1709 he was appointed professor of botany. His accomplishments in this field included the extensive cultivation of botanical gardens at Leyden, and he was tireless in his quest for new plants. He encouraged two new types of botanical research, plant morphology and sexual reproduction, and perhaps most significant, he sponsored Linnaeus.[4] He assumed the chair of practical medicine in 1714 and in this capacity introduced the modern system of clinical instruction, which is the basis of contemporary Western medical education. In 1719 he was also appointed to the chair of chemistry. He died on September 23, 1738, at Leyden, after thirty-seven years of instructing students from all of Europe and the New World. Because of the different disciplines which he both researched and mastered, Boerhaave was in a particularly advantageous position from which to disseminate the latest findings in all these fields to his medical students. Furthermore, perhaps because of his own extensive and wide-ranging knowledge, his medicine itself is eclectic, incorporating what proves useful from chemistry and botany.

Boerhaave's principal renown rests on his reputation as the greatest teacher in the eighteenth century. As the creator of the prototype of the present-day medical curriculum, his impact on medical instruction has endured. He advocated preliminary courses in sciences such as botany and chemistry, to be followed by a course in the structure and function of the human body, then courses in pathology and therapeutics, and finally extensive courses in clinical medicine. His three primary medical works all share the pedagogical concern to provide the student with a comprehensive description of basic physiology, diseases, symptoms, and treatments.[5] He felt that it was particularly important to publish the *Materia medica*, a collection of prescriptions, so that his students would be able to accurately apply his views in their treatment of disease. Most innovative and important, he restored bedside medical instruction to a central place in the medical curriculum.

Another factor in Boerhaave's influence in the eighteenth century was the vast international student body he was able to attract and inspire. These students returned to their own countries and effected changes in the medical curriculum in accord with Boerhaave's model. For example, it is generally conceded that Boerhaave was almost single-handedly responsible for the school of medicine at the University of Edinburgh; all of its outstanding teachers were at one time his pupils. And the University of Edinburgh was responsible for the training of physicians from the American colonies, making Boerhaave's influence as far-flung as the New World.[6]

The very character of Boerhaave's medicine may provide a key to both its impact and its modern neglect. His approach was flexible and firmly empirical, and his unwavering belief in the cumulative, progressive development of medical knowledge seems to have inspired his students, like Haller, van Swieten, and La Mettrie, to develop particular aspects of Boerhaave's legacy. As a result, his students contributed to the development of medicine in a number of different ways but did not form a distinct school of medical thought. This chapter will emphasize the parts of Boerhaave's legacy that La Mettrie invoked.

Boerhaave's Physiology

The late seventeenth century was dominated by two theories of physiology, both of which had developed to challenge Aristotelianism and Galenism, iatrochemistry and iatromechanism.[7] Iatrochemistry sought to apply chemical knowledge to the theory of medical practice. Rooted in an alchemical past, iatrochemistry was revitalized by Paracelsus's challenge[8] to Aristotelian university education and developed through the chemical research and experimentation of van Helmont.[9] François Sylvius de la Boë, the most famous seventeenth-century iatrochemist, described all physiological and pathological processes in terms of fermentation, effervescence, putrefaction, and by the theory of acid and alkali, which he considered the fundamental principle in nature. He posited an effervescence in the blood and thought that the processes of digestion could be explained by the interaction of acids and alkalis.

Inspired in part by the investigations of Galileo, iatromechanists based their understanding of physiological processes on the laws of mechanics. Thus outstanding seventeenth-century mechanists such as Borelli, Bellini, Pitcairn, and Descartes compared artificial machines to the human body, describing specific functions in terms of statics and hydraulics. The iatromechanists also generally relied on atomism as a basic theory of matter and were then able to explain changes in the body by changes in the configuration or movement of these small particles.

These fundamental conceptions were not rigid, and some physicians, attempting to understand human physiology, used elements of both theories. But Boerhaave was deeply disturbed by the tendency of followers of Hoffmann[10] and Sylvius to form schools, suggesting that either iatrochemistry or iatromechanism provided a complete explanation of physiological processes. Boerhaave forged a synthesis of these two theories that served as the foundation of medical thought and education throughout the eighteenth century. His importance resides not in the originality of the synthesis as a whole or any particular medical breakthrough it produced, but rather in the fact that he provided a compendium of the most complete contemporary physiological information in a nonpartisan manner, acknowledging the legitimacy of both methods of analysis. Boerhaave's synthesis also emphasized the pragmatic at the expense of the theoretical. His criterion for incorporation of an idea into medical practice was effectiveness, and empirical demonstration determined whether a tenet was acceptable medical theory. While Boerhaave saw the medicine of his day as being very enlightened, nonetheless he foresaw a need for continual revision and emendation, not only because there would be new discoveries in the future but also because he recognized that over the course of years the nature and the particular manifestation of diseases can change.

Physiology was not a separate field of medical study until 1700, when Boerhaave gave a definitive series of lectures published in 1708 under the title *Institutiones medicae in usus annuae domesticos*.[11] This work is part of a traditional genre, much on the order of a textbook, meant to provide comprehensive information that would enable one to practice in a particular field.[12] However, Boerhaave's *Institutiones* were more comprehensive, dealing primarily with physiology and pathology and providing some information on symptoms, hygiene, and therapy. Frequently reprinted and translated into many languages, this work was without question the most important medical text of the eighteenth century.

Dissatisfied with his students' knowledge of the basic sciences, Boerhaave sought to provide through these lectures a course in general physics and biology to prepare them for clinical studies. The text made extensive use of the most exact anatomical drawings by the best anatomists because, as Boerhaave contended, "there is nothing more agreeable, or more useful to those who examine the interplay of parts of the human body, than to know well its marvelous structure."[13] Boerhaave himself was one of the staunchest defenders of anatomy as a critical tool of the physician and therefore as an essential part of medical education as well. In his own independent study of medicine he dissected animals and assisted Anton Nuck in his anatomical demonstrations. As a professor, he continued to attend anatomical demonstrations given by Jacob Rau and Bernard Albinus and performed the autopsies on patients who died at Caecilia Hospital.[14]

In his preface, Boerhaave justified the scope of his study in answer to critics, who claimed that he restricted the field of medicine too narrowly. First of all, he included only what had been established through his own experiments or by incontestable evidence. Secondly, though he recognized that bodily states have effects on mental states and vice versa, Boerhaave refused to speculate further; one can perceive only the effects, he noted, and therefore no explanation is possible. He also contended that first causes, final causes, or any other metaphysical speculations were inappropriate areas for medical research, as it was "neither useful, nor necessary, nor even possible for a physician to study them."[15] Thus Boerhaave decisively exorcised metaphysics from medicine. He claimed that medicine must instead be concerned with the empirical and the useful.

In the prolegomenon to the treatise Boerhaave expressed his views on the history of medicine, a discussion which sets forth his relationship to both his medical predecessors and his contemporaries. Originally, he noted, medicine was merely a faithful record of what one observed. It had improved with more observation, more description of diseases and remedies, and more thorough autopsies and dissections. Because empirical observation was the crucial activity of the physician, Hippocrates, according to Boerhaave, was the first to merit the name of doctor. Later, as men began to seek out "by the paths of reasoning" the causes of what they observed, medicine lost sight of its true character. While observation is always "evident, useful, and necessary," Boerhaave noted, reasoning as to causes has been doubtful, uncertain, and subject to change according to the tenets of each sect.[16] Thus he praised Hippocrates for providing the model for the proper technique and derided Galen for trying to make medicine compatible with peripatetic philosophy. To

Boerhaave, who in all his medical writings tried both to provide a synthesis of opposing views and to establish an empirical base for medical instruction, Galen epitomized the greatest stumbling block to medical progress, sectarianism. However, with great optimism, Boerhaave hailed Harvey as the dawn of the modern age, for he had vanquished the sects by repudiating the sway they held over medicine. Boerhaave appreciated the history of medicine for the lessons it unfolded, the most important of which was that observation is always certain and reasoning as to causes always dubious.

Boerhaave was confident about the continued progress of medicine. He hoped that since Harvey had eradicated the accretions of false speculations, his contemporaries would be able, through the proper use of reason, to make rational medicine as certain as the empirical medicine of the ancients. Yet if Boerhaave was optimistic, he was not blindly so; he did not underestimate the difficulties. Medicine had to be founded on observation of the most scrupulous kind, "all that one can perceive of the well, the sick, the dying, and the dead."[17] And of all the medical research (or reasoning, as he sometimes called it) that attempts to understand what is hidden from our senses he was extremely demanding. "One can succeed in research of this kind only by sound reasoning, by maturely examining each experiment, by then comparing them carefully to see clearly how they agree or differ, and finally by noting with as much good faith as prudence, all the aspects of the experiment which remained locked away and that one cannot clearly deduce. Thus the path of reasoning will become as solid and sure as that of experience."[18]

In the *Institutiones* Boerhaave expressed his optimistic view that the medicine of his day was close to providing enough empirical evidence so that reasoning about what the senses could not perceive could be virtually certain. For example, he confidently based his physiology on the vascular injection experiments of his day. These experiments were technologically faulty, for they indicated that when a substance was injected into a vein it permeated the walls. But from them Boerhaave was led to speculate that the walls of the vessels in the body were composed of smaller vessels linked together. These vascular experiments and the demonstrable certainty that the laws of mechanics afforded the scientist were the building blocks of Boerhaave's physiology. He contended that the human body is composed of liquids and solids. The liquids are all the various humors, not restricted to Galen's four but including all the fluids in the body. The solids are the vessels which contain the humors and also the instruments which produce movement, that is, they form the pulleys and cords of the body. The movement of solids and the course of liquids through the body follow the laws of hydrostatics, hydraulics, and mechanics.[19]

Though his initial and fundamental physiological perspective was mechanical, Boerhaave also relied on other medical theories to substantiate his physiology. He admitted the atomic hypothesis, though its role in his physiology was not significant. He argued that indestructible atoms must exist since the universe has remained essentially the same for thousands of years. But since they are too small to be perceived by the senses, nothing more is known about them. Corpuscles were much more significant in his physiology; in addition to providing the basic structure of the human body, they seemed to him to explain a great deal about how liquids move through vessels.[20] For example, corpuscles explain why liquids in the healthy body are only found in the proper place—in other words, the size and shape of particles determine what path they will take through the body. Therefore, one never finds blood, chyle, or milk in urine because it is composed of small particles, and the urinary tract consists of small, convoluted canals to keep larger particles out.[21] Boerhaave also used the term "humor" extensively in his physiology. But he was not referring to Galen's four humors, which he discounted because he had determined that one could find all of Galen's four humors in the blood alone, that is, black bile was dried blood, yellow bile was blood serum, and phlegm was blood serum which had congealed. In Boerhaave's physiology "humor" was a term used to describe any liquids in the body. These categories of humors, corpuscles, atoms, and so on were conventionally tied to particular schools of medical thought; for example, humors were normally used by Galenic or Aristotelian physicians, atoms by iatromechanists, and corpuscles by iatrochemists. Boerhaave's use of all of these terms where he deemed them appropriate is an indication of his eclectic medicine and of his ability to take what he considered useful from a range of medical positions while detaching those positions from their sectarian connotations.

Despite his medical eclecticism, Boerhaave was sharply critical of the iatrochemists. He regarded them as "miserably mistaken in general laws, to which, from their particular experiments, they conclude all bodies to be subject." He chided them for "their cant of elements, fictitious ferments, effervescences, antagonistic salts, which they consider the only engine of nature."[22] He also tested their theories experimentally, subjecting the fluids of the body to acid/alkali tests with vegetable indicators such as syrup of violets, which turned red when exposed to acids and green when exposed to alkalis. The negative results of these tests (the bodily fluids that the chemists claimed were acid or alkali did not produce the expected results when treated with syrup of violets) were taken by Boerhaave to be a definitive refutation of the hypotheses of the iatrochemists as a comprehensive description of physiological processes.

Nonetheless, for Boerhaave chemistry was an essential part of physiology. He contended that "those vain trifling Chemists were certainly in the wrong when they claimed to explain physiology in all its parts by their art alone; however, neither are they who imagine that they can do the same thing without it less mistaken."[23] According to Boerhaave, chemistry was important to physiology because it was better able than any other science to investigate properties of bodies, especially those hidden under external appearances. Boerhaave claimed that "among all writers of natural philosophy, it has not yet been my fortune to meet with any that have more intimately examined and evidently explained the nature of bodies and the effects they are capable of producing than those that have gone by the name of Alchemist."[24]

Boerhaave noted that the assimilation of food could best be explained by recourse to chemistry. He also recognized that plants tended to ferment, turning sour and acidic, while animal flesh tended to putrefy and produce a volatile alkali. Boerhaave also felt he had to explain in some way the transformation of acidic food into alkali tissue. Heat was the solution—a clear indication of Boerhaave's debt to the chemical tradition of fire analysis. He recognized that in vitro the transformation of acid and alkali occurred with heat, and therefore suggested, since he explained bodily heat in a strictly mechanical fashion as the friction of fluids moving through vessels, that it was by means of this heat that food could be incorporated into the body to form tissues. This particular example illustrates Boerhaave's propensity for explaining phenomena by combining chemical and mechanical theories.

In general, Boerhaave was willing to invoke chemical analysis wherever he found that it could add to an understanding of the working of the body. Chemical analysis could explain to some degree the differences between humors such as bile and blood. An improper balance in the four chemical substances, that is, water, earth, salt, and oil, could explain some diseases. Though he vigorously objected to chemical systematizing and to the occult qualities the chemists sometimes used to explain physiological processes, Boerhaave did make use of chemical ideas and methods of analysis such as fermentation, putrefaction, fire analysis, and the subjection of bodily fluids and tissues to acid/alkali analysis.

However, Boerhaave attained renown as a mechanist, and for good reason. After all, he considered the evidence of mechanics sufficient as a basis for speculation about things one cannot observe. And from his preliminary statement of the nature of the human body in his *Institutiones*, his support for mechanism can be amply documented. Yet Boerhaave was not uncritical. He sharply criticized Cartesian mechanism because he saw it as mere analogy, the entertaining pastime of imagining that living organisms act as inanimate objects do. Although he relied on mechanism and mechanics to explain the functioning of the human body, he argued for an experimental approach, criticizing the mechanists for being too eager to apply general principles to all the particulars. Thus Boerhaave resisted mechanism as a comprehensive or systematic explanation of physiological functions. Nonetheless, he typically used mechanism to explain specific operations of the human body, and he had little tolerance either for his predecessors who were uninformed about mechanical principles or for his contemporaries who had not yet embraced them.[25]

Boerhaave gave purely mechanical explanations for many bodily functions. For example, urine is produced when the very tiny particles of urine are separated out of the blood by the force of its movement through the kidneys. Animal heat is generated by the friction of fluid moving through vessels. The lungs demonstrate the machine of Boyle. He also questioned nonmechanical theories about why blood is carried to the lungs, refuting by autopsies and the use of thermometers theories which contended that the blood was cooled in the lungs or that it moved to the lungs either to attract air or to expel murky parts.[26] Boerhaave specifically rejected the claim of Sylvius and the iatrochemists that the effervescence of the blood was transported to the lungs to be extinguished. Instead he claimed that the blood was brought to the lungs to be mixed with chyle. He posited a circulatory system for blood, lymph, and nerve fluid—an application of his belief that mechanism provided a secure enough foundation to be extended by analogy to what could not be seen, in this case the circulation of nerve fluids. All these fluids were propelled by the heart; thus, he considered that the whole body could aptly be called an hydraulic engine. Boerhaave's discussion of the action of the muscles, where he directed his reader to the mechanical demonstrations of Borelli and the hydrostatics and hydraulics of Mariotte, is perhaps the best indication of the critical role mechanics plays in his physiology.[27] In general, he claimed that mechanics provided the key to understanding the working of the human body, particularly its movement. While Galenic medicine or iatrochemistry could help the physician understand particular bodily functions, mechanism provided the best means to understand the functioning of the whole organism.

But Boerhaave found mechanism inadequate or inappropriate to explain sensation. He instead used as the basis of his discussion an epistemological framework which seems to be generally Lockean. Thus he assumed that all of our ideas are the result of the impression made on the senses by concrete physical objects. According to Boerhaave, ideas are clear and distinct not because they are innate, as Descartes contends, but rather because of the vividness of the effect of the object on the nerve. Or the idea might be clear because the object has often acted on the *sensorium commune* or because it is an unusual or distinctive object. Perhaps because Boerhaave was working within a medical tradition to try to explain physiological processes, he tried to draw explicit connections between those processes and the mind. For example, he understood sensation as the change occasioned in the surface of the nerve by the impression of a solid object and concluded that "the same action of the same object on the same organ always produces the same idea: from which it follows that the connection of these ideas follows the nature of the organ called sensitive."[28] Like Locke, Boerhaave noted that sensations were tied to pleasure or pain but used that association as an example of the effect of the completely physical "esprits de cerveau" on the muscle. He claimed that the *sensorium commune* was the repository of all the points of the brain which send out "esprits" (a term usually used to mean nerve fluid) to affect the muscles. The influence of the "esprits de cerveau" on the muscles is indicated by the muscular reactions that love or hatred produce.[29] Boerhaave also explained memory as Locke did, as an evocation of an idea by another similar idea, a process which unlocks a series of connected ideas and brings the memory evoked to the forefront of the *sensorium commune*. For Locke, this process takes place in the *sensorium commune*, but it is not an explicitly physical process as it is for Boerhaave, who described memory as *possibly* an entirely physical process: "This is what one calls memory, when one has previously had a similar idea. Thus an idea can equally be born of physical causes hidden within the body which affect the nerves, the 'esprits,' the brain in the same manner and consequently excites the same ideas, as these external physical causes."[30]

Although he was inclined to invoke Lockean epistemology and to apply Locke's terms, in so far as possible, to physiological processes, Boerhaave ultimately found ideas too complex to believe that he had dealt with them conclusively in his physiology. Despite the connections he drew between the body and the mind or, more accurately, between ideas and physiological processes, Boerhaave quite clearly backed away from any materialist implications, noting that "it therefore seems that this diversity of ideas does not depend solely on the different construction of the extremity of the nerve, but on still many more causes which, to tell the truth, are not influential as causes but as conditions established by the Adorable Author of Nature."[31]

Boerhaave's attempt to define sensation in terms of physiological processes makes his account more materialistic than Locke's. Yet he firmly believed that nature was the manifestation of God's plan and did not suggest that matter was capable of self-movement. For him, all movements are controlled and directed by "esprits de cerveau," which allow one to suppose that those "esprits" are directed by an immaterial soul. But beyond proclaiming his own faith, Boerhaave considered these questions to be idle and profitless speculation. However, his nondogmatic approach allowed his students to take many positions on this issue. They could ignore the whole question of the relationship of the mind or soul to the body, they could insert a vitalistic soul, or, as La Mettrie did, they could make the physiological connections much tighter and posit materialism as the end point of Boerhaave's sensationalism.

The connection between Boerhaave and Locke has not been treated by scholars. It is certainly true that Boerhaave's discussion of sensation is a very small portion of his physiology, and his use of Locke to discuss physiology is tentative. Nonetheless, this discussion was critically important to La Mettrie, and it no doubt also raised the specter of materialism for the pious Albrecht Haller. While it seems unlikely that Boerhaave met Locke (Locke's exile in Holland ended four years before Boerhaave assumed his first university position), there are several ways he could have come in contact with Locke's ideas. First of all, the University of Leyden, particularly receptive to new ideas, was the gateway to the rest of Europe for Cartesianism, Newtonianism, and Lockeanism.[32] Secondly, Locke spent part of his exile at the University of Leyden working with professors who were Boerhaave's immediate predecessors. Third, Locke and Boerhaave both sought to promulgate the ideas of Sydenham;[33] Locke's primary concern while in exile was proselytizing for the medical gospel according to Sydenham, a crusade Boerhaave later undertook with even greater effect.[34] Thus there are many ways Boerhaave could have come into contact with the ideas of Locke and significant reasons why he would have found Locke's epistemology appealing. Given that Boerhaave would have appreciated both Locke's campaign for Sydenham and the medical character of his philosophy, it is not surprising that Boerhaave used Locke's *Essay* as the foundation of his discussion of sensation.

Although Boerhaave was the most influential medical thinker of the eighteenth century, historians of medicine have been quite critical of him. Some of his explanations seem incredible; hence the view that Boerhaave must have been unthinking and uncritical. Medical historians are definitely out of sympathy with his use of mechanics in physiology because it was no longer novel or clearly progressive. They seem unable to understand the role that mechanism played in the intellectual climate of the time, the certainty it seemed to guarantee, and the universality of application it suggested to physicians of the eighteenth century. Most crucial, Boerhaave is not one of the heroes of medicine, that is, one associated with an important discovery in the annals of medicine and thus immune from the stigma of medicine in the benighted past.

Historians of medicine have tried to reconcile Boerhaave's immense reputation in the eighteenth century with his nearly complete neglect by the nineteenth and twentieth centuries and save for him some measure of esteem by extolling him as an early Newtonian. There seems to be little justification for this interpretation.[35] Lindeboom, the noted Boerhaave scholar and biographer, considers him to be a Newtonian not only because Boerhaave favored mechanism over iatrochemistry but also because Lindeboom equates an interest in empiricism with Newtonianism. Boerhaave was indeed a mechanist, but his mechanism is specifically indebted to the medical mechanists like Baglivi and Bellini, who provided the crucial examples of the applicability of mechanics to physiology, rather than to Newton. In fact, Boerhaave was critical of attempts to apply Newtonianism to physiology and was unconvinced that Newton's theory of gravitation had any application to it. In fact, he was inclined to see gravitation as a revival of occult forces and thus a return to the arcane, rather than as a force for medical progress. Specifically, he did not think that attraction could be used to explain the fact that corpuscles combined or the chemical reactions of substances.[36]

The source most often cited for the claim that Boerhaave was a Newtonian is his introductory academic lecture *De comparando certo in physicis*. In this work, Boerhaave instructed the young physician about what he must know to be a good physician. He began by claiming that a general knowledge of bodies was necessary for one who intended to study human bodies. Boerhaave certainly praised Newton but as a mathematical authority rather than as a thinker whose theories could be applied to medicine. The work itself is an indication more of Boerhaave's philosophical eclecticism than of his Newtonianism. For example, his general section on matter is the only extensive discussion of Newton, but Newton is only one of a host of references. In fact, Boerhaave's fundamental definition of matter was Cartesian, though he claimed Descartes should have added impenetrability to extension as part of his definition. He used Newtonian attraction interchangeably with Cartesian unity as terms to explain the cohesion of parts of bodies. He also used Huygens and Newton as the bases of definitions of mass. However, Boerhaave's fundamental theory of matter was atomistic. In fact, to learn about the nature of bodies, Boerhaave most strongly recommended that the young medical student study Lucretius, Diogenes Laertius's commentary on Lucretius, and Gassendi. He recommended the study of Newton, Keil, and Huyghens not as a prelude to medical study but rather to those few "who have a desire to penetrate the inmost recesses of Mathematics."[37]

Historians of medicine have most frequently found fault with Boerhaave's physiology, particularly his reliance on faulty injection experiments and his excessive use of mechanism.[38] Nonetheless, it must be kept in mind that Boerhaave used mechanism and injection experiments as the foundation of his system because they were based on the most recent, and what he saw as the most accurate, experimental evidence. He argued for adoption of his physiology not because it was conclusive but because it was clear, simple, and, most important, grounded in experiments and observation, which he emphatically advocated as the only means of furthering medicine. The fact that his basic physiology is founded on observations gleaned from faulty experiments is relatively unimportant, even to his physiology. Based on the interaction of fluids and solids in a body, a corpuscular notion of matter and disease, and so on, his physiology forms a very loose system. Once again, what Boerhaave consistently emphasized was the importance of what was observed. Neither a fluid-solid physiology nor any speculations about invisible corpuscles could in any way impede the incorporation of new observations into Boerhaave's system. It also seems inconceivable that Boerhaave's system would have in any way dissuaded his students from observation and experiment; quite the contrary!

Because Boerhaave thought he had established a sturdy foundation on which medicine could develop by incorporating new experimental studies into his basic physiology, he was optimistic about the future of medicine. Furthermore, he saw the progress of medicine to date as providing evidence for this view. According to his reading of medical history, Hippocratic empiricism gave way to Galenism and other sects that sought to make medicine conform to rationalistic principles that bore little relation to observable fact and inhibited empirical research. However, Boerhaave concluded that sectarianism did not characterize the corpuscularism of Boyle, the laws of mechanics, or the application of Lockean epistemology to physiology. They were principles which were not based on occult qualities, and Boerhaave could not imagine that their adherents could ever be considered members of sects. Hence, he perhaps rather naïvely concluded that at last physiology had been correctly grounded in certain principles; for in his view even the working of those parts of the body that could not be seen had been explained not by undemonstrable occult qualities but by the physical laws of mechanics. This naïve and overly optimistic view of the certainty of mechanics and the validity of its application to physiology has exposed Boerhaave to some criticism. However, his practice of medicine is measured in its use of various medical systems and firmly grounded in empirical observation.

Boerhaave's Practice of Medicine

Thus when Boerhaave castigates the moderns it is not the scientists of his day who are under indictment. Boyle, Harvey, the mechanists in general, and Locke are warmly praised. The clear implication underlying all of Boerhaave's work is that the science of his day has finally produced a clear and certain foundation for medical practice. It is the contemporary medical practitioner who presumes to build his medical theories on the sands of metaphysical speculation who is denounced. Boerhaave was certainly blind to the degree to which he had done the same thing in his physiology. But his ideas of medical practice were much less systematic than his physiology. In medical practice Boerhaave followed the path blazed by the modern he most admired, Thomas Sydenham, "the English Hippocrates." Hippocrates was Boerhaave's medical hero, and he considered Sydenham the modern who had most accurately followed the medical practices of Hippocrates.

When Boerhaave turned to the study of medicine he began with Hippocrates. Even though, as we have seen in his discussion of the history of medicine, he claimed that the moderns had made considerable advances, nonetheless the ideal of medical practice remained the Hippocratic method. In his first medical lecture, Boerhaave recommended the study of Hippocrates to his students. Hippocrates is the specific inspiration behind Boerhaave's *Aphorismes*: he provided the model for descriptions of disease, for the taking of case histories, and for the use of diet and exercise as therapy. As the observant physician par excellence, the example of Hippocrates suggested to Boerhaave the necessity of applying to medical education the model of Hippocratic practice. Thus Boerhaave revived bedside teaching and gave it a prominent place in the medical curriculum. Because Thomas Sydenham had also restored Hippocratic observation to medical practice Boerhaave saw him as his ally in the reform of medicine.

In his general approach and on many specifics of medical practice, Sydenham is very similar to Boerhaave, and the reasons that Boerhaave found him a kindred spirit are obvious. Sydenham praised the ancients and scorned the moderns for their reliance on systems, whereas Boerhaave scorned the unenlightened systematizers of an earlier age. Sydenham denounced systems as irrelevant to the practice of medicine. "And he that thinks he came to be skilled in diseases by studying the doctrine of humors, that the notions of obstructions and putrefactions assists him [with] the cure of fevers, . . . may as rationally believe that his Cook owes his skill in roasting and boiling to his study of the elements."[39] Sydenham was even more vehement on this issue than Boerhaave. Perhaps influenced by his Puritanism, Sydenham maintained that man's pride led him to form systems and then to expect nature and even God to act according to them.[40]

Boerhaave and Sydenham also shared similar concepts of disease. Sydenham's method of learning about diseases and their cures was to take careful case histories and then to compile them into a "history of the disease," very much according to Francis Bacon's suggestions. He considered that many diseases occur seasonally. Certain diseases attack certain types of people. Sydenham distinguished these types by age, vague terms such as "loose habits," and a Galenic sense of one humor as preponderant and thus temperament-determining. Boerhaave considerably expanded and clarified the notion of the effects of disease on "types." His definition of a type is a person of a certain disposition, prone to certain particular habits of eating, drinking, and exercising, of a particular age and sex, and residing in a certain kind of climate. In the treatment of disease, in addition to relying on careful description preceding diagnosis, Sydenham's practice was dominated by the overriding idea that theory must give way to observation, a principle that Boerhaave, too, adamantly advocated. Sydenham also relied on moderate and sensible prescriptions as remedies and recommended the mildest sorts of remedies and in small doses, as Boerhaave did later. He also suggested exercise, fresh air, and changes in diet. In addition, Sydenham and Boerhaave shared a notion of disease as particulate.

There are, however, great differences between the two that account in large measure for their different contributions to the history of medicine. Boerhaave was *the* medical establishment of his day and as such was able to effect great changes in medical education and practice. Sydenham, on the other hand, was very much outside the medical establishment and rather defensive about it. He was almost entirely self-taught, he had a private practice, and some of his medical remedies were widely ridiculed. Sydenham's defensiveness and alienation from the medical community is evident in this remark to a friend about his treatise on gout: "If this dissertation escapes blame both from you and those other few (but tried and honorable men) whom I call my friends, I shall care little for others. They are hostile simply because what I think of diseases and their cures differs from what they think. It could not be otherwise. It is my nature to think where others read; to ask less whether the world agrees with me than whether I agree with the truth, and to hold cheap the rumors and applause of the multitude."[41]

Part of the reason for Sydenham's defensiveness was that his simple remedies found little favor with his medical colleagues. For example, the common way to treat smallpox in seventeenth-century England was to prescribe exotic, expensive cordials and to keep the patient very warm to hurry the crisis of the fever. Sydenham, believing essentially that a cure should follow the course of nature, thought that in the case of smallpox one should engage in normal activities as long as possible, and when one finally took to one's bed one should simply remain loosely covered. This method was called the "cooling down method," and it was widely ridiculed by doctors who claimed that Sydenham packed his patients in ice.

Sydenham's unorthodox (though very effective) medical practices kept him out of favor with his medical contemporaries. It is also no doubt true that several opinions he held had the same effect, for Sydenham argued that most forms of medical research and experimentation carried on in his day were unfruitful and misdirected. He contended that the study of anatomy was unlikely to produce "improvement to the practice of physic." In conjunction with his dismissal of anatomy, he argued that autopsies could not instruct the physician. Microscopes he considered useless because they could not tell us "what organicall texture or what kind of ferment separate any part of the juices in any of the viscera, or tell us of what liquors the particles of these juices are, or if this could contribute to the cure of the diseases of those parts which we so perfectly know."[42] Sydenham claimed that the studies of his day which were directed towards determining the functions of organs in the body would never disclose how an organ functions or correct its malfunctions.

His opposition to the medical establishment has cast Sydenham in the guise of a medical hero. Nonetheless, because of his extreme antagonism toward all these areas of medical research, Sydenham can seem a bit the irrational and irascible fanatic, especially since so much of his opposition stems from the religious conviction that these sorts of scientific investigations overstep the bounds that God set for human knowledge. But it must be acknowledged that his argument was also based on his recognition of the in vivo-in vitro problem, that is, the problem of applying results gained from experiments in test tubes to living organisms.[43] The depth of his conviction that medical theories were irrelevant is illustrated by a story that, though it may be apocryphal, ironically makes this point. Once Sydenham was asked by a friend which books he should read to gain a knowledge of medicine; he replied: "Read *Don Quixote*. It is a very good book. I read it myself still."[44]

But despite his skepticism about medical theories, Sydenham was unable to completely avoid giving some causal explanation for disease. He seemed to acknowledge the merits of the iatrochemists when he said that spring produces a livelier ferment in the blood and summer the greatest effervescence in the bile. Probably because of his friendship with Robert Boyle, he loosely adhered to a particulate concept of disease and used Boyle's corpuscles to explain their epidemic spread. But in explanation he generally fell back on the four humors. He uncritically accepted the entire Hippocratic corpus and used it as the theoretical backdrop, albeit an unobtrusive one, to his medical observations.

Sydenham has become one of the heroic figures of medicine in part because his descriptions are painstaking and easily recognizable to one trained in modern medicine. Sydenham also acknowledged his debt to Francis Bacon, and thus the historian of medicine does not even have to try to postulate a resemblance. And Sydenham passes a crucial acid test for inclusion in the ranks of those who form the straight line of scientific progress: his work is readable!

Yet to his contemporaries Sydenham's legacy was problematic. He had provided a model of accurate and painstaking medical observation. However, his unwavering support of the ancients and disparagement of the moderns produced idiosyncrasy and distortion. For example, his research on dropsy was faulty because he refused to take Harvey into account and expected the course of epidemics in London to be analogous to those of ancient Greece. He had also argued vehemently that contemporary research and technological advances were irrelevant to medical practice. Thus there was little likelihood that his contemporaries would have combined modern research discoveries with his empirical observations, especially in light of his extreme alienation from the established medical and scientific communities. However, the support of two men within that community, Locke and Boyle, gained a hearing for his ideas. Above all, Boerhaave's enthusiastic praise of Sydenham and his incorporation of Sydenham's work into both his own writings and the medical curriculum assured a place for Sydenham among the moderns he had so disdained.

In keeping with his ties to the medical observations of Hippocrates and Sydenham, Boerhaave's thought is much richer, far less rigid, and clearly less mechanistic when he instructed his students on how to diagnose and treat disease than in his more theoretical works. His *Aphorismes sur la connaissance des maladies* perhaps best indicates this.

The *Aphorismes* themselves are pithy statements upon which he elaborated in his *cours particulier*. In the prolegomenon, he clearly states his fundamental ideas on medicine. His conception of disease is derived from the physiology set forth in the *Institutiones*. Hence, disease equals the natural functions "deranged," that is to say, a disturbance of the solids and liquids or an improper balance between the two. For example, solids can be too weak, soft, or lax, or they can be too stiff, firm, or rigid. Fibers which are too soft can be corrected with an iron diet and exercise. Fibers which are too rigid can be corrected with a watery diet. An improper assimilation of food can produce humors which are alkaline and thus tend toward putrefaction. The remedy for this condition is the ingestion of acidic foods. Inflammation is produced by an improper flow of liquids in the body, the result of both an obstruction of small blood vessels and an increased velocity of blood flow. Inflammation can therefore be corrected by a redistribution of humors that is brought about by drawing them away from the affected area with warm baths, mustard plasters, and so on.

In the *Aphorismes*, Boerhaave was concerned with practical medicine, which he defined as that medicine which allows us to know and cure disease. Thus, although his physiological explanations remain at the core of his consideration of disease, Boerhaave relied most on his own observations and experiments. In his attempt to treat disease, he was far more willing to employ the methods suggested by those schools whose physiological ideas he stridently criticized. In line with this pragmatic approach, Boerhaave stated that knowledge about diseases and their cures was best obtained by observation and analogy. Observation entailed a thorough case history of the patient, a careful enumeration of those things that seem favorable or harmful throughout the course of the disease, and an autopsy.

To explain disease, Boerhaave used medical theories he had criticized. For example, even though he severely castigated Galen for his metaphysics and discredited his four humors, when the remnants of Galenic theory could account for disease, Boerhaave did not hesitate to employ it. Thus he was perfectly willing to allow that melancholy might be caused by an excess of black bile or that a disposition towards certain disease might be inherent to those individuals of a phlegmatic or sanguine temperament. Even though Boerhaave decried the excesses of the iatrochemists, he nonetheless incorporated their theories into his account of how food is absorbed by positing the transformation of acidic food matter into alkaline tissue through the agency of bodily heat. So, too, in his theory of disease, an incomplete assimilation of acidic matter could be cured by eating alkali foods to redress this imbalance. In addition to relying on the acid/alkali distinction of the iatrochemists, Boerhaave also invoked in this case the age-old idea of cure by contrary.

It cannot be overemphasized that although Boerhaave disagreed with the extreme views of the iatrochemists, who he thought had uncritically applied chemical ideas to medicine, he nonetheless considered the study of chemistry to be one of his most important activities. Through his lifelong work of chemical experimentation and his twenty-seven years of chemical instruction, Boerhaave not only increased the standing of chemistry as a science but also gave it a permanent place in medical education. He advocated a new method in chemistry, which meant that the principles and rigid exactness of physics and mathematics should be applied to chemical experiments. He expected others to follow the high standard he set for himself: "I report of my experiments and their results simply and without verbosity; things that have no bearing on the matter should not be added inconsiderately; therefore, I do not wish to include anything that is not borne out by the result. Consequently my work can offend no one except perhaps those who are fighting for a preconceived opinion."[45] Boerhaave also carried out extensive experiments on fermentation and putrefaction, milk, urine, albumen, and blood serum. With the methods at his disposal, he went as far as possible in the field of biochemistry. The results of these experiments were given a prominent place in his physiology.

Boerhaave attempted to put the claims of the alchemists to the test of experiment without in any way prejudging the outcome. To this end he carried out a series of experiments on metals, some of them lasting over fifteen years. He also extolled the medical remedies found in the writings of Paracelsus and van Helmont. In his correspondence he often sent chemical remedies taken from the works of these authors to those who had written to describe their symptoms and seek his counsel. He had a particularly high regard for van Helmont, whose work he had read seven times, committing large sections of it to memory. Yet despite his praise for some of the chemists and his use of their remedies, Boerhaave found the veiled language of chemical writings particularly frustrating. "I rest neither day nor night in my efforts to isolate from the ore the hidden medicinal properties that are highly praised by the Chemists . . . and it is my ardent wish that the Hermetics would describe their unsuccessful experiments truthfully instead of filling their empty works with idle promises and fictitious words."[46]

Boerhaave was generally wedded to his notion of a solid-fluid physiology as the determining factor in sickness and health, but where he dealt with practical medicine, as in the *Aphorismes*, he recognized that a disease can have a great many causes, some of which strike the modern reader as highly improbable. For example, in discussing epilepsy, he suggested that the cause could be hereditary, often skipping a generation; or the infant could acquire the disease from his mother's milk if the mother saw an epileptic during her pregnancy;[47] or the brain could have been "wounded on the surface, in its substance, or its ventricles, by wounds, contusions, abscesses, pus, blood, a bitter, putrid lymph, by bony growths in the cranium."[48] In cases like this Boerhaave assigned equal weight to all possible causes, recognizing that he did not have enough information to discriminate among them.

His views on the treatment of disease also show an epistemological modesty. Recognizing that some diseases and some types of wounds are inevitably beyond the skills of the doctor, he readily acknowledged what he could not know. For example, in discussing fevers he concluded that he did not really know the nature of a fever, and the only thing he could determine as common to all fevers was rapid pulse.[49] (The thermometers of the day were not exact enough to measure slight variations in temperature.)

His particular treatments were guided by general principles. He believed that remedies should vary according to the symptoms of the disease, and thus every discussion of disease included lengthy sections on the symptoms. He had a marked preference for organic remedies over chemical ones. In fact, in his *Traité de matière médicale*, a companion piece to the *Aphorismes*, Boerhaave gave the exact recipes for remedies he had suggested in the *Aphorismes*. He listed remedies in order of the gravity of the symptom they were to treat, from weakest to strongest. This arrangement corresponds to remedies from the vegetable, animal, and mineral kingdoms. Chemical remedies, many of them taken from Glauber,[50] should be employed, he insisted, only in the most severe cases of the most serious diseases. He also used autopsy findings to support his conclusions about diseases and appropriate remedies.

Another crucial factor in Boerhaave's treatment of disease was the role that the particular constitution of the sick individual might play in the manifestation of the disease. Therefore, one must prescribe remedies according to the temperament of the patient, the season, and the degree of complication of the disease. He claimed that certain "types" of people (by which he seems to have meant a combination of Greek temperaments and individual habits) are more prone to diseases. For example, in discussing pleurisy, he said: "This disease principally afflicts those adults who are of a sanguine temperament, who are overweight, drink much expensive wine, get much exercise, who are rarely subject to acid belches, who have some tendency towards inflammatory diseases, above all in the spring when a great heat succeeds a great cold and in winter when one is exposed to a cold, piercing, and burning wind."[51] In diseases like frenzy the emotional causes outweigh the physical. In such cases, part of the recommended treatment is to "distract the spirits of the sick."[52]

Boerhaave also invoked Lockean explanations to account for certain types of diseases. For example, in his description of delirium, Boerhaave contended that it resulted from ideas produced inside the brain which did not correspond to sense perceptions. (By inference, ideas are normally produced in the brain in direct correlation with sense perceptions.) However, in cases that dealt with the effect of the mind on the body, Boerhaave was unwilling to commit himself to a particular cause. For example, a heartbeat that is too rapid and too strong may be caused by too many "esprits," or the result of the "passions of the soul or sorrow," or it may have a purely physical cause, "bitter matter, salt, or purulent alkali salts in the blood."[53]

Hermann Boerhaave, the teacher of all Europe in the eighteenth century, bequeathed a formidable heritage to his students. He provided a complete system of medical education. His work in physiology synthesized the reigning currents of thought and made available to his readers the most recent anatomical illustrations and experimental results. The sciences of physics, chemistry, and botany were incorporated into the study of medicine insofar as was possible. His work on the diagnosis and cure of diseases relied on and advocated careful, extensive observation and experimentation. It brought once again to the forefront of medical practice the teachings of Hippocrates and his English follower, Thomas Sydenham. Perhaps most important, Boerhaave's teaching reinstated clinical practice as a vital part of medical education.

As important to the development of his students as the information he provided was the spirit in which it was presented. Boerhaave bequeathed his legacy to his students in a manner that was undogmatic and empirically modest, and he encouraged his students to emend and build on his medicine. He gave to his students a thorough presentation of the medical knowledge available in the eighteenth century, combined with a great deal of specific experimental results and general information about the other sciences Boerhaave considered essential to medicine, especially chemistry and botany. Because this heritage was so rich, his students could choose to develop certain portions. For example, his students from Great Britain tended to concentrate on Boerhaave's medical curriculum and clinical instruction. Gerard van Swieten applied Boerhaave's curricular innovation to the teaching of medicine, chemistry, and botany at the University of Vienna. Albrecht Haller used Boerhaave as a foundation for his more extensive investigations of organic functions. Particularly important to La Mettrie was the way Boerhaave prefigured an Enlightenment methodology: his work was ordered and systematic rather than rigidly attached to a system of thought, and he advanced utility as a standard of knowledge; for example, despite a loose adherence to iatromechanism, Boerhaave used iatrochemistry and even Galenic medicine where appropriate. Boerhaave advanced a view of medicine which criticized the role of metaphysics in medicine and instead argued that medicine must be based on what was empirically demonstrable and useful, an inheritance fundamental to the development of La Mettrie's medical theory and practice and ultimately to the development of his philosophical positions.

4

La Mettrie's Practice of Medicine

Boerhaave was the most important influence on La Mettrie's practice of medicine. His exposure to Boerhaave provided the structure for his own medical work and a path for career development, and his studies with Boerhaave provided him with the best understanding of the working of the human body available to an eighteenth-century physician. With that understanding as the basis of his medicine, further refined by his sense that the progress of medicine demanded the most stringent criticism, La Mettrie brought the works of Boerhaave to the French reading public, modified in accord with his own perceptions.

La Mettrie's own medical treatises acquainted both the public and the scientific community with conclusions he had drawn from his medical practice and a theory of disease largely indebted to Boerhaave. In treatises about venereal disease, smallpox, and dysentery[1] he developed his understanding of the cause of disease. He relied on both the Galenists and the mechanists in his theory of imbalances in the constituents of the human body. His treatments followed logically from his ideas of causation. The most complicated and problematic discussion of the nature of disease occurred in his treatise on vertigo, which raised crucial problems that he addressed in more detail in his philosophical writings.

By seeking to enlighten the public about the dangers of some popular remedies for these diseases, La Mettrie demonstrated his concern with preventive medicine. Keenly aware of the limits of contemporary medicine, he sought to acquaint the French reading public with the writings of Hippocrates and George Cheyne, works which took note of the environmental and dietary factors involved in health and disease.[2] His concern with public health issues was motivated by his conviction that it was much more effective to try to educate people about the steps they could take to remain healthy than to try to cure them once they were ill. The treatises also provided case studies to inform his fellow physicians about cases which defied conventional treatment or seemed to indicate new manifestations of a disease;[3] they show La Mettrie to have been a very cautious practitioner himself who used chemical remedies but emphasized care in determining dosages and who qualified every prescription by noting all the facets of the individual constitution which must be taken into consideration.

The Critical Assessment of the Practical Inheritance

Though La Mettrie was aware of the problems and shortcomings of Boerhaave's synthesis,[4] he deeply admired Boerhaave as a model of medical practice, and his medical writings can be firmly placed within the context of Boerhaavian medicine. He consciously modeled his writings on the heroic triumvirate of Boerhaave, Sydenham, and Hippocrates. He defended Boerhaave's treatise on venereal disease and Sydenham's method of treating smallpox, and he used Hippocrates' work *Airs, Waters, and Places* as a standard for public health. Though he criticized particular points of Boerhaave's physiology, La Mettrie was to a large degree wedded to Boerhaave's liquid-solid physiology as an effective way to understand how the human body functioned in both health and disease. He used both the mechanists and the chemists according to Boerhaave's definition of their proper relationship to medicine—that is, he used mechanism as a useful descriptive analogy and chemistry as a source of some effective remedies and a few descriptions of physiological processes. He generally favored the methods of Sydenham and Hippocrates in the treatment of disease. But La Mettrie rigorously applied the critical sense espoused by Boerhaave to all issues of practice, even those advocated by his medical models.

La Mettrie's debt to Boerhaave is explicit in the *Observations sur les maladies vénériennes* (1735), which is in large measure a translation of Boerhaave's treatise on venereal disease, originally published in Leyden in 1728. La Mettrie interjected some of his own ideas about the disease in the preface, used footnotes to emend specific points of Boerhaave's text, and added his own treatise, which expanded upon Boerhaave's discussion of venereal disease by considering the debates of his own day about the nature of venereal disease and by taking into account new developments in its treatment. However, La Mettrie waxed indignant with others who criticized Boerhaave's practice of medicine more overtly.[5] For example, he defended Boerhaave as an outstanding observer, experimentalist, and practicing physician against Jean Astruc, who had in his own scholarly treatise on venereal disease challenged Boerhaave's notion of the treatment of the disease.[6] Astruc's pedantry divorced medical scholarship from observation, whereas, according to La Mettrie, scholarship must always yield to observation.

Although La Mettrie defended the value of Boerhaave's observations over Astruc's scholarship, he recognized, as Boerhaave had, that the continued progress of medicine depended on an ongoing process of criticism and revision. But La Mettrie was more inclined to criticize medical heroes than Boerhaave had been. For example, La Mettrie was part of the seventeenth- and eighteenth-century Hippocratic revival. He accepted the necessity of incorporating concerns about the environment and the individual constitution into medical practice; his prescriptions were often Hippocratic, recommending a particular diet and regimen of exercise; he also deliberately modeled his treatise on practical preventive medicine on Hippocratic writings. Nonetheless, his assessment of Hippocrates was somewhat less than deferential. Though he found most of Hippocrates' remarks in *Airs, Waters, and Places* credible, he considered Hippocrates' observations about the customs, habits, and physiology of faraway peoples to be "very curious and amusing," and his overall assessment of the text is ambiguous. To Hippocrates' work in general he gave only qualified praise: "Although fundamentally erroneous, the magnificence of his writings and the genius which pierces through the errors and certain superstitions always excites in connoisseurs sentiments of esteem and admiration sworn in almost all centuries."[7]

La Mettrie considered Sydenham's legacy even more problematic. He recognized, as Boerhaave had, the value of Sydenham's treatment of smallpox and admired his meticulous case studies. However, he was also much more critical than Boerhaave had been of Sydenham's failings, chiding him for his failure to appreciate the significance of recent medical texts and the importance of chemistry and anatomy in medicine.

In his work on smallpox, La Mettrie praised Sydenham as the source of the most accurate and precise information about the disease. He considered Sydenham's case studies especially admirable, noting, for example, that Sydenham's description of the two types of smallpox, discrete and confluent, were so complete that those who had seen both types, himself included, acknowledged that "they lack, in my opinion, not the least essential circumstance." La Mettrie claimed that Sydenham provided an important service for physicians, because, as he put it, "nothing gives as much security to the physician as to know well the course of the disease, to follow nature step by step, and to be warned early about what it will be necessary to do."[8]

But La Mettrie felt quite free to take issue with Sydenham's analysis and treatment of dysentery. He criticized Sydenham for never having opened a cadaver. As has been noted in discussing La Mettrie's satires, the failure of a doctor to consider anatomy was sure to provoke his harshest condemnation. He also criticized Sydenham's treatment of dysentery because Sydenham categorically refused to use chemical remedies; owing to blind prejudice he persisted in the use of his preferred treatment, opium, despite the fact that, according to La Mettrie, it suppressed bodily functions and thus augmented inflammation. Most importantly, he called into question Sydenham's entire approach to discussing disease, claiming that simple description was not sufficient, "because so many observations which will not provide information as to the character and the cause of maladies appear to me to be quite frivolous and serve only to make apparent an analogy between those diseases which appeared at a certain time and those which appeared in another time."[9] Sydenham is often praised as a model of Baconian science, and his descriptions of diseases are so painstaking that they can be readily identified by a modern physician. However, La Mettrie, in contrast to most eighteenth-century physicians, was quite uninterested in nosology[10] and found both the cataloguing of diseases and description for its own sake to be of very little value. If from his descriptions and classifications the physician could make no recommendations for effective treatment, then, La Mettrie contended, they were a pointless exercise.

La Mettrie deliberately resisted any attempts to lionize medical heroes, even those he personally admired, because he was acutely aware of the danger of endowing any medical thinker with so much authority that his medical practices and prescriptions could not be questioned. He contended that to point out the failures of great men of medicine was only to treat them as human beings, and, more importantly, to fail to do so could have disastrous effects.[11] In treating his own case of cholera, La Mettrie realized the ineffectiveness and positive danger of Sydenham's use of narcotics and concluded: "It is greatly to be wished that doctors would have all the diseases they treat in books or at the bedside of the sick. Better instructed at their own expense, they would make fewer errors whether with pulse or pen in hand."[12] For La Mettrie the continued progress of medicine depended on a rigidly critical methodological stance which must challenge every authority, defeat popular prejudices against innovative practices, and evaluate every medical theory in terms of its concrete, practical applications.

The Crusade for Public Health

As a direct application of his notion that medicine must be useful, La Mettrie sought to promulgate Boerhaave's medicine and his own observations and experiences as a physician by making his writings accessible to the literate public; he deliberately made his medical works readable. Furthermore, each work was undertaken to direct specific information to a particular medical constituency or to the general public. In addition, they were motivated by several fundamental principles. First, medicine must be useful, deliberately directed to the prevention and most effective treatment of disease. Second, medicine must be reformed, and this could be accomplished if medical information were more widely disseminated. Third, medical information must be extended to the public so that they would be able to take better care of themselves and understand some of the issues involved in the treatment of disease. Finally and most importantly, the public must be informed so that they could participate in medical reform. Just as his satires revealed the failings of contemporary physicians in order to provoke the public to demand better physicians, so his medical works were intended to acquaint the public with good practice and to warn them about dangerous practices. This attempt to raise public awareness of health issues can be seen as part of the reform efforts of the Enlightenment. By making the private knowledge of the medical corporation public, La Mettrie could hope both to inform the public and to further his quest to break the Faculty of Medicine's power, which was based on a monopoly of medical education.

As an application of his conviction that medicine must be useful, La Mettrie sought to disseminate what he considered to be the most authoritative evidence—his case studies. For example, he presented in great detail a case study of a hysterical catalepsy in one of his Saint-Malo patients[13] because this particular case had unique symptoms and because it failed to respond to orthodox methods of treatment. He also gave a careful description of normal manifestations of this disease and evaluated the different remedies commonly employed in its treatment.[14] In addition, he presented a detailed account of his own case of *cholera morbus*.[15] His discussion of the epidemic reveals his debt to Hippocrates, since he believed that specific climatic conditions gave rise to epidemics. He remarked that the conditions in Brittany in 1741 were ideal for producing a cholera epidemic, that is, a very harsh winter followed by a rainy spring and a hot, dry summer. The heat of the summer was, in his opinion, the determining factor because cholera is produced by a bile which is dry, abundant, and bitter and produces in the intestines an "irritation which attracts all the fluids from the viscera." In his own case a burning heat in the ventricle indicated to him that the disease had inflamed his blood, and therefore bleeding was the appropriate remedy. So he bled himself seven times. He also tried laudanum as a remedy, since Sydenham recommended it so highly, but discovered to his discomfort that laudanum was not to be employed until the symptoms had abated, because otherwise the bile, "so dangerous in cholera, would remain unaffected and continue to irritate, inflame, and tear with even greater efficacy."[16]

La Mettrie also discussed the problems of diagnosing and treating new manifestations of diseases. Having seen several cases of a new type of smallpox, La Mettrie concluded that *rougéole nouvelle* was a form of *rougéole* complicated with "scurvy or, more frequently, with a great gangrenous dissolution in the blood."[17] To determine the appropriate treatment for the disease, La Mettrie consulted the physicians of Normandy and relied on their advice because the disease had been epidemic and successfully treated there. He also confirmed that his observations about this disease had been borne out by the autopsies he performed.

These particular case studies were directed to other physicians who, far from centers of medical research, might be unaware of new developments in the treatment of disease, peculiar cases, or new manifestations which would warrant unusual treatment. This desire to be of service to his fellow practitioners and the citizens of his country is the expressed purpose of all of La Mettrie's medical works. For example, he said that he had translated Boerhaave's text on venereal disease both to make himself useful to his country and to render a specific service to the surgeons, "as they are consulted every day on diseases which often have their site in the marrow of the bone; it is left to a zealous citizen to put at their disposal the works of a physician which will guide them unerringly in the cure of these diseases."[18]

La Mettrie also conducted a vigorous campaign to warn the public about ineffective and dangerous remedies[19] by publishing his medical works as serials in popular journals such as the *Journal des savants* and *Lettres sur quelques écrits*. Even if some remedies could be considered harmless in themselves, the public had to be warned against them because using ineffective remedies meant a delay in using effective ones. Such a delay could allow a disease to spread throughout the entire circulatory system, a development La Mettrie considered dangerous and difficult to combat. Just as he argued against "society physicians" in his satires, he condemned remedies which were used simply because they were in vogue. He also meant to warn the public against the sorts of physicians who would use ineffective remedies.

Thus, in discussing the treatment of dysentery, La Mettrie argued both against those physicians who used astringents, because he claimed that astringents halt the flow of humors which nature so wisely produces to rid the body of an irritant, and against those physicians who claimed to cure the disease "par quelque prétendu spécifique," which he denigrated as nothing but the promises of charlatans.[20] He claimed that specific remedies such as rhubarb, ipecacuanha, and simaruba, so loudly touted by the public, owed their reputations for success in the treatment of dysentery to the fact that a number of cases of dysentery are mild enough to cure themselves. He noted that though ipecacuanha was once the rage of Paris, it was ultimately discredited. Helvétius provoked La Mettrie's ire in his satires because he claimed to treat the disease successfully with this remedy. Instead of these remedies, La Mettrie argued in favor of the use of an emetic, a harsh chemical remedy which physicians were disinclined to use. He denounced their reluctance as frivolous prejudice which could be discredited by experience. "If physicians most zealous for the progress of the art of medicine are prejudiced against the best medicines, either because they don't dare use them or because the public is doubtful about them, medicine will take a century to advance a single step. A sad reflection, because it is true!"[21]

La Mettrie's specific purpose in his own treatise on smallpox was to dissuade the public from ineffectual remedies. He discussed the use of cordials, which were very much in vogue as a remedy for smallpox. Their popularity rested on the idea, which La Mettrie claimed was not borne out in practice, that cordials contribute to the cleansing of the blood. The argument was one of analogy: the natural progress of the disease reveals its tendency to move from the center to the circumference, or from the inside of the body to the outside. What could be better therapy than to imitate the course that nature follows, that is, to do everything possible to make the eruption prompter and more complete? La Mettrie was harshly critical of this line of reasoning. The public, "who can't see further than its nose," was enamored of this reasoning, which was confirmed by "vulgar physicians." Most deserving of scorn, in La Mettrie's opinion, were the *femmelettes* who took upon themselves the treatment of their husbands, children, brothers, and sisters and gave medical advice to friends. They made the traditional treatment even more dangerous with their advocacy of greater heat. They confined their patients to bed, with windows and curtains closed, under the weight of many covers, in a room with a fire—all to hasten the eruption of the disease. La Mettrie proclaimed this to be a "cruel method more likely to disfigure, to say nothing of making the entire human species perish."[22]

The fundamental tenets of La Mettrie's medicine, stringent criticism and painstaking observation, might seem to make him an outstanding eighteenth-century practitioner. Especially because of his concern with public health issues, it is tempting to consider him in the forefront of Enlightenment medicine. But despite the fact that La Mettrie's medical works seem to be outstanding examples of the work of a well-informed, critical medical writer and an observant, cautious medical practitioner, nonetheless his work is also indicative of the problems and limitations of eighteenth-century medical practice and analysis. Despite the critical acumen he brought to bear in evaluating cases, the remedy he most often recommended was bleeding, and some of his explanations of disease strike the modern reader as ludicrous.

In particular, La Mettrie cannot be connected to the chief medical crusade of the Enlightenment, inoculation against smallpox. In fact, he argued vehemently against inoculation.[23] In his day inoculation was the practice of inserting matter from smallpox pustules into an open vein of a healthy person (variolation). Though this practice usually produced a mild case of the disease that also gave immunity against further smallpox infection, it sometimes produced severe or even fatal cases. Even more dangerous, in La Mettrie's opinion, was the fact that the inoculated person was able to transmit the disease; he was as contagious as if he had naturally acquired the disease.

The preparation for inoculation "consisted in bleeding, purging, bathing, to dilute the blood and, in a word, to make the blood circulate with all the tranquility and slowness possible."[24] The reason for these preparations was the belief that an inflammation caused the blood to flow more quickly, and since inoculation introduced inflammatory matter into the blood one had to take means to slow the blood flow. However, despite many successful cases of inoculation and the use of these precautions, there were cases, La Mettrie noted, of robust men who were well prepared for inoculation but nonetheless died from it.

Evidently La Mettrie felt that in the case of an inflammation one employed certain means to moderate its effects, and if some unexpected property in the blood produced an unforeseen resolution of the disease, the doctor could be certain that he had done all that he possibly could. However, in the case of inoculation, one took unnecessary risks because the doctor could not assume that his best efforts to allay the effects of inflammation could be guaranteed successful. Thus La Mettrie concluded that the practice of inoculation was pernicious and ought to be abandoned, as the English had done.[25] But La Mettrie's conclusion that the English had abandoned inoculation was mistaken. In England in the 1720s inoculation was practiced in some noble families and by a few physicians, with the result that there were several well-publicized deaths in noble households. After 1728, discussions of inoculation disappeared from English periodic literature, and it was widely assumed that the English had abandoned it. In fact, inoculation continued to be performed, but only in small numbers, because England did not experience a severe epidemic in the period from 1727 to 1746. After the epidemic of 1746 there was a large public demand for inoculation, and it became a common practice. The philosophes in France made a crusade for inoculation the focus of their medical concerns after 1750.[26]

Though in retrospect the benefits of inoculation seem evident, La Mettrie was not completely mistaken in his critical assessment of variolation. Statistics from the 1720s and 1730s showed that one in six persons who contracted the disease died, while one in fifty died after variolation.[27] The question that La Mettrie raised was whether it was legitimate to infect someone who might not contract the disease or to increase the spread of the disease (because those who were variolated actually contracted the disease and were contagious).

Despite La Mettrie's crusade for public awareness of health issues and his critical appraisal of medical practices, he nonetheless proselytized for bleeding. Although bleeding is often singled out as a failure of early medicine, there were reasons for its use that rested on critical observation and experience. Lester King suggests that bleeding became established as a therapeutic technique because it was effective often enough to justify confidence in it.[28] It was advocated so often by La Mettrie because he shared the notion, common to eighteenth-century physicians, that inflammation was caused by an obstruction in a blood vessel that could be resolved or disengaged by bleeding. It was the appropriate treatment for an inflammation, as indicated by La Mettrie's definition of fever: "Fever is only a wave which pushes that which won't go any more."[29] Bleeding produces a void in the blood vessels which allows the blood to move faster through them, making it possible for the obstruction that produced the inflammation to be worn away or set loose into the bloodstream. "By that means the stagnant blood takes its course again with facility."[30] Thus, for La Mettrie bleeding is a logical therapeutic outgrowth of Boerhaavian physiology that considers the balance of solid and liquid to be fundamental to questions of health and disease. Because La Mettrie had concluded that smallpox was the result of a particularly virulent inflammation, he considered bleeding to be the remedy of choice. He was frustrated by his inability to sway public opinion from the use of cordials in favor of bleeding. In fact, La Mettrie contended that one of the principal responsibilities of the practicing physician was to overcome the prejudices of the people against necessary and efficacious medical practices, despite the fact that the most effective way for a physician to ensure that his practice would flourish was to prescribe according to the prejudices of the people, in other words to be "the slave of the vulgar way of thinking."[31] In general, La Mettrie argued that prejudices against bleeding must be overcome in those cases where the symptoms were a strong pulse, *symptômes pressants* like the oppression of breathing, convulsions, swellings, and so on. And he insisted that these prejudices against bleeding be given no quarter at any sign of inflammation.

Although La Mettrie's general advocacy of bleeding and his opposition to variolation does not set him apart from his contemporaries as a medical innovator, neither do those positions irretrievably consign him to the ranks of the unenlightened or the uncritical. His opposition to variolation was based on his understanding of the risks involved, especially the risks to public health that further spread of the disease would entail. His support for bleeding was his response to the puzzling phenomenon of fever, and the remedy he advocated was logically consistent with his understanding of the physiological cause of the symptoms, heat generated by the friction of obstruction in a blood vessel. (Unfortunately logical consistency does not always produce an understanding of a disease or provide effective treatment.) Bleeding was also demonstrably safer in the treatment of smallpox than the more popular treatment of cordials. So while in light of the subsequent history of medicine these positions may not seem to be the most enlightened, La Mettrie took them because he was concerned with public health, the empirical observation of the course of disease, and the response of diseases to remedies.

La Mettrie also sought to inform the French reading public about means to avoid the dubious remedies of some physicians. His *Lettres sur l'art de conserver la santé*, which first appeared in serialized form in the popular French periodical *Lettres sur quelques écrits de ce temps* (1734), acquainted the French reading public with the medical advice of Hippocrates and Cheyne.[32] This text demonstrates La Mettrie's continued concern with one of the crucial aspects of his Leyden medical education, the revival and promulgation of Hippocratic medicine. No doubt, too, because it was substantially based on Hippocrates' *Airs, Waters, and Places*, this treatise concentrated on external causes of disease and environmental factors in the maintenance of health. Its goal was preventive medicine rather than the determination of the causes of disease and the appropriate cures. This text was explicitly directed towards the public; its purpose was to inform his fellow citizens so that they would be able to know what ought to be required of the physician and to have some control over their own state of health.

La Mettrie claimed that his interest in preventive health care was motivated by the fact that it was more effective medical practice to instruct on how to maintain health than to cure the body once it was diseased. Maintaining health requires simply that one know what to take and what to avoid, whereas curing disease "requires that one have recourse to other men, who know the activities of our machine and have made a long and careful study of its diverse arrangements." La Mettrie took upon himself the task of a "good citizen and zealous physician" to provide rules of life so simple and clear that they would make it possible for one to distinguish immediately between what was beneficial and what was detrimental to the preservation of health, "because medicine is at best uncertain, and it must, with regret, be conceded that most diseases are incurable."[33]

The first letter on *Airs* was meant to alert the average person to the ways air that is too cold, too humid, too dry, too heavy, or too light can affect one's health and to indicate what steps could be taken to circumvent these harmful effects. For example, too great a heat dries up bodily fluids, "elongates, relaxes, weakens the solid fibers which make up our vessels, and, in a word, makes the body soft and effeminate, as one observes in warm countries." La Mettrie claimed that residence in a humid climate is not healthy because of exhalations of "corrupted vapors." He also advised that when the air is heavy and humid those who have weak chests should not leave the house until the fog has been evaporated by the sun. This advice, he noted, is a critical concern to the residents of London because so much carbon is burned there that the city is covered with a nitrous-sulfurous smoke from November to February.[34]

La Mettrie also recognized that the habits of the individual certainly affected his susceptibility to diseases. For example, he noted that those who regularly drink wine can expose themselves with impunity to cold air and yet do not seem to catch colds or epidemic diseases. His explanation gave some indication of his concept of contagion and the role of the individual physiological constitution in influencing susceptibility to disease: "Why so? It is thanks to their naturally strong circulation which has become more rapid through the use of good wines, the vapors of which transpire in abundance across the pores of their skin, preventing the entrance of particles of air which could derange the animal economy. In contrast, these same harmful particles pass easily into the vessels of sedentary, studious people who have weak fibers, blood poor in spirits, and whose weak transpiration must yield to the pressure of external air."[35]

This letter on air also had some practical applications. For example, La Mettrie intended to make the general reader aware that he should take into account the air quality before building a house. One should specifically avoid building near chemistry laboratories, dye or vinegar factories, or mines, especially those producing mercury, antimony, and sulfur.[36] He also intended to alert the physician to the importance of understanding the effects of the climate in treating his patients.

In his second letter, La Mettrie wanted to acquaint his readers with George Cheyne's general rules of diet, rules like: foods and animals which mature earliest are easiest to digest, animals and vegetables with a strong taste are less easy to digest than those with a weak taste and, "in general, it is necessary that foods be proportional to the strength of those who take them as much in quality as quantity." Other authors who had treated this subject, La Mettrie claimed, were merely content to indicate the effect of a certain type of food, as if the effect of a particular food were completely independent of the body on which it acted. In other words, these authors had failed to consider, as Cheyne had not, the effect of "age, temperament, habits of exercise, and the strength or elasticity of fibers."[37]

Concern with the nature of the individual constitution was a fundamental characteristic of La Mettrie's practice of medicine. For example, in discussing cholera, he noted that the treatment varied according to the constitution. He made the distinction between his case of cholera and that which afflicted an old man. First of all, the causes of disease were different in the two cases. His own case was brought on by too much study, too little exercise, and insomnia. The old man's case was brought on by grief at the death of his daughter, which, combined with his age, produced a massive buildup of bile. The constitution of the old man required a treatment different from that employed for a younger man, especially since age slowed the circulation. Narcotics such as laudanum would have been too strong, and bleeding would have been too dangerous. Though he did not ordinarily prescribe cordials (a legacy, no doubt, from Thomas Sydenham), La Mettrie found them to be appropriate in this case. In general, he contended that the medical history of the patient, his general health, age, and habits must be considered.[38] Constitutional factors also played a critical role in determining the best method of treating smallpox. Certain temperaments, La Mettrie argued, must signal to the physician the need to employ the most drastic remedies. For example, "those of sanguine temperaments with warm, salty oils, burned as much by their own ardor as the fire of wine, all night revelry, and the pleasures of love, exact an entirely different approach. Smallpox, which in these cases appears at first to be mild, can have the cruelest consequences in people of this temperament."[39] Even bleeding, one of his most frequently suggested treatments, required an appraisal of the individual constitution "based on the violence of the fever, the nature of the symptoms, the age and temperament of the patient."[40] The appropriate dosage of medications must be based on the physician's assessment of the patient's strength, an assessment determined by the state of the fibers and the nature and proportion of liquids in the patient.

The Notion of Disease

La Mettrie applied his inheritance from Boerhaave and the findings of his own medical practice in his discussion of the nature and the appropriate treatment of three diseases—smallpox, dysentery, and vertigo. He was concerned with smallpox and dysentery because they were epidemic in his native Brittany. He also worked against the backdrop of Sydenham's and Boerhaave's discussions of these diseases, attempting to address the practical applications of Boerhaavian physiology and to apply Hippocratic notions of practice to these specific diseases. In his treatise on vertigo, La Mettrie was venturing into less explored areas of medicine. This disease seemed to defy the possibility of a single cause or remedy. La Mettrie's pugglings over vertigo developed his notion of causation and raised problems he later addressed in his philosophical works.

In discussing the nature of smallpox, La Mettrie, invoking his loosely corpuscular sense of matter, contended that smallpox consisted essentially of "diverses particules venimeuses" of an extreme subtlety prevalent in the air we breathe. The virulent effect of smallpox on the body was not to be wondered at, for even if one was in a perfect state of health the smallest corpuscle transmitted to veins was able to disturb the entire *oeconomie animale.* Thus the venomous character of smallpox is able to excite a fever "and disturb the liquors as much in their flow as in their substance." The circulation will also be increased if the venom reaches the heart and irritates the cardiac nerves, for this venom will "strain, contort, and irritate every fiber of the body it is carried to by the circulation." After the eruption of the disease the symptoms calm and the skin is stretched with heat, pain, and inflammation. Thus the circulation and breathing "are restrained and consequently the humors are more strongly pushed back."[41]

Because the disease had such small particles that it circulated easily throughout the body, La Mettrie concluded that remedies must be evaluated by whether or not they moderated the effect of smallpox in the blood. He quarreled with the popular use of cordials, which, instead of producing a beneficial change in the composition of the blood, actually rendered the disease more virulent.[42] And since the net effect of the disease was to reduce the pulse to such "an extreme debility," bleeding was the only remedy because "insofar as the blood flows, a constricted circulation develops, and the pulse becomes more vigorous again."

La Mettrie was more explicit in describing the nature and course of dysentery. His determination of the nature of the disease showed him to be a true disciple of Boerhaave. He invoked both a mechan-

ical and an iatrochemical explanation: "All this venomous deprava-
tion comes only from the excess of mechanical movement of this
humor mixed with other fluids in the vessels. This venom owes, in
my opinion, its origin to this extreme alkalescence of the bile." La
Mettrie claimed that he had been able to isolate the nature of
dysenteric bile; its smallest particles "are composed of a rancid, fetid
oil and of saline, alkaline, fiery principles, forming by their close
mixture a sort of arsenical amalgam which by its viscous tenacity
remains in the lining of the intestines where it burns, stings, and
tears."[43]

La Mettrie's guide to the treatment of dysentery was the operation of nature itself. Nature, he noted, when threatened by dysentery will put into motion a force shared by all *corps animés*; "It will
try to rid itself of its bilious adherences, and to repair itself from the
effects of this caustic substance which caused it to suffer."[44] La
Mettrie contended that this was an automatic movement of the sort
denied by the Stahlians. In other words, this sort of movement was
characteristic of the organism itself and not directed by Stahl's
anima. Though La Mettrie did not yet have Haller's study on muscular irritability, which was such a catalyst in the development of his
philosophical ideas, nonetheless he saw this automatic movement
everywhere as the organism naturally sought to rid itself of irritants.
For example, he noted that nature produces a humor to wash a
cinder out of the eye. In many cases this automatic movement is
sufficient to remove the irritant, but this is not the case in a disease as
virulent as dysentery. Hence the practitioner must seek to augment
the practice of nature by prescribing powerful purgatives.

For both smallpox and dysentery, La Mettrie was able to isolate
what he considered the essential character of the disease, to describe
its course through the body, and to determine a remedy which
would logically attack the disease. But in investigating vertigo La
Mettrie found neither the nature, the course, nor the remedy for the
disease to be clear-cut. Yet because the complicated nature of this
disease prevented La Mettrie from deducing one mechanism of its
cause and treatment, his *Traité du vertige* is both the best example
of the clarity and consistency of La Mettrie's medical reasoning and
the most striking demonstration of the limits of his method of
analyzing and treating disease.

La Mettrie was bemused by the great number of completely

divergent circumstances which produced visual distortions. He was ultimately able to group these disparate manifestations under two probable causes. He concluded either that the fibers of the brain in general, or those of the optic nerve itself, had been disturbed ("the apparent movement of a still body depends on the slightest derangement of the fibers of the retina or the optic nerve"),[45] or that a direct action of the imagination had produced the symptoms of vertigo. Thus, when discussing specific manifestations, he gave equal weight to disturbances in the eye and to the action of the imagination.

Vertigo as a result of an action of the imagination was not easily discussed, documented, or classified. Furthermore, the manifestations of vertigo are more extreme when the imagination is the cause; it is not simply the case that still objects appear to move circularly but rather that "it [vertigo] can also represent an image of ourselves to ourselves, ascending in the sky, turning like a *tourbillon* in the atmosphere at the least wind, precipitating into deep chasms, as happens in dreams." What distinguishes vertigo from delirium and other diseases of the brain is that in delirium reason is taken in by the imagination, while with vertigo one is able to recognize these perceptions as errors. Thus he placed the site of vertigo in "la partie fantastique du cerveau."[46] The role of the imagination in disease raised difficult questions about mind/body relationships or, as La Mettrie would insist, brain/body relationships, and perhaps because of his work on vertigo he was particularly aware of the role of imagination and inclined to give it a prominent role in his discussions of mental processes.[47] La Mettrie also tried to use his observations about vertigo to address causes and remedies for other mental disorders.

La Mettrie's notion that vertigo was caused by disturbed fibers is consistent with his other medical works; it too reveals his debt to Boerhaave's liquid-solid physiology as an effective way to understand the workings of the human body in both health and disease. Within this physiological framework, La Mettrie tried to connect specific visual distortions suffered in vertigo with disturbances in the solid-liquid balance within the eye. For example, one sees two objects instead of one because the axis of vision turns towards different points and thus pictures the object on two different points of the retina. Since this same phenomenon can be artificially produced when one presses with the finger on the eye, La Mettrie concluded that the ultimate cause of seeing double is that "as the humors of the two eyes are not always equally rarefied, the vessels of one eye sometimes swell more than those of the other, and consequently, since the retina is unevenly agitated, the axis of sight can be deranged."[48]

La Mettrie also discussed internal causes of vertigo as the result of the rarefaction of liquids that increased their movement, distending, dilating, or being pushed outside the vessels in which they were normally contained, and thus acting on neighboring organs. To explain the symptoms of vertigo produced by alcoholic consumption, La Mettrie argued that the level of alcohol in the two eyes was not the same, so that sometimes the blood vessels in one eye were significantly more swollen, which disturbed the retina.[49] This explanation seemed so ludicrous to the only biographer of La Mettrie who has dealt with his medicine that he dismissed all of his medicine as equally absurd.[50]

Although La Mettrie did not specifically use mechanical analogies to explain the causes of diseases, his view of the relationship between health and disease is clearly indebted to the mechanical tradition. The body is described as a very delicate machine which, at the slightest provocation, will go out of proper working order, but which can be repaired by a readjustment that is generally quite simple once the proper cause has been determined. His idea of the states of health and disease was based on a conception of the human body as composed of solids and liquids in perfect equilibrium, essentially the view of the human body suggested by Boerhaave. Any disturbance of the equilibrium produced disease. This is particularly the case for diseases like vertigo that involve the very delicate tissues of the nerves and the brain.

It is rather ironic that this concept of disease and the way in which an appropriate remedy was determined seems to have entailed the same sort of thinking on which the Galenic system relied. That is to say, despite the fact that throughout his medical work La Mettrie only mentioned Galenic medicine as a completely irrelevant myth from the past, his thinking about disease seems remarkably similar to the Galenic system, in which disease was the result of a humoral imbalance of too much or too little of one of four substances. In La Mettrie's medicine the causes are both more complex and more mechanical: There can be too much or too little blood, or nervous fluid; there can be an inflammation which causes liquids to flow too fast, or the balance of fluids within the body can be disturbed; there can be too much blood in the arteries and not enough in the veins. Because there are so many factors involved in the explanation, it can seem, at first glance, that this sort of explanation is far more complex and of a different kind than that used by the Galenists. However, the problem is essentially one of imbalance and the remedy suggested essentially that of a rectification of that imbalance. La Mettrie's discussion of causes reveals, of course, that he was familiar with all of the physiology since Galen, and hence his explanation of disease was not simply a question of four humors that can go awry but rather the contention that any one of the vast multitudes of liquids and solids can be out of healthful proportion, or that the whole relationship between solids and liquids can be askew. And of course La Mettrie would have no doubt claimed that his concept of disease as an imbalance derived from Boerhaave rather than from Galen.

La Mettrie's treatment of these disorders also reflects his exposure to the mechanists. Although he did not rigidly or consistently apply their principles, nonetheless his treatments rely on what he understood of the movements of fluids through the body. For example, heat or friction will increase their speed, bleeding will diminish their quantity and thus pressure, speed, and friction can make the solid "more solid, more elastic, and stronger." Horseback riding, a remedy La Mettrie noted was so frequently employed with good results by Sydenham, is also helpful in cases of vertigo. La Mettrie's remarks on why this was so are very revealing of the way he thought about remedies for disease. All types of exercise increase transpiration and appetite and decrease the amount of fecal matter produced, "which proves that it [exercise] more effectively separates chyle from food and consequently solids acquire more strength and elasticity." La Mettrie also acknowledged that the remedies he suggested were not out of the ordinary. In fact, he conceded, "so true is it that medicine is nothing other than judgment enlightened by physiology." For example, in diseases that are the result of a debility of fibers or of *esprits*, La Mettrie suggested attention to diet and recommended the white of the egg as the best nutrition for human beings. He argued from analogy: according to the observations of Malpighi, in twenty-one days the white of the egg, by virtue of the heat of the chicken sitting on the egg, forms the entire body of the chicken. Because a thermometer shows that the heat of man is similar to that of the chicken, an egg white eaten by a human being "should therefore transform itself in the body of man into very solid parts."[51] In addition, the chemical experiments Boerhaave did on lymph, the material of human nutrition, showed the analogous characters of lymph and egg white. La Mettrie also suggested the chemical remedy of iron filings, presumably because of the analogy between the strength of iron and the rigidity of healthy fibers.

La Mettrie also discussed more complicated causes of vertigo. Thus a blow to the head can communicate that motion to the nerve or brain tissue, producing distortion. He noted, for example, that a blow delivered at the point of origin of the nerves can make the most intelligent man an imbecile. To explain this change, he said, "it suffices to conceive that in the movement of a violent commotion the *esprits* which are too agitated could carve out for themselves new routes and thus disturb the organ of intelligence." This led La Mettrie to speculate about the relationship between intelligence and nerve fluid. He claimed that there was such an extensive analogy or sympathy between the two that it seemed to him that intelligence depended entirely on the circulation, quantity, and quality of this subtle nervous fluid. Despite this inextricably close connection, La Mettrie disclaimed any certain knowledge; "it must be admitted that the properties of matter are so unknown that one can never perceive any connection between the traces of *esprits* and the ideas which result from them."[52] Nonetheless, La Mettrie here began to discuss the relationship between mental states and physiological processes. Because vertigo involved the brain and perceptions, he applied a Lockean epistemology, which Boerhaave had suggested as the most reasonable theory of knowledge, to his specific discussions of this disease. La Mettrie thought that there were "sympathetic" causes of vertigo, meaning a sympathy between the ideas and bodily states. For example, not eating for a long time or engaging in scholarly activity for too long can produce symptoms of vertigo.

In conclusion, La Mettrie claimed to have isolated the causes of vertigo as being of three types: "all that which weakens, exhausts, troubles, or fixes the spirits, all that which irritates mediately or immediately the nerves or the substance of the brain, and finally all that which prevents the blood from circulating can cause vertigo."[53]

Ultimately he considered disease to be a disruption of the normal proportions of constituent parts of the body. In addition to its resemblance to Galenic medicine, his view of disease is indebted to the mechanists in that the rectification of any imbalance need not involve recourse to a mysterious agent. It instead involved an operation that, after having assigned the proper cause, was so simple and natural as to be self-evident. Ultimately his treatment of diseases applies Boerhaave's physiology and explicitly carries out Boerhaave's eclectic approach to medical practice.

La Mettrie's medical works suggest philosophical issues which he would treat in more detail in his later works. These issues were initially only peripheral to his fundamental concern to disseminate medical information. For example, the action of the body in divesting itself of disease was evidence of automatic movement, which he called irritability. His investigation of the causes of disease produced more evidence of the effects of physical states on mental states. His discussions of therapeutics exposed the problem of the primacy of the individual constitution—variables in human physiology which made the treatment of disease complicated and severely limited the efficacy of the physician.

La Mettrie was not able to transcend the inherent limits of eighteenth-century medical practice. He did not advance the frontiers of medical knowledge, nor is his name associated with particular breakthroughs in the treatment of disease, and as a result his medicine has gone virtually unnoticed in the annals of medical history. But perhaps in part as a result of this neglect, La Mettrie is a particularly useful figure for examining the relationship between medical theory and practice in the eighteenth century, a particularly useful mirror for observing the application of Boerhaavian physiology.

La Mettrie is also a good example of a committed, careful medical observer who diligently tried to eschew medical systems that might cloud his observations of disease. His concern with describing diseases led him to emphasize both unusual aspects of diseases and the relationship between the disease and the constitution of the individual. Although he wanted to disseminate information about disease to his fellow physicians, La Mettrie was particularly concerned to bring information to the public, to warn them of dangerous remedies, and to advise them on what means to take to remain in good health. In general, La Mettrie's own medical treatises further the crusade of his satires; they too seek to undercut the stranglehold over medical information of the Faculty of Medicine, and in them La Mettrie insisted, as did so many other Enlightenment attacks on corporate power, that the private knowledge of the corporations must become public. In other words, Boerhaave's physiology gave La Mettrie the information with which to direct a campaign for public health to the public. But, more important to La Mettrie's development as a philosophe and to establishing the connections between medicine and the Enlightenment, he felt free to modify and criticize Boerhaave's physiology, just as he had recast his teacher's medical practice in an Enlightenment mold by modifying Boerhaave's notion of the physician. While Boerhaave had claimed that the physician must have a thorough knowledge of his art and be willing to use it in the service of the sick, La Mettrie portrayed the doctor as a medical reformer. The physician must not only be a critical observer well educated in both the theory and practice of medicine, he must also seek the reform of his art. That reform entails stringent criticism of conventional methods of treatment and a concerted effort to educate the public on issues of preventive medicine and public health. And those concerns provoked La Mettrie to critically reappraise Boerhaave's physiology.

5

La Mettrie and Boerhaave

Medical Theory Reappraised

Boerhaave was not only indisputably the greatest medical influence on La Mettrie's practice of medicine, he was also the crucial influence on La Mettrie's understanding of medical theory. In 1740 La Mettrie published his two-volume translation of Boerhaave's *Institutiones medicae* as part of a campaign to make his mentor's writings more widely accessible, and in 1743–48 he republished it in an edition expanded by six volumes of his own commentary. The six volumes of commentary on Boerhaave's text are the most important source of exploring La Mettrie's debt to Boerhaave and the critical text for understanding La Mettrie's development as a *médecin-philosophe*.

La Mettrie's commentary on the *Institutiones* has never been considered for its role in the dissemination of Boerhaave's medicine nor on its own merits. Scholars, influenced by the outrage of Albrecht Haller, have generally assumed that La Mettrie's work is entirely plagiarized from Haller and without merits of its own. But the two texts are dramatically different. Haller's commentary is essentially a series of Latin footnotes explicating particular words or phrases of Boerhaave's numbered, aphoristic remarks. La Mettrie incorporates much of the content of Haller's notes, so Haller certainly had grounds for his vehement complaints and outraged charges of plagiarism.[1] (La Mettrie acknowledged his debt to Haller, freely admitting that he had inserted Haller's "excellent notes" into his own commentary.) However, La Mettrie's commentary is different in both style and substance. La Mettrie did not simply replicate a disjointed series of Latin footnotes. Instead he provided a connected commentary written in French in a conversational style and designed to be accessible to a much broader audience. He adapted the text to his audience, claiming that "I would have believed that I had ill-served the taste and delicacy of the French, if I had not thrust aside a great many thorns and brambles." He noted that a very frequent defect of the work of foreign scholars, especially their commentaries, "was that their works bent under the burden of materials which strangle them and the citations which piteously crush them; which do not make the text more accessible, except to those who need their explications to understand the original text, and which disgust or revolt others."[2] La Mettrie also altered the substance of his commentary, incorporating accounts of meetings of academic societies, recent experiments, and contemporary scientific events which would have been familiar or intriguing to his audience. His text, as he points out, includes his own notes from Boerhaave's classes based on lectures he attended ten years after Haller.[3] Most striking is the way La Mettrie's text advances his philosophical and reformist agendas. As a result, its significance to the development of La Mettrie's medicine and philosophy cannot be overstated. La Mettrie used the commentary to distinguish his own medical views from those of Boerhaave. Specifically, he defined a stringently critical and rigidly clinical perspective from which to examine the uneasy synthesis of iatrochemistry and iatromechanism which Boerhaave's *Institutiones* promulgated. La Mettrie ultimately rent that synthesis asunder by indicting all contemporary medical theory for its failure to eschew the metaphysical and to wed theory to empirical demonstration. Moreover, within the context of Boerhaave's discussion of brain physiology and his own critical assessment of that discussion, La Mettrie began to raise questions which would lead him to rewrite Boerhaave's epistemological position as materialism. Thus the commentary on Boerhaave's *Institutiones* must be considered a crucial work in the formulation of the epistemological position which underlies all of La Mettrie's philosophical works.

The translation was in the first place directed to a popular audience. Given his scorn for and distrust of most of the medical practitioners of his day, especially the medical trend-setters in Paris, La Mettrie seems to have felt called upon to alert the public through his satires on the Faculty of Medicine and to try to inform them about the workings of the human body through his translations of

Boerhaave. This concern is particularly well reflected in his commentary on the *Institutiones*, for he clearly took great pains to make it readable. Though the work presupposed some medical knowledge and an acquaintance with the names and ideas of leading men of science and medicine, La Mettrie did everything possible to make it relevant to the everyday experience of his reader.

By way of the commentaries, this translation of the *Institutiones* also produced a work quite different in tone and conclusion from the original. La Mettrie felt perfectly free to build on the original text and to criticize it, in keeping with Boerhaave's own expectation that the progress of medicine required a tradition of continuous reappraisal. However, one cannot help wondering whether Boerhaave, when he advocated this tradition of criticism, had La Mettrie in mind—someone who devoted so much attention to criticism of Boerhaave's synthesis, had such a pessimistic view of the history of medicine, and was willing to use Boerhaave's modest sensationalism as the basis of a materialist philosophy. La Mettrie, the disciple of Boerhaave, the French custodian of his words, used them to produce a very different idea of the prospects of medicine and the direction it must take. Optimism had led Boerhaave to postulate a synthesis upon which he confidently expected the future to enlarge, incorporating new discoveries in medicine and the other sciences. La Mettrie's pessimism, or perhaps his sense of mission as a guardian of medical truth, led him instead to undermine that synthesis by subjecting it to criticism wherever he felt it erred.

La Mettrie and Boerhaave

As La Mettrie himself gratefully acknowledged, Boerhaave taught him that the practice of medicine required that one seek the mean between the empiricist and the metaphysician. The physician who restricts himself completely to what he has observed is left without an understanding of the working of the human body and is incapable of determining the causes of diseases. The metaphysical physician, on the other hand, relies too heavily on theoretical constructs, using meaningless, or at the very least nonobservable, terms like "the immortal soul" to describe the working of the human body. These he compared to Icarus: "they let nature escape to embrace only phantoms." Boerhaave, according to La Mettrie, stood out from both types. But even more praiseworthy was his epistemological modesty;[4] Boerhaave completely avoided useless research into first or final causes and concentrated instead on the study of the actions of living bodies. Boerhaave opened La Mettrie's eyes to the possibilities for medical practice and reform that clinical experience, dissection, and the study of comparative anatomy offered.

Despite La Mettrie's enthusiastic admiration for Boerhaave, his commentaries reveal some marked differences in their views of the state of medical knowledge and the prospects for reform. Perhaps as a result of his personal sense of mission at Leyden and the progress he could see in medical education as he reintroduced bedside teaching, Boerhaave was decidedly optimistic about the future of medicine. He recognized that medicine had experienced a dark period illuminated only by great men like Hippocrates and some of the Arabs. However, he claimed that since Harvey medicine had banished metaphysics and was founded on the certainties of mathematics and mechanics.[5] Imbued with this confidence, Boerhaave postulated a synthesis of leading medical theories, a synthesis he confidently expected the future to enlarge by incorporating new discoveries in medicine and the other sciences.[6] But, perhaps as a result of *his* firsthand knowledge of the abuses of medical practice and medical scholarship at the hands of his Parisian contemporaries, La Mettrie emphatically disagreed with Boerhaave's sanguine description of the progress of medical history. Whereas Boerhaave saw medicine as moving towards greater certainty, La Mettrie described medical history as a series of inappropriate and unsubstantiated hypotheses, one succeeding another. He thought it abundantly clear that Harvey's discovery of the circulation of the blood had not banished metaphysics from medicine. "One has seen ferments, archei, sieves, and strange gases boldly insert themselves into medicine since Harvey."[7] In fact, he claimed, Harvey's discovery had been used specifically as the foundation of ridiculous hypotheses advanced by the Cartesians and the chemists to explain the action of the heart.

Nor did La Mettrie see developments in other sciences as the foundation of medical progress. He acknowledged that advances had been made in individual sciences: the microscope had led to anatomical discoveries; chemistry had taken great strides, particularly through the experiments of Boyle and Boerhaave; and developments in physics had produced more exact quantitative determinations. But perhaps in reaction to the unbridled enthusiasm for physics in the eighteenth century, La Mettrie advised skepticism toward the wide application of quantification.[8] He was even more vociferous when he contemplated its application to medicine. "Nothing, therefore, is more certain than the general axioms of mechanics, and nothing more deceptive than that which the mechanists, deducing from their rules, apply to the human body."[9] He argued, for example, that it was ridiculous to claim to explain everything about the humors of the body in terms of mechanical laws which apply to other fluids: "it follows that we are very far from claiming that we could ever explain all the phenomena of medicine mechanically."[10] He also noted that in the works of those who espoused "la médecine mécanique," such as Malpighi, Bellini, Borelli, and Pitcairn, there were a great many errors and contradictions even in their figures.[11]

Furthermore, La Mettrie did not base his hope for medical progress on the incorporation into medicine of new scientific findings but rather on the dissemination of medical information. He delighted in the fact that literary commerce, especially through journals, allowed many to become familiar with new discoveries. Scientific societies enabled scientists to keep in contact with each other and to cultivate a taste for experiment. His belief that the hope for medicine lay not, as Boerhaave thought, in the application of the findings of other sciences to medicine, but rather in raising public awareness of health issues explains La Mettrie's interest in popularizing Boerhaave's medicine (and in large part the course of his own medical career).

Just as La Mettrie and Boerhaave had different hopes for medical reform, so too they set their different tones according to the audiences they wished to affect. Boerhaave sought to educate the medical community; La Mettrie conducted a campaign for medical reform by addressing the public. His edition of Boerhaave's *Institutiones* is clearly meant for a popular audience. It is full of anecdotes from the contemporary Parisian scene, used to describe disease and methods of treatment or simply to illustrate arguments. The findings and reports of French medical and scientific societies are also cited. Written in a lighter manner than the original text, it offered the reader not only a translation but also, in the interest of increasing public understanding and appreciation, a thorough explication and amplification of Boerhaave's text.

La Mettrie and the Chemists

While La Mettrie's commentary on Boerhaave's *Institutiones* disputes the basis of Boerhaave's hopes for medical progress and reform, it also attacks the substance of Boerhaave's physiology. That attack was motivated by a sense that medicine had remained too tied to schools of medical thought and was too intent on using experiments for the express purpose of substantiating theory. Despite the new commitment to clinical and bedside medicine Boerhaave advocated, medicine was too esoteric, the abstract philosophy of the armchair physician. La Mettrie raised general doubts about the applicability of the findings of other sciences to medicine, but he was especially skeptical of the role chemistry might play. He could, based on discussions of specific chemical explanations of physiological functions, point to chemistry as an outstanding example of a theoretical science that too often made claims that it had resolved ultimate questions about the nature of matter. And, most damning in La Mettrie's opinion, chemistry was far too limited in its scope of practical applications to be of use to the physician.

La Mettrie was no doubt constrained by his great respect for Boerhaave to give some credence to the chemists, though he did ask, "What was this science, before he [Boerhaave] had carried into its shadows the torch of physics and geometry?"[12] He thought that Boerhaave had done his utmost to discredit the Paracelsians and had steered chemistry in a new direction, out of the musty laboratories of secretive old men and into the light of experimental science as practiced and shared by an international community of scientists. In effect, what Boerhaave had done was "to strip from this science all the barbarism it had before him,"[13] and therefore La Mettrie was willing to accept as conclusive the chemical experiments Boerhaave had used to illustrate certain points of his physiology.

La Mettrie's assessment of the role of chemistry in the history of medicine was otherwise mixed. For example, he spoke of Paracelsus as the true father of chemistry, who had so much influence that, within a comparatively short time, one had to become a chemist in order to be a doctor; "it became an absolute necessity to cure, or rather to kill by chemistry." He did, however, greatly admire van Helmont both for his contentiousness and for the way in which he discredited the schools. (La Mettrie could perhaps see in van Helmont's challenge to the medical establishment a parallel to his attack on the Parisian faculty.) As far as the use of chemical remedies was concerned, La Mettrie certainly did not share the "extravagant prejudices,"[14] as he called them, of those like Guy Patin, who considered all chemical preparations to be poison. Nor would he have been as tentative in the use of chemical remedies as Sydenham, for he thought that Sydenham's very limited knowledge of chemistry prevented him from using chemical remedies to good effect.[15]

However, La Mettrie raised fundamental questions about the legitimacy of applying the results of laboratory experiments to the workings of living bodies. He cited the in vivo-in vitro problem as particularly characteristic of chemistry. "Properly speaking it [chemistry] is only the remains of bodies after their destruction, above all in the plants, where fire shows us the principles of its fabric, that is to say, those to which it gave birth, in changing the principles of the substance which it demolished."[16] He did concede that what we can know about bodily fluids we know through chemical analysis, a methodology "without which one could not know how to judge the value of foods and remedies."[17] But if La Mettrie granted that there was some benefit from chemistry, he was vehement in his denunciations of the chemists' distorted notions of physiological processes. He argued that the claims of the chemists could not be substantiated by experiments. For example, Sylvius de la Boë supposed that the blood in the heart was alkaline and combined with other blood rich in chyle and pancreatic juice to produce a ferment which explained bodily heat and circulation. La Mettrie argued that none of the tests he had performed on blood showed it to be alkaline: it had no alkaline taste; it did not produce a painful reaction if applied to a wound or to the eye; it did not ferment when combined with acids. Nor did it turn violet-colored tincture of flowers green, as alkaline salts do. In fact, La Mettrie claimed, the chemical operations of fermentation, effervescence, and ebullition could be discovered not in the circulatory system but in the "prejudiced imagination"[18] of the chemists. These specific experiments discredited the chemists as systematizers and called into question their methods of analysis.

La Mettrie was equally vehement in denouncing chemical explanations of the workings of particular bodily organs. His discussion of the working of the glands, the actions of the muscles, and the formation of urine are only three examples of his objections to the chemists, but they are particularly effective illustrations of the nature of his criticisms. For example, since the chemists believed that no change occurred in the body without a ferment, they explained the secretions of the glands by supposing that a specific ferment in each gland changed the juices (meaning blood and chyle) that arrived at the gland into the specific glandular secretion.[19] La Mettrie argued that if these ferments were to exist they would have to be either in the glands or in the blood. He found the glands to be too small to contain the requisite amount of ferment and he could not conceive that the ferments could exist in the blood itself. If they were assumed to exist, he wondered how then the ferments could be restricted to the transformation of a limited quantity of blood and then direct this transformed blood to the proper gland. And finally, he considered that the chemists' view of the glands seemed to necessitate an "infinite progression of ferments."[20]

La Mettrie found the chemical hypothesis no better able to explain the action of the muscles. He cited Thomas Willis, who had observed that pure spirit of niter mixed with alcohol produced a sudden explosive effervescence; he had inferred that animal spirits had to be of an acid nature and the blood full of oil particles, and that the mixture of oil and acid produced muscular action. La Mettrie objected that this supposed mixture does not allow any role for the mind in muscular action, nor is it clear, if the mind were allowed a role, how it could control an explosive force in such a way as to produce the regular geometric motions associated with muscular action. He found it inconceivable that such a force could exist, for it would destroy the fabric of the muscles; furthermore, "sulphur of the blood and the acid of the spirits are the mere products of imagination."[21]

La Mettrie's arguments against the chemical explanation of the production of urine are a forceful indictment of chemistry. He claimed that "the Chemists, not content with the simple fabric of the parts, must have the secretion of urine accounted for by some operation better known to themselves than to the nature of the animal: and therefore they suppose every animal juice to be derived from another which is more gross, and this in the manner of precipitation. . . . But to what purpose is it for us to lose our time in searching into obscure and precarious notions, when the fabric of the parts is sufficient to account for all appearances?"[22] In this remark La Mettrie revealed his hostility toward the secrecy and the self-invested authority of the chemists. He found that many of their explanations were consistent only with their own system of reasoning and bore no relation to the actual nature of what was being considered. Equally objectionable was the way in which the chemists universally applied their chemical procedures, such as ferments and precipitations, to the workings of the human body, which La Mettrie found to be based on an insufficient, questionable, or even entirely objectionable rationale. Finally, and most telling for La Mettrie, there was a simpler, more convincing argument to be gained from a mechanical approach. In this particular example, the choice is not presented as being between mechanical and chemical explanation. Were that the case, La Mettrie would have endorsed the mechanical explanation because of what he saw as its greater accessibility to the senses and the fact that it did not resort to mystery. But here the choice was between fiction and truth![23]

Most objectionable, in La Mettrie's opinion, was the chemists' fabrication of a mysterious agent to explain what could not be seen: the archeus, "a being between that of a conscious mind and inactive or common matter that directed all the functions of the human body in health, cured diseases, etc."[24] La Mettrie could not understand why van Helmont supposed the existence of an archeus. He personally admitted to being far more comfortable with epistemological modesty, preferring to acknowledge a cause as unknowable rather than to attribute it to an unknown power. Emphatically disallowing the intervention of anything mysterious into physiology, La Mettrie attempted to circumscribe all the activities attributed to the archeus under the more comprehensible rubric of the mechanical functioning of the human body. Even if the first cause of this mechanical functioning could not be explained, it could at least be taken out of the realm of the mysterious by likening it to the winding of a clock or some other, more acceptable and rational mechanical analogy.

Thus La Mettrie's strongest objections to the chemists focused on epistemological issues. It might be said that La Mettrie saw the chemists as the metaphysicians of the natural sciences. The chemists did not display sufficient epistemological modesty. They were too wedded to chemistry as a systematic explanation. They made unwarranted assumptions and drew analogies too widely between observable and hidden physiological processes. Most reprehensible of all, in their quest to provide chemical explanations of physiological functions, the chemists were not averse to suggesting occult qualities.

It must be wondered at this point whether La Mettrie's vehemence against the chemists was not produced by his sense that chemistry inevitably led to vitalism. Though his criticisms of the chemists on vitalistic grounds were never made explicit in his medical works, in his philosophical works Sylvius the iatrochemist is replaced by Stahl the vitalist as the brunt of his ire and his prime example of improper methodology and illogical conclusions.[25] Thus it seems that either the vitalists were the real target in the violent denunciations of the chemists of the medical works, or the arguments he developed against the chemists were equally appropriate against the vitalists. In either case the arguments he directed against the chemists were crucial to La Mettrie's subsequent medical works, which repudiated the metaphysical and theoretical concerns of the chemists in favor of clear descriptions of the manifestation, course, and treatment of particular diseases. To address these issues he used extensive case studies as the basis of his medical work and wrote treatises on preventive medicine and hygiene designed to educate the public.[26] The arguments against the chemists also shaped La Mettrie's philosophical works, enabling him to work toward an Enlightenment epistemology in the sense that his arguments are staunchly opposed to *esprit de système* or any sense of the occult and rigorously modest in their sense of the limits of human knowledge. And more specifically, he consistently upheld the claims of the empirical scientist over the metaphysician.

La Mettrie and the Mechanists

In his discussion of the production of urine, La Mettrie made a distinction between chemical and mechanical explanations, which he reduced to the difference between truth and fiction. His objections to chemistry make it clear why he would have seen the distinction in such black and white terms. At least in the example cited earlier, the mechanistic explanation referred, as far as La Mettrie was concerned, to the actual working of the body. It described what one could see, or, as in the case of the supposed circulation of nerve fluids, it properly applied reason and analogy based on what one could know. In contrast, the chemists had become too enamored of their hypotheses and thus were inclined to apply those hypotheses to the human body without verifying that it was appropriate to do so. Also, much to La Mettrie's almost perceptible relief, the mechanists did not hypothesize mysterious agents like the archeus. In his commentary on Boerhaave's physiology, where La Mettrie set forth both the mechanical and the chemical explanations for certain functions of the body, his bias in favor of the mechanical is evident.

Part of the reason for this bias is that La Mettrie accepted certain basic tenets that allowed the application of mechanism to the human body. At one point he defined the body as "a compendium of all manner of machines most advantageously disposed."[27] He also considered the use of mechanical analogy to be valid, that is, that the application of mechanical models can be an effective means of understanding the workings of the human body. He claimed that "if the several parts of the human body agree thus with the structure of mechanical instruments, they must also necessarily act by the same laws. . . ."[28] He was willing to assume that parts of the body do in fact correspond to mechanical instruments. Beyond this acceptance of the general tenets of mechanical philosophy, La Mettrie used, wherever appropriate to his physiology, the theory of matter generally advocated by the mechanists, that is, corpuscularism.

The functioning of the brain and the nervous system could also be discussed in mechanistic terms. To La Mettrie, as to most medical men of his day, it seemed logical to suppose a circulatory system with vessels too small and fluids too subtle to be perceived. The argument is a telling example of Boerhaave's "rational medicine," or one of the ways in which mechanics offered such a clear foundation that reason and analogy could be justifiably extended beyond the observable. It was simply a case of applying what was clearly known about the circulation of fluids in the body to a fluid which could not be perceived. Hence La Mettrie described the circulation of nerve fluids with what may seem to the reader unwarranted certainty.

"Though the nervous juice of spirits separated in the brain are the most subtle and moveable of any humor through the whole body, yet are they formed like the rest from the same thicker fluid of the blood, passing through many degrees of attenuation, till its parts become small enough to pervade the last series of vessels in the cortex, and then it becomes the subtle fluid of the brain and nerves."[29]

La Mettrie also used mechanical analogies to explain the working of the muscles. "It is through the use of pulleys that mechanists raise the heaviest bodies; and in man nature conducts itself in the same way."[30] Even human flexibility could be explained in mechanical terms, for the vessels of the human body function as elastic cords. Mechanism could also be used to explain growth and decay. Decay occurs as particles are worn away from the vessels of the body by the passage of liquids through them. Growth occurs when more particles of fluids attach themselves to vessels than are worn away.[31]

Thus La Mettrie was as willing as Boerhaave had been to invoke mechanical explanations for certain operations of the body, and, no doubt because his work was an elaboration of Boerhaave's text, he gave much more detailed accounts of exactly how these mechanisms could be shown, or supposed, to operate. Yet he was also far more skeptical than Boerhaave about the relevance of mechanics to the human body and nature as a whole. La Mettrie's skepticism about Boerhaave's assumption that mechanism was the crucial turning point in the history of medicine has already been pointed out. He also had specific disagreements with explanations the mechanists had given. This is particularly evident in his long rebuttal of the mechanical account of the functioning of the glands. Essentially, the mechanists argued that the glands were sieves with holes of particular sizes that separated out from the blood particles of the appropriate size to form glandular secretions. "But," La Mettrie claimed, "this is far from giving a just solution of the problem why different juices are secerned in different parts of the body of a determinate nature."[32] First of all, he argued, as the use of the microscope has proven, all the vessels of the human body are circular in cross-section; their shapes therefore do not explain the diversity of glandular secretions. Secondly, even if the great diversity of shapes needed to explain the diversity of glandular secretions were supposed to exist, these vessels would still be so soft that they would conform to the shape of any particles which presented themselves. Finally, "[e]ven granting immutable pores of various figures, and particles of the blood of various figures, it will not follow that some pores will receive one kind of particle and refuse the rest, for whatever be the figure of a pore it will admit all sorts of particles."[33]

The overriding impression of this denunciation of the mechanical explanation of the functioning of the glands is, first, that mechanical analogies are not always appropriate explanations for the functioning of the human body, and second, that the mechanistic view that the location of each fluid in the body is determined by the size and shape of particles that make up that fluid is too simplistic to explain glandular secretions.

According to La Mettrie, the effort to apply mechanism to diseases and cures had also produced some absurdities. For example, if a physician wished to explain inflammation he could refer to the mass and movement of "animal spirits," which he could compare geometrically to the force of the heart; obviously, however, none of this led to any real understanding of inflammation or gave the physician any idea of how to cure it. La Mettrie facetiously suggested that the physician use geometry to determine prescriptions by "a curve of dosages or remedies appropriate to every age and temperament."[34]

La Mettrie also made several attempts to qualify or restrict the application of mechanism to medicine. He noted that the human body presented such a complex series of interactions among its parts that mechanics could not hope to deal with it in terms of its principles. For example, in discussing a tertian fever, he explained that "the manifest cause of all this disorder is apparently an obstruction in the smallest vessels; but no mortal will ever explain all these appearances by the principles of hydraulics and hydrostatics because they arise from a change made in the constituent particles of the blood."[35] This led him to wonder whether the laws of mechanics, based as they were on inanimate machines made by the successive addition of parts, could explain animate machines. Finally, he argued that the application of mechanics to medicine is questionable because of the uniqueness of the human body, an argument which severely undermined the applicability of mechanism to medicine. He enumerated a series of telling qualifications to be considered in using mechanical analogy:

Were the fluids of the human body possessed of no other properties but those common to pure water, and were its vessels metal tubes infinitely resisting, the aforementioned principles would then be sufficient to explain their actions; but many of our fluids contain elastic globules, and all of them are compounded of oil, salt, earth, and water, variously attracting and repelling each other; their containing vessels are also made up of elastic fibers admitting reciprocal elongation and contractions; therefore, the fluids in the human body do not strictly follow either hydraulic or hydrostatic laws but they stray from those principles in proportion to the difference between them and common water.[36]

The preceding remarks obviously call into question the validity that La Mettrie had seemed to grant mechanism in explaining human physiology. However, his denunciations of mechanism were not intended to revoke his earlier acceptance. They were instead meant to rule out the possibility that mechanical explanations could completely account for the working of the human body. The fact that the mechanists nonetheless made such claims to certainty exposed them, in La Mettrie's opinion, as idle speculators and metaphysicians, terms of the harshest condemnation in the eighteenth century. But he himself was willing to continue to use mechanical analogies, and they serve as a descriptive tool in all of La Mettrie's philosophical and medical writings.

La Mettrie's use of mechanical analogies has often been cited to support the claim that he was fundamentally a mechanist and that mechanism alone is sufficient to explain his science and his view of nature. But his criticisms of mechanism challenge this interpretation and separate him from many of his contemporaries, who, while accepting fundamental limits to human knowledge, nonetheless saw mechanical analogy as the best means of understanding physiological processes. La Mettrie's assessment was much more critical because he was acutely aware that mechanism provided a severely limited and often flawed analogy for physiological processes. Furthermore, mechanism, especially as extended into a system, was not a useful tool for the practicing physician who needed to diagnose or treat disease.

Physiology and Epistemology

La Mettrie modified all aspects of Boerhaave's synthesis; he was more harshly critical of the chemists and much warier of mechanism than Boerhaave had been. It was from this critical perspective and from within his assessment of Boerhaave's physiology that La Mettrie developed some of his fundamental epistemological concerns.

First of all, La Mettrie intended to limit the proper area of research for the physiologist in line with Boerhaave's assertion that first causes were beyond the scope of the physician. Boerhaave's contention was intended to keep metaphysics out of medicine. It was also a humble acknowledgment that man must concede ultimate ignorance before the works of the Creator. La Mettrie's epistemological modesty was of a different sort, reflecting entirely different concerns. For one thing, he specified, in far greater detail, the areas of physiology about which the physician can know nothing. For example, Willis tried to parcel out the faculties of the soul to different parts of the brain, but La Mettrie contended that "nothing until now has been able to locate these supposed departments."[37] He also took care to note his objections to both the chemical and mechanical explanations of the functioning of the glands and conceded that "there are probably many artifices concealed from us in this branch of nature, which we have not so much suspected or thought of."[38] In these instances he seems to have conceived of the unknowable as a temporary condition, that is, men have not yet been sufficiently perceptive to determine the causes. But ignorance does not justify the introduction of occult qualities.

La Mettrie also pointed out to the reader all the cases in which reason and analogy were used beyond the evidence of the senses, because he thought that such knowledge was highly questionable. In this respect his translation and commentary are strikingly different from the original, for Boerhaave's optimistic view of the state of medicine inclined him to accept arguments from analogy as equally certain as those based purely on the evidence of the senses.[39] La Mettrie, however, was concerned to point out uses of analogy made by the chemists and the mechanists that he considered to be illegitimate. Even cases where he considered the use of analogy to be appropriate, or the only means of incorporating what could not be seen into physiology, he emphasized that knowledge gained by this means is merely probable. So, for example, he considered the circulation of nerve juice, supposed to be an extremely subtle form of lymph, as only probable, because "we are not led thereto by the full evidence of our senses and experiments, but barely by reason and analogy."[40] He also claimed that the entire science of embryology was only probable, as it was based merely on analogy between parts of the adult and parts of the fetus.[41]

La Mettrie's commentary on Boerhaave's medical texts allowed him to refine his own methodology. While he approved of Boerhaave's attacks on medical sects, La Mettrie considered Boerhaave's own medicine to be too wedded to metaphysics. As a result he sharpened Boerhaave's antimetaphysical attacks and directed them against Boerhaave's own medicine, thereby demonstrating that criticism was a crucial tool for medical progress and that an empirical, nonsystematic approach was even more important than the content of Boerhaave's physiology.

La Mettrie circumscribed the proper area of research for the physician in another way, not because, as Boerhaave might have claimed, such knowledge was not intended for so lowly a creature as man, but rather because it was completely irrelevant. For example, in the case of vision, Aristotle had argued that it is the mind and not the eye which sees. La Mettrie responded, "But it is not the business of a physician to inquire what vision is in the mind, for let the eye be found to be duly formed, and the inhabitant will see by it."[42] So even if it is the case that the mind sees, the physician, through the study of the eye, will be able to explain vision completely. Another example is provided by the mistaken search for the way in which the muscles obey the will—mistaken, La Mettrie thought, because the information it might provide was unimportant. "If I know that B moves A, what does it matter to me, the physician, to know what moves B?"[43] These restrictions on the physician's area of inquiry are essential for understanding La Mettrie's philosophical works because, in his opinion, the proper area of inquiry for the physician and the philosopher were one and the same. In fact, he argued in the *Discours préliminaire* that the physician was best able to discuss philosophical questions and that medicine was the surest foundation for philosophy.[44]

In working through his interpretation of Boerhaave's physiology, La Mettrie examined specific issues which were crucial to the development of his philosophy. From Boerhaave's modest sensationalism he began to develop materialism. He took the tentative and inconclusive connections Boerhaave had drawn between a Lockean epistemology and the physiological processes of the brain and tried to strengthen them.[45] First of all, he was emphatically unwilling to consider immaterial causes of physiological processes such as movement: "Even at the present time there are many eminent physicians, who admit of no other cause than that of the impulse of the will to move the muscles. I readily admit, that the mind is the first mover or cause of motion in the muscles; but then I place the exercise of its action only in the common sensory: For in muscles themselves the moving cause must be corporeal which was not residing there before the contraction of the muscles, as is evident from the hardness and resistance perceptible in a muscle by the touch."[46] La Mettrie admitted that the relationship between the functioning of the brain, nerves, and muscles was impossible to determine. But although the supposed nerve fluid or the "corporeal cause" mentioned in the citation above could not be demonstrated, La Mettrie was intent on disallowing an immaterial will and emphasizing material force in the muscle itself. Thus, even before Haller's findings on muscular irritability, La Mettrie began to argue that individual fibers were capable of self-movement.[47]

Though La Mettrie did note the effect of the emotions on the functioning of the body, he was much more interested in pointing out, as he would later do so thoroughly in *L'Homme machine*, the effects of physical states on the mind.[48] La Mettrie also gave several examples to suggest that the channeling of ideas through the brain could be explained in purely physical terms. For instance, he claimed that if one poses a particularly difficult problem to a geometrician while walking with him, he would stop walking while solving the problem because "all the other passages to the common sensory are shut up so that the only thing sought for by the mind may appear more distinct." Similarly, mental labor is so fatiguing because "all the passages from the common sensory to the voluntary motions are shut up, and the spirits are retained in the brain so that they cannot flow into the muscles."[49]

La Mettrie was concerned to describe the functioning of the mind in completely physical terms. For instance, he noted that mental capacity can be correlated to brain size. He also suggested that if one were to find two people with completely identical configurations of the brain, it would be highly probable that, given the same education, they would think exactly alike. In other words, differences between individuals were, according to La Mettrie, more reasonably the result of differences in the organization of brain matter than the effect of an individual immortal soul.

La Mettrie also tried to tie behavior or disposition to completely physical states. For example, he noted that there are certain characteristics of temperament common to men at each stage of life. He pointed out that some have located the source of certain emotions in specific organs of the body. For example, the ancients thought the spleen caused laughter. La Mettrie refused to speculate on the specific location but did argue that physical states affect the emotions: "But this is certain, that joy depends much on a free circulation of the blood through all the viscera and vessels of the body which being obstructed produces anxieties and an uneasy sense of the mind."[50] La Mettrie investigated the physiological causes of happiness more thoroughly in his philosophical works, *La Volupté* and *Discours sur le bonheur*.[51]

Ultimately La Mettrie, through his commentary on Boerhaave's *Institutiones medicae*, produced a work which diverged considerably from the original. He redefined the area of research open to the physician-philosopher. He denied that the physician should attempt to deal with first causes and questioned information based on mechanical analogies. He used physiology as the basis of his discussion of the relationship of the mind to the body and attempted to correlate the activities of mind with the physiological processes of the brain. And he suggested that individual differences were the result of different organizations of brain material. La Mettrie's commentary also effectively cast doubt on Boerhaave's carefully constructed synthesis of iatrochemistry and iatromechanism by his stringent criticisms of these theories as applied to medicine. He faulted the chemists as abstract metaphysicians who sought to explain all phenomena in terms of chemistry, and the mechanists he chided for failing to consider crucial differences between living organs and the parts of machines and for being too enamored of quantification for its own sake.

But La Mettrie's reexamination of Boerhaave's synthesis did not simply hone his critical acumen. Boerhaave's legacy also provided the foundation of his conception of medical practice and his notion of the ideal physician, an amalgam of the zealous, reform-minded philosophe, the adept empiricist, and the well-educated, idealistic man of medicine. This ideal, epitomized by Boerhaave, became the goal sought by La Mettrie in his medical and philosophical works. More important, his reexamination of Boerhaave's synthesis was crucial to the development of La Mettrie's philosophical perspective. La Mettrie's conception of scientific method was the direct result of his medical heritage. Unlike most would-be Newtons of his day, La Mettrie was extremely skeptical about the practical value of mathematics, especially as a model for understanding human physiology or man in society. Instead, La Mettrie's science was empirical, clinical, and firmly rooted in the biological sciences. Although he criticized attempts inspired by Bacon to make the natural sciences a catalog of nature, he nonetheless concurred with Bacon that the essence of science must be practical, deliberately directed towards the amelioration of the human condition. La Mettrie's sense of the proper method of science is eclectic, reflecting the Enlightenment rejection of the metaphysical *esprit de système* in favor of a less rigid *esprit systèmatique*. His sense of science is also moderately optimistic since, insofar as one is always stringently critical of received ideas and willing to incorporate new findings, one can further the progress of science.

La Mettrie's work within the Boerhaavian corpus provided much of the substance of his philosophy. Like Boerhaave's medicine, La Mettrie's philosophy was eclectic and based on a physiological system little more specific than the balance of liquids and solids. This loose formulation allowed the incorporation of new experimental data. In the context of La Mettrie's philosophy, it was flexible enough to allow him to advance plausible explanations of the physiological processes which could connect the mind to the body. Boerhaave's use of the Hippocratic constitution as a primary consideration in therapeutics was also crucial to the development of La Mettrie's medicine and philosophy. In La Mettrie's medicine it was the crucial factor in limiting the efficacy of the physician. The individual constitution made each case unique and gave the physician a host of imponderables to consider. In philosophy it was the key to understanding the problematic relationship of some individuals to society as well as a critical limitation on hopes for reform. Perhaps most important, Boerhaave's moderate Lockean sensationalism was the key to La Mettrie's development as a materialist philosopher. La Mettrie was able to rework Boerhaave's tentative connection between mind and brain function into a much closer connection by building on Boerhaave's suggestion that Locke provided the most convincing epistemology in terms of which to discuss mental states. Furthermore, Boerhaave, in La Mettrie's hands, must be acknowledged as a crucial figure in defining objections to Cartesian physiology and as a primary source for the interpretation of Locke as a materialist and a medical figure; these themes will be considerably extended in La Mettrie's philosophical texts.

The French Inheritance

The assumptions which govern the conventional understanding of the intellectual tradition of the Enlightenment acknowledge the impact of the great seventeenth-century metaphysicians or assume the overriding importance of Newton on the development of the French Enlightenment. When an explicitly French context for the Enlightenment is explored the political and financial crises of the ancien régime are discussed with an occasional mention of Fontenelle or some of the clandestine literature of the period before the Enlightenment. But La Mettrie worked through physiological issues to develop a reformist campaign, to define an epistemological stance, to redefine nature and human nature, and to contribute to discussions about the nature and the role of the philosophes. While this method is perhaps not the most usual route for a philosophe to travel to reach the concerns of the Enlightenment, nonetheless La Mettrie's use of physiology to define philosophical perspectives is not foreign to the physiological texts written in the first half of the eighteenth century, when a number of physicians, including Guillaume Lamy, François Maubec, Antoine Louis, Louis Moreau de St. Elier, and Antoine Le Camus,[52] sought, like La Mettrie, to investigate the physiological bases of human behavior. In other words, when La Mettrie worked through physiological texts and came to radical philosophical conclusions, he was invoking a French physiological tradition.

Eighteenth-century physiologists set their works explicitly within the parameters of philosophical debates and addressed the philosophical implications of virtually every aspect of their physiology. This philosophical concern can be explained in part by the very nature of physiology in the eighteenth century. Biological sciences were divided into physiology and natural history.[53] Natural history, based on a system of Baconian classification and considered as a function of memory on the encyclopedic tree of knowledge, used natural phenomena to oppose the aridity of mechanism and to demonstrate the glory of God.[54] Physiology, however, was a different kind of discipline. Classified as a part of physics, its place on the tree was under reason, its realm was the investigation of function, and its practitioners were inclined to place their investigations within a philosophical context. Several other factors contributed to the affinity between philosophy and physiology: physiologists of the period were almost invariably physicians well trained in Aristotelianism;[55] they pursued or were fully aware of investigations of brain physiology; and their investigations inevitably challenged metaphysical assumptions that could not be empirically demonstrated.

Physiologists, unlike natural historians, sought to distance scientific question from theological issues in order to conduct investigations into all aspects of human behavior unfettered by theological or metaphysical constraints[56] and informed instead by empirical observations. Regardless of their specific philosophical positions, they also shared assumptions about their endeavor which suggest their import for the Enlightenment. For example, they assumed that the workings of the body and the soul, at the very least the sensitive soul, must be studied empirically, especially through anatomy, and that anatomical studies substantiate the comparability of man and animals. They also recognized, some with enthusiasm, some with reluctance, that their concern with empirical research and comparative anatomy served to subordinate mental processes to physiological functions.

Despite these critical assumptions held in common, one issue was common to every text, fundamental to subsequent discussion of moral issues, and deeply divisive: the nature of the soul. This issue invariably provoked further discussion of the relationship of the soul to the body and impelled each author to take a stand for or against materialism, a critical test of philosophical, physiological, and religious orthodoxy. Another less controversial but significant aspect of these texts was the position their authors defined for themselves within the philosophical tradition, especially their response to Descartes. These two issues are fundamental to these texts and afford a convenient way to address their philosophical content.

The nature of the soul and related questions provoked extensive discussion and controversy. Guillaume Lamy,[57] physician, physiologist and frequently cited author of the *Discours anatomiques* and the *Explication méchanique et physique des fonctions de l'âme sensitive* written in the 1680s, insisted that physiology conclusively demonstrates that the sensitive soul is a "very subtle body, always in motion, whose reservoir is in the brain" and suggested further that, since perception only involves the movement of matter, "all bodies are capable of thought and perception as well as movement."[58] Lamy extended the realm of the sensitive soul into the traditional domain of the rational soul, discussing its "internal senses," which included the sensorium commune, the imagination, and memory, but going beyond these faculties, which were the traditional preserve of the sensitive soul, to make all rational faculties dependent on memory.[59] Thus the sensitive soul becomes the source of all intellection. Lamy defended his materialism as an inevitable conclusion, responding ironically to his critics on this point: "so much the worse for those who have so little faith in their religion that they abandon certitude for reasonable doubt."[60] He, like other materialists, attacked Descartes's *bête machine* hypothesis, claiming that animals, conceded by everyone to be simply corporeal bodies with only sensitive souls, nonetheless give the same signs of cognition and evidence of the passions as a stranger who does not speak our language. He also used the comparability of human and animal brains to refute the Cartesian understanding of thought as immaterial.[61]

François Maubec's treatise of 1709, *Principes physiques de la raison et des passions des hommes*, took a more conciliatory tack on the question of materialism, claiming ignorance about the nature of the spirit and focusing his attention strictly on observable results of investigations of brain physiology and the senses. Although he denied that matter can think, he nonetheless emphasized the role of traces of "esprits animaux" on brain matter in thought processes and ultimately concluded that we think only because of the vibrations of brain fibers. But he inserted the crucial caveat that this relationship exists solely by virtue of the will of God.[62] Maubec was equally vehement in his critique of Descartes. He rejected Descartes's definition of thought and insisted that mental phenomena must be explained by physical causes. He compared human and animal brains to suggest that because similar structures support similar functions they must both generate thought.[63]

Antoine Louis, the prolific eighteenth-century surgeon, proclaimed in his *Essai sur la nature de l'âme, ou l'on tâche d'expliquer son union avec le corps, et les lois de cette union* of 1747 that his purpose was to bridge the gap between reason and metaphysics, whose purest forms he considered to be physiological observation and religion.[64] Since religion was to be reinforced by physiology, materialism was the enemy to be defeated. Nonetheless, Louis claimed as an undeniable premise that "the diverse alterations of the spirit which derange the entire body of man and the different disorders of our machine which diversely affect the spirit are truths which cannot be subjected to doubt and establish, between body and soul, a liaison so intimate and a dependence so mutual that it seems that these two substances make only one."[65] This close relationship suggested to Louis that the soul must be located in a specific site in the brain (which he identifies as the corpus callosum).[66] But he dogmatically denied that his conclusions supported materialism. He maintained that the soul is both extended and immaterial and was thus led into direct conflict with Cartesian metaphysics. Descartes, Louis claimed, confused the properties of things with their essences. The Cartesian assumption that thought is the essence of the soul Louis considered absurd because, he insisted, thought is simply the effect of sensibility and activity, and an effect cannot be an essence.[67] Although Louis dogmatically opposed any claim that the soul is simply the result of the mechanics of the body, he nonetheless also thought that Cartesian dualism had opened the door to materialism by making all extended things material and by making thought the essence of a soul whose existence could be proved only by the light of revelation.[68]

Physiologists who were not materialists condemned Descartes because he had placed them in the uncomfortable and untenable position of either declaring in favor of materialism or accepting a complete break between rational and physiological functions. The arguments of both Maubec and Louis are weakened by their conflicting desires to discredit Descartes, to argue for an empirical understanding of mental processes, and yet denounce materialism. And, ironically, whether they were materialists or not, these physiologists, as part of their critical response to Cartesian dualism, treated all aspects of human behavior, including intellectual and moral activities, as functions of a mind that they considered an organ of the body. They also repudiated Cartesian mechanism as an inadequate model for any living body, especially the human body. Ultimately they could find no way to correlate Descartes's positions with physiological observation. Although these physiologists disagreed as to whether the close conjunction of body and soul led to materialism, they were all harshly critical of the distortion Descartes had wrought in physiology. But they were equally perturbed by his epistemology and metaphysics. Just as his physiology robbed the body of life by making the body a machine divorced from rational processes, so, they suggest, his arbitrary definition of matter as extension and the soul as thought made philosophy inimical to physiology.

These physiologists not only considered it essential to define their philosophical tenets but were also led, as La Mettrie would be, to address the moral implications of their physiological views in part because of fundamental assumptions they shared about the nature of physiology. For example, because of their own observations as practicing physicians they accepted the decisive argument that physiological states affected all human behavior, including intellection, acts of will, and moral behavior. But they did not simply accept a correlation between mental states and physiological processes; they also analyzed the physiological roots of moral behavior and suggested treatments for moral ills or behavioral problems.

Lamy's text explicitly indicates the way in which physiologists were led to address moral psychology. Because the senses are assumed to be inclined or disinclined towards objects of sensation in a way that corresponds to pleasure or pain, then those inclinations are defined as the passions or the fundamental physiological cause of human behavior, including moral behavior. Antoine Le Camus, in his three-volume work *Médecine de l'esprit* (1752), went much further, saying that "the desire to be useful to men has made me bold."[69] He assumed that the functions of understanding and the "springs" of the will are produced by mechanical, physical causes that have an incontestable power over the spirit. He intended to study those mechanisms in order to determine what specific causes impair or enhance them.[70] By understanding the physical causes of behavior "the vices of the understanding and the will"[71] could be corrected. It was simply a question of uprooting the defects in the organism that one previously assumed to belong to a soul impervious to medical treatment. Medicine was to be the vehicle for reform, as only the experience of physicians could reveal the vices of organs which impede the function of the soul. The cure to both mental illness and aberrant behavior was to be sought in medical treatment, in the same way, he insisted, that physicians cure chest fluxions.[72]

Moreau de St. Elier, who as Maupertuis's brother might have exerted a direct influence on the philosophes, wrote a treatise entitled *Traité de la communication des maladies et des passions. Avec un essai pour servir à l'histoire naturelle de l'homme* (1738) in which he was led to espouse radical philosophical positions in his quest to polemicize against breast feeding and in favor of wet-nursing. (Wet-nursing provided an influence on the health of the baby to counter that of the mother, which was likely to be detrimental or even evil and had already, through pregnancy, been excessive.) Having remarked on the ill effects of breast milk on the human body, Moreau de St. Elier examines its evil effects on the soul. To make this argument, he assumes that the passions are dependent on the state of nerve fibers, which in turn are fundamentally affected by the liquids that nourish them.[73] Thus "all that modifies the body influences the way of thinking or feeling"[74] to such a degree that, he claimed, "the slightest difference in the composition of the blood is capable of changing our passions, our manners, and our reputation."[75] Although the passions exist to preserve the body and to seek its well-being, the body, if its nerve fibers are irritated, will seek well-being in "the greatest follies, the most cruel vengeances, and the most monstrous impurities."[76] In essence, according to Moreau de St. Elier, the union of the body and the soul obliges the soul to feel the needs of the body and the body to seek passionately its own well-being.[77] For Moreau de St. Elier, the effect of temperament or the physiological condition of nerve fibers on human behavior is akin to concupiscence, and remedies are to be sought by careful medical control of fluids like breast milk.

These early eighteenth-century physiological texts provide a particular understanding of the philosophical tradition that bequeathed to the philosophes a source perhaps comparable to the clandestine literature of the period. Although they were less polemical than writers of clandestine tracts, physiologists were equally forceful in

indicating the materialist implications and unflinching in acknowledging the moral dimensions of their physiology. They provided a
stringent analysis and critique of Cartesianism grounded in empirical rather than epistemological issues (and perhaps more attractive
on that ground than a Lockean or sensationalist critique of Descartes). These criticisms of philosophical authorities offered the
philosophes a position from which to assail metaphysics as irrelevant to the pursuit of knowledge. Physiologists also provided a body
of scientific opinion that not only argued the virtually complete
identity between body and soul but also recognized that this view
had important implications for morality. This would have allowed
the philosophes either to dismiss the immortal soul as scientifically
undemonstrable or to claim that, since the correlation between body
and soul was so thoroughgoing and persuasive, the immortal soul, if
it existed, was reduced to a negligible role in human behavior. If the
influence of physiological states on moral behavior as suggested by
physiologists was accepted by the philosophes, then they had a
stance from which to attack Christian morality and to argue for
toleration. Philosophical reflections on physiology suggested that
the moral and social improvement of man was possible through an
understanding of physiology. In other words, physiology provided a
reworking of the philosophical tradition, which in turn offered a
distinct scientific foundation for Enlightenment programs for social
reforms.

La Mettrie is a pivotal figure in developing this argument about
the connections between physiology and philosophy. He not only
worked through Boerhaavian physiology and produced physiological works that addressed philosophical issues but also wrote philosophical works in which physiology provided much of the essential
structure and evidence. La Mettrie built upon Boerhaave's tentative
correlations between Lockean epistemology and the physiology of
mental processes to develop a materialist philosophy.[78] Materialism
led La Mettrie to emphasize Aristotelian substantial forms, to use
the sensitive soul as a way to discuss mental processes,[79] and to
denounce Cartesian physiology and metaphysics.[80] He rehabilitated the senses as the only way to knowledge and rescued the
empirical method from the disparagement of the Cartesians. He
argued that the soul must be completely identified with the physical

functions of the body, and any claims about its existence or function could only be substantiated through physiology.[81] La Mettrie emphatically insisted that just as sensation and motion are inherent to matter, all the functions of the soul can be circumscribed under matter.[82] To refuse to espouse materialism, according to La Mettrie, is to take refuge in metaphysical constructions which only distract us from truths readily available through the senses.[83]

Like other physiologists, La Mettrie looked to physiology as the appropriate context within which to discuss moral issues. He sought to determine whether our notions of virtue and vice correspond to human nature as revealed by physiology. He used the physiological comparability of men and animals as the basis for his argument about the natural state of man and concluded that society was not only unnatural but also arbitrary, and that its notions of virtue and vice, while socially useful, were fundamentally at odds with nature and simply the result of socialization.[84] This conclusion overtly challenged the natural law tradition by arguing that our ability to conform to the social notions of virtue and vice is ultimately determined by our particular physical constitution, that is, the particular way our senses are inclined towards pleasure or pain. In much the same way that physicians work within the parameters set by the individual constitution, La Mettrie sought to gauge the limits of the efficacy of the moral reformer. Just as the physician must acknowledge the effects of the individual constitution on health and disease, so too the moral reformer must recognize the limits that an individual's constitution imposes on his ability to behave as society demands. The moral imperative that physiology suggests is toleration for those whose constitution makes them unable to conform to social standards of virtue and a reexamination of society to ascertain whether its admittedly arbitrary standards could, without harm to the social order, be modified to reward a greater array of human behavior. But La Mettrie was not only taking the perspective of the physician, that is, concern for the well-being of the individual; he extended his conclusions about the relationship between physiology and moral behavior into the social sphere. By using physiology explicitly to challenge Christian morality and the theory of natural law and applying physiological conclusions about the individual to prescriptions for society, La Mettrie radicalized the correlation between physiology and morality drawn by physiologists, and he specifically used the philosophical context of contemporary physiology as the basis for arguments for social reform.

The philosophical content of the physiological tradition must be acknowledged as a source of La Mettrie's philosophical development. While Boerhaave gave him the most basic philosophical orientation, that is, an explicit physiological guide to materialism, the French physiological tradition, because of the issues it treated and its approach to epistemological issues, offered palpable evidence that physiology could comment on philosophical issues. It thus led La Mettrie to understand the intimate relationship between physiology and philosophy, to appreciate the free rein physiology could give to philosophical speculation, and to use empirical findings to undercut metaphysics. But all of these uses of the physiological tradition become more forceful, explicit, and polemical in La Mettrie's philosophical works, where he issues no cautious disclaimers and does not retreat from unorthodox conclusions. These works were not directed to the restricted and specialized audience of physiological texts but were rather undertaken with an intent to proselytize in the cause of Enlightenment.

6

Materialism and Lockeanism

The Medicalization of Metaphysics

Those who wish to know the properties of the soul must above all investigate those properties which are clearly manifest in bodies . . .
—La Mettrie, *Histoire naturelle de l'âme*

When La Mettrie turned to philosophical writing in 1745 with the publication of *L'Histoire naturelle de l'âme*, he took the treatment of philosophy in physiological texts a step further by discussing philosophical issues in terms of medicine and physiology. He reappraised philosophical issues, working toward new evidence, new authorities, new methods. But the style of this work is much too close to that of a metaphysical treatise to appeal to historians of the Enlightenment who, accustomed to the wit, style, and grace of writers like Diderot, Voltaire, and Rousseau, do not expect to be confronted by arid metaphysical treatises. In studying La Mettrie they have more usually attempted to wrestle with the contextual complexity but stylistic delights of *L'Homme machine*, and thus, in part for stylistic reasons, *L'Histoire naturelle de l'âme* has not been considered important to the Enlightenment or even to La Mettrie's corpus. Why, when *L'Homme machine* is the source of La Mettrie's reputation, would one turn to a problematic metaphysical text?

Furthermore, La Mettrie's style and the substance of this text are not sufficiently metaphysical to seem credible to philosophers; they are frequently discomfited by Enlightenment notions of philosophy, which might be summarized as a lack of methodological rigor and a kind of irreverence or playfulness in treating philosophical issues. However, if the philosopher turned his attention to *L'Histoire naturelle de l'âme*, he would be rewarded by a particular French interpretation of Locke's *Essay on Human Understanding*.[1] But even this might not persuade him of the worth of La Mettrie's philosophical writings. For La Mettrie's intention is to recast the nature and grounds of philosophical discourse. As a result, even though he began his text in an orthodox philosophical manner, arguing clearly from one point to the next and grounding his arguments firmly in the context of Aristotelian-Thomistic tradition, he was able to maintain that philosophical rigor of both form and argument for only a few pages at a time. Throughout the work he strains to leave behind the uncomfortable and confining metaphysical morass to rush into what is for him the crux of any argument, the empirical evidence of case studies. Physiological evidence weighed far more heavily than metaphysical conventions. And he could not resist deliberately distorting the arguments of other philosophers so that they might foreshadow or support his conclusions.[2] As a piece of philosophical writing, *L'Histoire naturelle de l'âme* is too unorthodox to be taken seriously by philosophers.

Serious historical or philosophical analysis of La Mettrie's text is hampered by several unresolved and fundamental questions. Why would an eighteenth-century thinker, especially one inclined to chafe at the constraints of traditional systems of thought, provide an Aristotelian framework for his own philosophy? Why did La Mettrie invoke substantial forms and Aristotelian categories of the soul when he, like most of his contemporaries, could and did regard Scholastic thinkers as men so beclouded by theological concerns that their philosophy could be dismissed as nonsensical and futile linguistic disputation? And why, when all of his other works are so unconventional in style and content, would La Mettrie cloak his arguments in the guise of an orthodox metaphysical treatise? In sum, why did La Mettrie write *L'Histoire naturelle de l'âme* in the way he did?

Placing La Mettrie's philosophical works within the context of his medical concerns suggests several answers to these questions. Perhaps after he had followed the path through the entire human body as marked by Boerhaave's *Institutiones*, adding his own clarifications and emendations, La Mettrie wanted to investigate the mind or soul and to amplify, in a more conventional style and form, his brief but suggestive remarks on spirits in the *Institutions*.[3] Perhaps he intended to bring medicine to bear on philosophy as he both interjected medical issues into his philosophical works and used Locke's *Essay* as the epistemological foundation for materialism.

While these general, medical concerns do inform this text to a considerable degree, I would like to suggest that La Mettrie's purpose was much more radical: he intended to discredit metaphysics as a way of understanding. He levelled against the entire endeavor of philosophy the same criticisms he had directed against the encroachment of metaphysics into physiology: system building, lack of practical application, pointless distinctions, linguistic quibbling, and, most damning for the empirical scientist, a lack of relevance to reality. For La Mettrie, empirical studies must replace metaphysics, and the findings and the methods of medicine and physiology must be used to critically reappraise philosophy. He wrote *L'Histoire naturelle de l'âme* as a physician committed to the practical application of empirical physiology to investigations of man and his soul. The only acceptable terms in which to discuss the soul are those which can be empirically demonstrated.[4]

If La Mettrie's purpose is to discredit metaphysics, his own adherence to the form of a metaphysical treatise obscured his intention. But this may be a case of applying the methods of the enemy to undo him. To build support for his materialism, La Mettrie uses the philosophical tradition in three distinct and rather unconventional ways. First, he manipulates the philosophical canon against itself. For example, the arguments of some orthodox thinkers (quotes from the church fathers are especially effective)[5] are pitted against the Scholastic position on the soul, and, in general, theological disputations are used to discredit all theological opinion as groundless. Second, he legitimates his materialism by finding philosophical antecedents for materialism within the established philosophical canon; his most important source is Aristotle. Third, he maintains that the only credible philosophical position on the human soul is that it is material and mortal. Any other position, to the extent that it cannot be forced into some conformity with his materialism, is absurd. By this tactic, he denounced the opinions of seventeenth-century metaphysicians, Leibniz and Descartes in particular, as arrant nonsense.

These aims, fundamentally those of the polemicist, do not afford La Mettrie an opportunity to analyze thoroughly other philosophic positions or even to make important distinctions in his own view of matter and motion. But La Mettrie is not concerned to present a careful philosophical argument; he intends instead to drive home his materialist stance. To carry out this goal La Mettrie brought to the fore some of the polemical skills that he developed in his medical satires (and that he honed by continuing to write the satires concurrently with his philosophical writings). Materialism is presented in the staunchest of terms as obvious and irrefutable; other opinions are exposed as contradictory, absurd, or nonsensical quibbling over definitions. Similarly, the stylistic tools of the polemicist allow him to distort the thought of his opponents and to cloak it in convoluted and obscure language from which the reader will be eager to flee to the clear and forthright expression of La Mettrie's materialism. La Mettrie's purpose and his stylistic conventions, then, are obviously responsible for the failure of this work as a metaphysical treatise; he does not, after all, wish to discuss the nature of the soul constrained by the metaphysical debates and issues of his day but rather to shed the light of empirical medicine on the obscurity of metaphysics.

In this first of his philosophical works, La Mettrie used the philosophical tradition to define and support his own philosophical and scientific concerns—specifically, to develop a new philosophy of man based upon empirical studies by physicians, surgeons, anatomists, and physiologists. His use of that tradition is designed to serve a specific polemical purpose—to discredit all metaphysics insofar as they do not serve his notion of a new philosophy and to salvage what is useful to that end. As such, this text, designed to persuade or convert, takes an extreme position on issues that occupied his contemporaries. While many of them blanched before La Mettrie's materialism, they could not fail to notice the ways their own positions lent support to La Mettrie's more extreme arguments. Because he made no compromises, he played an unusual role in these debates. He horrified the devout, exposed the weaknesses of moderate positions, and blazed a trail for French materialists. By taking an extreme polemical position so early in the Enlightenment, more flamboyant than subtle and more controversial than persuasive, La Mettrie played a crucial role in setting the terms in which philosophical issues would subsequently be discussed.

La Mettrie and the Philosophical Tradition

La Mettrie did not hesitate to proclaim his most radical conclusions and assumptions. The very first sentence is a bold, clear statement of his initial premise that the nature of the soul is unknowable. "Neither Aristotle, nor Plato, nor Descartes, nor Malebranche can teach you what your soul is."[6] He singled out these particular ancients and moderns to criticize their notions of the soul and to suggest that metaphysics is an insufficient or defective tool for investigating such questions. More important, this statement reaffirms the position he developed in response to medical theories, namely, an absolute horror of systems and an unwavering epistemological modesty bordering on skepticism. Thus his ultimate claim is that the soul will remain *as unknown* to us as the essence of matter and bodies. Epistemological modesty is very much in keeping with his physiological investigations, and the virtual equivalence of bodies and souls is meant to suggest that bodies and souls are unknowable in exactly the same sense, and, by extrapolation, that what *can* be known about *both* can be known by the same means, that is, by empirical, scientific investigation. In other words, any conclusions about the soul must be supported by empirical, physiological evidence, and whatever notion of the soul one might advance, it must be inextricably connected to the body because the notion of the soul without a body is like that of "matter without form, absolutely inconceivable."[7] Because the immaterial soul has thus been summarily discounted, La Mettrie's discussion of souls becomes a discussion of matter. This facile equivocation of terms undercuts the philosophical strength of his argument but furthers its development, pushing the reader inexorably towards an acceptance of materialism.

Instead of looking to metaphysical systems to discuss the notion of matter, La Mettrie claimed to rely on the findings of empirical investigations of the body because there can be no surer guide to truth than the senses. "Whatever ill one may say of them [the senses], they alone can enlighten the reason in the search for truth."[8] These initial premises are both the heart of La Mettrie's philosophical perspective and the result of his medical investigations. He specifically rehabilitated cognition through the senses and the empirical method from the disparagement of the Cartesians. In general, he repudiated the overextended application of systems, be they scientific or metaphysical, and steadfastly maintained that there can be no understanding of first causes or essences. Thus any argument about these unknowable essences can be nothing but idle speculation. This perspective does not promote despair, but rather sounds a clarion call for empirical investigation, for the clear understanding of man, his environment, and his society that the evidence of the senses invariably and unquestionably produces. The optimistic assessment of the possibilities inherent to materialism is characteristic of all of La Mettrie's works and explains in part the appeal of his particular brand of materialism. Bereft of certain knowledge but thereby liberated from the chimeras of established authorities, man nevertheless has a productive, if narrowed, area of inquiry.

La Mettrie's stated purpose in this treatise is to examine "what we can discover in matter, in the substance of bodies, and above all in organized bodies, but seeing only what is there, imagining nothing."[9] This premise begins La Mettrie's attack both on the immaterial and immortal soul of man and the elevated position in the natural order which that soul has traditionally merited for man in the eyes of theologians, philosophers, and even scientists.[10] La Mettrie refused to countenance such a distinction. "It is demonstrated that the human body is nothing more in its origin than a *worm*, whose metamorphoses have nothing more surprising about them than those of an insect. Why should it not be permitted to research the nature or the properties of this principle, unknown but evidently active and sensitive, which makes this worm, puffed with pride, raise himself up from the surface of the earth."[11] La Mettrie used this Pascalian image of the insignificance of man as compared to the majesty of the universe to challenge boldly the Christian theory of matter and to rule out implicitly the Biblical account of creation. Without providing any real justification or context for the following remark, La Mettrie nonetheless unequivocally stated:

All the diverse properties of matter that one notices in the unknown principles [the essence of matter] demonstrate a being in which exist these same properties, a being which consequently should exist by itself. Furthermore, it is impossible that a being which exists by itself cannot create and destroy itself. Evidently it can have only the form of which its essential properties make it susceptible, which enable it to destroy itself and reproduce itself *tour à tour*. Thus experience forces us to avow that nothing makes itself from nothing.[12]

These conclusions cleverly undermine orthodox belief about the nature of matter and God's role in creation without having it appear that that was La Mettrie's intent. In fact, La Mettrie cites the Scholastic philosopher Goudin to support these conclusions.[13] While on the face of it he has simply stated properties of matter, La Mettrie has also claimed that a being with extension, the power to acquire motive force, and the faculty of sensation must be assumed to exist by itself. By making movement and sensation characteristics of matter, he first of all is denying that these powers are granted by God or infused into matter; they are instead simply qualities intrinsic to matter. Second, he is claiming that the faculty of sensation is certainly not limited to men, as Descartes would have it, but common to all living matter. Implicitly, then, there is no essential distinction to be drawn between men and other living matter. Third, this definition makes matter self-sufficient; it does not require the constant, active intervention of God to preserve it in existence. By drawing a further implication from his argument, that one cannot conceive of a being which can exist by itself but cannot create or destroy itself, La Mettrie has also attacked creation. This definition of matter precludes the possibility of ascribing either creation or death to the intervention of God and denies a divine role in the preservation of matter. Fourth, the acquisition of an immortal soul is made to seem a logical impossibility because, by his definition, a being can take on only those properties to which it is made susceptible by its essential properties. As if deliberately to inflame the orthodox, La Mettrie further claimed that all philosophers, Christian or not, have come to these same conclusions about the nature of matter, with all their strongly antireligious implications.

While La Mettrie was generally content to treat the Christian conception of the soul ironically, he returned to the theme at the very end of this treatise and challenged the authority of theologians overtly in a chapter entitled, "That faith alone can fix any belief in the nature of a reasonable soul." Although the title seems conciliatory, conceding an area for faith (which has sometimes been taken to deny that La Mettrie was a dogmatic atheist or to suggest that he was at worst an agnostic), the chapter reflects not moderation but rather La Mettrie's explicit desire to avoid the fanaticism which characterized discussions of religious issues.[14] He also used in his own behalf the traditional defense of the freethinker, the irreconcilability of faith and reason.[15] He assumed that all scientists and philosophers recognized two standards of truth, one based on faith, the other grounded in reason or science. His point was not to lend credence to faith but to argue the authority of reason in dealing with the things of this world.

But certain sections of the work seem more belligerent towards religion. Like Galileo and Bacon before him, La Mettrie demanded an independent science. Scholastic and theological meddling in scientific questions particularly provoked his ire because it impeded empirical science and produced metaphysical chimeras. The mixture of religious and scientific issues by both Descartes and the Scholastics led La Mettrie to choose quite purposefully to refute their views of matter together, for part of his violent objection to Descartes was his feeling that Descartes had made the serious mistake of trying to reconcile religious and scientific truths.[16] La Mettrie consistently used Descartes throughout his philosophical works as the last credible, but completely ineffective advocate of the immortal soul.[17] He believed that by making the immortal soul part of his metaphysics Descartes had violated this unspoken but universally acknowledged dichotomy between religion and science that made scientific progress possible and had, as a result, permanently involved religious authorities in a misguided quest for *one* truth. Descartes had also invited religious authorities to scrutinize his own works, seeking the approval of Scholastic philosophers for his own metaphysics in order to get it accepted as part of a university curriculum.[18] The perils of that strategy must have weighed on La Mettrie's mind, as he was clearly aware that subsequent objections to Cartesian metaphysics focused on transubstantiation.[19]

Throughout his text La Mettrie consistently applied his empirical standards to both ancient and modern theories of the soul and matter. He specifically chided proponents of traditional science (Aristotle) and the new science (Descartes, Leibniz) for their failure to adhere to empiricism and for their introduction of metaphysical or occult qualities into theories of matter. La Mettrie reduced all theories of matter to two: Aristotelian matter as the power to receive different forms that produce themselves in the matter itself and through which the matter can acquire motor force and the faculty of sensation, and Cartesian matter as extension. Other theories were dismissed as the result of theological squabbles of the Middle Ages or the misguided metaphysical systems of seventeenth-century rationalists.[20]

La Mettrie stringently criticized the second theory. For example, in order to arrive at Descartes's innate ideas, it is necessary that we "consultons nos connoissances," the antithesis of an empirical investigation. Opposed to this interior knowledge are "connoissances qui viennent toutes des sens."[21] Because one cannot conceive of matter as simple extension without form, Descartes's definition is absurd. Ultimately, according to La Mettrie, Descartes's theory of matter created a self-contained system which is not grounded in phenomena; once his definition that matter equals extension has been accepted, all his other corollaries follow, but what has then been established is geometrical knowledge "which the spirit cannot know." In other words, "the extension of matter is thus only a metaphysical extension which offers nothing sensible." Despite his own concerted attack, La Mettrie then blithely dismisses Descartes's theory of matter as insignificant and frivolous, a more suitable subject for a Scholastic than for an enlightened man of the seventeenth century![22] Although he treats Descartes cavalierly, his blatant disregard is intended to discredit someone he sees as a serious threat to his own materialism and to forestall Descartes's anti-empiricism and the a priori truths of innate ideas.

La Mettrie's most violent criticism of Descartes is provoked by the *bête machine* hypothesis, a theme he developed in *L'Homme machine*. Because Descartes restricted sensation to those endowed with an immortal soul, La Mettrie claimed that Cartesian metaphysics constructed "un labyrinthe dont ils ont cru sortir par cet absurde système que les bêtes sont de pures machines." La Mettrie found the *bête machine* hypothesis ludicrous because "experience proves to us that there is not less of this faculty of sensation in animals than in men."[23] If one assumes, as Descartes does, that other men feel because they use the same affective language, there is no reason, according to La Mettrie, to deny sensation to animals since they too give the same signs, even if the comparability of the affective language of animals and men has escaped the notice of the "sectateurs de Descartes," who rely on "sentiment intérieur." But philosophers who apply themselves to the study of comparative anatomy acknowledge the extensive correspondences between men and animals. Anatomy, La Mettrie suggests, puts the philosopher on much more certain ground than metaphysics and is the most fruitful area of study for the "true philosopher." In fact, La Mettrie completely dismisses the *bête machine* hypothesis as "an opinion so laughable it has never been accepted except as *badinage d'esprit* or as a philosophical amusement."[24]

Though he charged that Aristotle's theory of matter was riddled with metaphysical terms, La Mettrie found Aristotle's notion of matter less objectionable than Cartesian extension and used it to argue his own theory. He invoked, for example, the ancient distinction between passive and active forms of matter. For the ancients passive forms like size, shape, and situation had extension as their source. They were also convinced that matter potentially contained in itself all forms. For La Mettrie this is a logical failure in their theory that he can put to good use in arguing his own. If simple extension makes matter susceptible to an infinite number of forms, matter cannot then receive any specific form without its proper motive force. If matter sometimes takes on a certain form and not another, that cannot be the result of its nature as defined by the ancients because it is too inert. Therefore, if matter acquires a form it must be the result of a "new form, which merits here the first rank because it plays the greater role in nature. It is the active form, or the motor power; the form, I repeat, by which matter produces those [forms] it receives."[25] In other words, what La Mettrie found useful about Aristotle's theory of matter was its emphasis on *motive force*.[26] La Mettrie also uses the Aristotelian categories of vegetative, sensitive, and rational souls, only to collapse them all into the sensitive soul. He also appreciates the frequently cited Aristotelian maxim, "nothing in the intellect which is not first in the senses." Ultimately, La Mettrie concludes, Aristotle's *De Anima* supports his own conclusion that there is no soul without a body, because "Aristotle says too that those who claim that the soul is not a body are right: because, he adds, the soul is not a body but it is something of the body."[27]

Though the ancients made distinctions that were based on metaphysical speculation rather than empirical evidence and that were thus inadmissible by La Mettrie's empirical standards, they had, to their credit, made a crucial distinction of distinguishing matter with only the power to be moved from matter with the power to move; they called the latter a substance. But La Mettrie professed not to be able to understand why, once this distinction had been made, the ancients did not espouse materialism. "It is clear that the ancients should have easily recognized an intrinsic force of movement within the substance of bodies, because finally one can neither prove nor conceive any other substance which acts on it."[28] Because the moderns were too eager to blur this important distinction, La Mettrie claimed, they failed to recognize the crucial role that the *force motrice* and the *faculté de sentir* must play in any understanding of matter.

La Mettrie admitted that it is difficult for man to accept that his sensitive faculty is simply an attribute of matter because of his *amour-propre*. But, challenging the Cartesians, he asked whether sensitivity as an attribute of matter is any more difficult to understand than how extension flows from its essence or how extension is related to matter. And to those who might posit a quality in living bodies that belongs to a being distinct from matter, La Mettrie responded, "Does the light of reason permit us to admit in good faith such conjectures?"[29] This query might be said to be the Occam's razor[30] that La Mettrie's entire philosophy and much of Enlightenment philosophy rigorously applied: if there is no empirical basis for a belief, no matter how comforting or socially useful, there is no reason to allow it. In this respect, La Mettrie went much farther than other philosophes. He was personally much more comfortable with the admission that certain things are unknowable, and he would not tolerate the supposition of any hypothetical being because he considered that such suppositions impeded empirical research.

For La Mettrie, physiology provides convincing evidence of the material nature of the sensitive soul because the senses act through the nerves. (Note that without any discussion of his use of terms, the *faculté de sentir* has become, for purposes of discussion, the sensitive soul.) Numerous experiments inform us that the sensitive soul receives the sensation *propre à l'animal* in the brain. Once again arguing the authority of the physician over the metaphysician, La Mettrie noted that while philosophers debate the nature of the soul, *all* physicians since Galen have acknowledged that the sensitive soul is only affected in the brain and that the soul has as much sensation as it receives actual impressions of nervous fluids. By implication, the fact that all these distinct nerves feed into the *sensorium commune* leaves, both literally and figuratively, no room for something occult, the immortal soul, for example.

Thus no aspect of the sensitive soul justifies or supports Cartesian dualism. Regardless of what might be hypothesized about the soul, La Mettrie claimed, "it is absolutely necessary that it is not itself unextended, as Descartes purports." According to La Mettrie's reading of Descartes, body and soul are entirely opposed; the body is capable only of movement and the soul only of understanding, and it is therefore impossible that the body acts on the soul or the soul on the body. And if one supposes a mind/body dualism, how can the effects of sensory deprivation or diseases of the brain upon thought processes be explained? In direct opposition to Descartes, La Mettrie maintained that there is only one *reasonable* conclusion: the connection between the body and the soul is so close that they form a single entity which must be material and extended. In other words, the soul, by definition material and active, now conforms to La Mettrie's definition of matter and can be analyzed empirically. So close is this connection that all the modifications or varieties of human behavior that we consider the result of the soul are, La Mettrie suggests, actually due to temperament, not in the classical sense but rather simply "la disposition des organes."[31] In other words, those things formerly held to be the activities of the soul can effectively be studied medically as physiological phenomena.

To refuse to follow his argument thus far, La Mettrie claimed, was simply to interpose metaphysical constructs, distracting us from the direct path to truth available through our senses. He berated most of the great philosophers for having resorted to chimeras. "You see that to explain the union of the soul and the body, it is not at all necessary to put the spirit to such tortures that the great geniuses Aristotle, Plato, Descartes, Malebranche, Leibniz, and Stahl have devised. It suffices to go directly to the correct path, to look neither behind nor to the side when the truth is directly in front of you."[32] The prejudiced, "who will not even bend over to gather up the truth if they find it where they do not wish it to be,"[33] are even more culpable. This statement highlights the belligerent tone that characterizes much of La Mettrie's philosophy. He intended to get to the truth no matter where it was to be found, radically redefining the areas in which one ought to search for truth away from metaphysics and towards medicine and physiology. This remark also suggests an obvious affinity between the quest of La Mettrie and the much vaunted motto of the Enlightenment, *sapere aude*. However, most of the writings of the philosophes set limits on their daring, limits La Mettrie was all too willing to transgress, boldly asserting that the only conclusion one can accept, once one has overcome the prejudice of the systems-makers, is that the soul must be material.[34] Metaphysicians have not only refused to accept the true premises but they have burdened the notion of the soul with qualities that cannot be empirically demonstrated. He attacked the Cartesian *cogito* because "my soul constantly shows, not thought, which is accidental to it, no matter what the Cartesians say, but activity and sensibility." Leibniz, who did recognize these two qualities of activity and sensitivity as inherent to matter, nonetheless also supposed "a subject at the base of them which exists by itself and to which belong by rights these same properties. Thus, one concludes, the soul is a being separated from the body, a sort of spiritual monad." To reject Leibniz's contention, La Mettrie queried: "Why would one wish that I imagine a nature absolutely distinct from bodies, when I clearly see that it is the organization of the nervous system itself, from the beginning of the nerves to the end of the cortex, which freely exercises in a healthy state all the properties?"[35]

No doubt aware of the opposition his materialism would provoke, La Mettrie made the force of his argument revolve around probabilities. For example, those who argue that behind matter there lurks an immaterial soul can only bring metaphysical arguments to bear, while his evidence is based on observation and experiment. Therefore it is no *more* improbable that matter should be able to think and feel than that something immaterial acts on the material. Since all experimental data support the former, it is the more probable.

It is sometimes assumed that in *L'Histoire naturelle de l'âme* La Mettrie's materialism was dogmatic and therefore uninteresting, but that in *L'Homme machine* his position softened and his materialism became merely heuristic.[36] However, his probabilistic argumentation in the former suggests that La Mettrie's position is more consistent than generally believed and that his materialism is heuristic only in the sense that all knowledge is heuristic once you have limited the grounds for certainty in the way characteristic of much of Enlightenment science: that is to say, one must deal with what can be known and not seek to fathom what cannot, for example, first causes or essences. The difference in the tenor of the claims for materialism in the two works reflects their different purposes: *L'Histoire naturelle de l'âme* is more dogmatic because it intends to destroy the ground of conventional metaphysics; *L'Homme machine* is a more positive effort that builds a new philosophy and demonstrates what conclusions can be drawn on the basis of empirical, physiological evidence.

La Mettrie's discussion of the philosophical tradition occupies some thirty pages of *L'Histoire naturelle de l'âme*, only about a quarter of the whole text, yet it is the most problematic portion of the work. In part the problems are of La Mettrie's making. He is inclined to change terms, to alternate an ironic and a serious tone, and to employ a convoluted style. His tendency to discount opponents through the use of polemical devices also makes this text less than straightforward. But interpretations too have muddied the waters. Scholars have been inclined to discount the scorn heaped on Descartes as of passing significance, since they assume in light of the standard interpretations of *L'Homme machine* that by 1747, a mere two years later, La Mettrie was a rigid and confirmed Cartesian mechanist.[37] And the use of Aristotle in a materialist, quasi-metaphysical treatise has seemed so uncharacteristic that the work has been considered a satiric attack on the Scholastics or as a first philosophic mistake written in an aberrant style.

While it is true that La Mettrie does use the Scholastics against themselves, and very cleverly, the argument that the text itself is a satire directed against them makes the Scholastic tradition far too important to La Mettrie and mistakes a subtle and persistent stylistic thread for the substance of the work. The notion that his use of Aristotle makes the entire treatise a youthful philosophical indiscretion gives too much weight to this particular section of the treatise, fails to consider the role it plays in defining his philosophical perspective and philosophical allegiances, and neglects important and consistent connections between this work and his other philosophical writings. Furthermore, La Mettrie's own sense of the importance of this treatise must be acknowledged. He wrote it in 1745, reissued it in 1747, and gave it a prominent place in his collected philosophical works, wherein he provided a key, the *Abrégé des systèmes*, to explain the work. So while La Mettrie never took up the form of *L'Histoire naturelle de l'âme* again, he obviously intended the work to be seen as an integral part of his philosophical corpus.

An interesting, if perhaps unresolvable, question is what La Mettrie thought his reconstruction of the tradition added to his materialism. Specifically, what benefit did he think he derived from his discussion of Aristotle? Obviously it suited La Mettrie's polemical purposes and diabolical sense of fun to use the figure at the heart of the Thomistic synthesis to support materialism and to argue against an orthodox and immaterial view of the soul. But more central to La Mettrie's purpose was the use of Aristotelian naturalism and empiricism against the seventeenth century metaphysicians, who, La Mettrie suggests, could be discounted as neither naturalists nor empiricists. Aristotelian empiricism and naturalism are what La Mettrie considered salvageable from the philosophic tradition, and they can be connected to the proper epistemology and method, that of John Locke.

How La Mettrie Read Locke

Once La Mettrie had dealt with his philosophical predecessors, albeit in a less than orthodox manner, he dramatically changed the tenor of his treatise. His style is no longer obscure or ironic; the polemicist retreats before the serious medical writer. La Mettrie had worked through the philosophical tradition and found much to be repudiated and little to be retained, but he was much less ambiguous about the merits of John Locke's *Essay on Human Understanding*. While he may legitimately be charged with failing to grapple with the metaphysical issues of Locke's *Essay*, he did not deliberately distort Locke to serve his own ends. His intent is clear and his style equally forthright; Locke was a philosopher whose epistemology he read as supporting his own materialism. His purpose then is to lend substance to Locke's epistemology by providing physiological evidence.[38] But La Mettrie's natural history of the soul also provides evidence of a closer anatomical or physiological correlation between mental states and physiological processes than Locke allows. The sources La Mettrie invoked as the appropriate foundation for a new philosophy were physiologists, doctors, and anatomists. Although he considered Locke a timid materialist, he saw no difficulty in connecting Locke's epistemology to the increasingly weighty (from his point of view) evidence of eighteenth-century physiology and anatomy in order to develop an explicitly materialist philosophy.

Several questions come to mind at this point: First, why did La Mettrie consider the question of Locke's materialism such an open-and-shut case? That interpretation is, after all, clearly at odds with the philosophical tradition which maintains that Lockean empiricism is more likely to lead to Berkeley's idealism than to materialism. Second, why did La Mettrie see Locke as such a kindred spirit that he became the philosophical anchor for his materialism? Finally, to what end did La Mettrie use Locke in his own work?

The first question deals with the issue of the reading of Locke prevalent in the eighteenth century. Most modern philosophers claim that Locke's discussion of whether God could have added thought to matter is hypothetical and parenthetical and in no way indicative of a hidden materialist agenda. Indeed, the more accepted reading of Locke leads to Berkeley's idealism, and Locke's contribution to the Enlightenment is considered to be Condillac's sensationalism, which explicitly avoids materialism. Nonetheless, Locke's *Essay* raised a furor in England about its deistic and materialistic implications.[39] And in eighteenth-century France, there was another prevalent and influential reading of Locke that took it as a foregone conclusion that he was a materialist. John Yolton has pointed to several factors which help to explain this transmutation of Locke's philosophical legacy in France.[40] Voltaire's "Letter on Locke" emphasized Locke's suggestion that matter might think and noted his affinities with the English Deists and materialists. The notion of Locke as a materialist was also highlighted in the clandestine tract, *L'âme matérielle*.[41] But in addition to these routes into France of the propagation of Locke as a materialist, La Mettrie could see in Locke's epistemology the clear possibility of such a strong correlation between physiological and mental processes that the mind or soul must be an active force. Furthermore, as I have suggested earlier, La Mettrie had a clear precedent of a cautious use of Locke to support these correlations in the works of Boerhaave.

In the *Abrégé des systèmes*, attached as an explanatory key to the *Traité de l'âme* (as *L'Histoire naturelle de l'âme* is called in his collected works), La Mettrie left a forthright discussion of his position vis-à-vis other philosophers, and he is quite explicit in his praise for Locke and clear about the affinities between Locke's position and his own. First he assumed that Locke's approach to knowledge was the same as his own; Locke too proclaimed his ignorance of the nature of bodies in lieu of developing an imaginary (read metaphysical) notion of the essence of bodies; he proved the uselessness of syllogisms, destroyed innate ideas, and renounced Descartes's notion that the soul is always thinking. These are the sorts of arguments La Mettrie himself used against Descartes.

La Mettrie appreciated Locke's appeal to commonsense experience and his discussion of case studies. "What is quite certain is that the opinion of this subtle metaphysician is confirmed by the mutual progression and decay of body and soul, and principally by the phenomena of illness which demonstrate clearly, even against Pascal, that man can very well be conceived without thought. And consequently, thought does not make the being."[42] These are important points for La Mettrie's own philosophy. As a result he was inclined to see Locke's concerns as his own and to overlook quite considerable differences as insignificant in light of these fundamental affinities. La Mettrie read Locke as a fellow physician, someone whose interests were, like his own, empirical and antimetaphysical. In fact he stated that "thus it is true that M. Locke was the first to dissipate the chaos of metaphysics, the first to give us true principles by recalling things to their first origin."[43] Referring no doubt to Descartes, La Mettrie noted that the errors of others put Locke on the right path, for, unlike Descartes, Locke thought that "sensible observations were the only ones which merited the confidence of a *bon esprit*, and he made them the foundation of his meditations; the torch of experiment served him as an accurate compass. His reasonings are as severe as they are remote from prejudice and partiality and one does not see in them the sorts of fanaticism of irreligion."[44] This quotation praises Locke at the expense of Descartes. Sensible observations were not the basis of Descartes's *Meditations*; it is no accident that La Mettrie uses that word to characterize Locke's *Essay*. And, to his credit as far as La Mettrie is concerned, Locke did not invoke God to anchor his metaphysics. La Mettrie's understanding of Locke as sharing his concerns explains both the fact that there are no satiric references to Locke and that he is accorded such a prominent place in the *L'Histoire naturelle de l'âme*.[45] La Mettrie did not distort but rather cautiously stated Locke's position on the material soul: "He appeared to have believed the soul material although his modesty did not permit him to decide it."[46] Nonetheless, based on the connections Locke drew between body and mind, La Mettrie confidently assumed, as some of his contemporaries also did, that Locke was a materialist, or at the very least that Lockean epistemology, by being rooted in physiology, could provide the foundation for his materialist philosophy.

It is likely that La Mettrie turned to Locke as a fellow physician. Intrigued by Locke's commonsense observations, he assumed that Locke too would be interested in substantiating physiological correlations in order to diagnose and treat disease. Boerhaave had established the crucial precedent, using Lockean psychology as the foundation for his explanations of sensation and cognition, reproducing Lockean accounts of memory, imagination, and reflection and then suggesting the patterns of *esprits de cerveau* which might correspond to the thought processes Locke described. But while Boerhaave retreated before the materialist implications of his conclusions, La Mettrie showed no such hesitation.

La Mettrie's fundamental understanding of Locke as approaching philosophical issues from the same background of medicine and physiology explains both the way he used Locke and the ways he deviated from him. La Mettrie reproduced Locke's particular definitions of mental processes, but he was intent on connecting all such definitions, insofar as he was able, to accounts of explicit physiological processes.[47] (When he had no concrete evidence, he was willing to hypothesize about how the physiological process might work.) Because he thought that physiological processes ultimately provide the only basis for knowledge about mental states, La Mettrie was unwilling to grant to the mind an explicitly active power such as Lockean reflection. Instead, he placed the power of mind in the physical organs involved in sensation and the transmission of sensation. For example, all the physical organs involved in sensation affect the nature of the sensation itself. Because each nerve has an effect on sensation, it cannot be assumed that the sensations themselves correspond directly to physical reality, since they are affected by the nerves. Thus at the outset of his sensationalist analysis La Mettrie redefined Locke's epistemology, making it both materialistic and much more skeptical than the *Essay*.

Because mental states are to be investigated physiologically and because sensation is the basis of all mental processes, La Mettrie discussed what anatomy and physiology, supplemented by analogy when necessary, could tell us about how sensation works. For example, his observation of how we see led him to the following conclusion about sensation: "The diversity of sensations varies according to the nature of the organ which transmits them to the soul . . . each nerve produces different sensations, and the *sensorium commune* has, to put it this way, different territories, of which each has its nerve and receives and focuses the ideas brought by this tube. . . . Not only do different senses excite different sensations, but each varies to an infinite degree in those it transports to the soul according to the way in which they are affected by external bodies."[48] La Mettrie also provided additional physiological evidence for his conclusions about the process of sensation by discussing a dissection of the eye.[49] The eye provided the best evidence because it is the only sense organ which visibly represents the actions of the exterior objects and is therefore the most useful for conceptualizing the effects of objects on nerves. La Mettrie then used his notion of animal spirits and mechanical analogy to suggest the way in which impressions made on the retina were transmitted to the *sensorium commune*: "These small cylinders of a diameter so narrow can only contain a single file of globules. From which follows the extreme facility with which these liquids move at the least shock. And from the regularity of their movements follows the precision, the fidelity of the traces or the ideas that are produced in the brain: all effects which prove that the *suc nerveux* is composed of round elements."[50] This quotation indicates an important point at which La Mettrie's philosophy differs from Lockean sensationalism. Locke thought that sensation was transmitted from the sensory organs to the *sensorium commune* in the mechanical-corpuscular fashion La Mettrie suggested. (Locke and La Mettrie both used the same billiard-ball analogy as part of their discussions.)[51] But whereas Locke refused to speculate on the connection between the *sensorium commune* and the brain, La Mettrie, chiding Locke for lack of courage, did not fail to emphasize at every point that they are identical and material. The quotation also illuminates the connection between La Mettrie's science and philosophy. La Mettrie, under the influence of Boerhaave, espoused a loosely corpuscular view of matter and found mechanical analogies heuristically valuable. At every juncture he was interested in emphasizing links between physiology and Lockean sensationalism, and he insisted that sensation, as a physiological process, could be completely explained without reference to the occult or to the immaterial.

But in considering the physical organs of sensation, La Mettrie was led to a critical break with the sensationalists. In a chapter entitled, "That the sensations do not make known the nature of bodies and that they change with the organs," he espoused a radical epistemological modesty and articulated an extreme individualism that is both the product of his criticism of mechanism and his medical emphasis on the individual constitution and the force behind his discussion of morality.[52] Although La Mettrie consistently pointed out that knowledge of first causes and essences is denied to us, here he seriously questioned the knowledge gained by way of the senses with the claim that "sensations do not enlighten us on the nature of either the active object or the passive organ."[53] He also scrutinized all the areas where the senses might fail and only grudgingly conceded that shape, movement, mass, and hardness are attributes of bodies "on which our senses have some hold." "Some hold" can scarcely be construed as expressing great confidence. Perhaps influenced by Locke, La Mettrie was aware of the problematic nature of sensationalist epistemology, as indicated in the following quotation: "But how many other properties are there which reside in the final elements of bodies and which are not seized by our organs with which they have a confused connection or none at all? Colors, heat, pain, taste, feel, etc., vary to such a point, that the same body can appear sometimes hot and sometimes cold to the same person. Consequently the sensitive organ does not retrace on the soul the true state of bodies."[54]

La Mettrie did not use the problems inherent to the process of sensation to argue, as Descartes had, that one must look somewhere other than to the sensations for certain knowledge. The senses are the only access to knowledge we have. He seems to have felt that it was misbegotten to seek for absolute truth at all. What the senses offer is a pragmatic truth: they are meant to preserve us in existence, not to gain for us a metaphysical truth. They cannot misinform us about danger to our well-being unless we mistake the signals they offer by acting too hastily. It is ironic that La Mettrie ultimately drew the same conclusion Descartes had about the practical value of sensation. However, he went much further in his skepticism about the senses than Descartes, who ultimately accepted their evidence as informing us about the nature of the external world because his God does not have the character of a practical joker perpetrating an enormous hoax.[55] La Mettrie, without this convenient guarantor, was much more skeptical about the relationship between the object and the information conveyed by the senses, and even questioned the concession noted earlier: "I say more: one does not know the first qualities of bodies any better,"[56] that is, the ideas of height, hardness, and so forth are only determined by our organs. Like other perceptions, we have different ideas of the same attributes because of the effect of the physical organs of sensation on the sensation itself. "Thus our ideas do not come from a knowledge of the properties of bodies, nor in what the change which affects our organs consists. They form themselves by this change alone. . . . Sensations thus do not at all represent things as they are in themselves, since they depend entirely on the corporeal parts which offer them transit."[57]

In other words, what remains uncertain for La Mettrie is the correlation between sensations and the external world, not the correlation between physical and mental states. In order to deal with the individualized, nonprescriptive character of sensations and their problematic correlations to mental states, La Mettrie provides as thorough a description as possible of all the physiological factors involved. He also attempts to explain the diversity of sensation and some of the problems involved in describing the effects of sensations on our organs. Most difficult to ascertain is the individual character of each nerve, since "Each nerve differs from the others in its beginning and consequently appears to carry to the soul only one kind of sensation. In fact, the physiological history of all the senses proves that each nerve has a sentiment relative to its nature, and even more to that of the organ across which it modifies the external impressions."[58] The condition of the brain itself is also crucial to the transmission of sensation: each sense has its own small department in the medulla of the brain, and the acuity of the sense can therefore be affected by "the tissue of the nerve sheaths which can be more or less solid, their pulp more or less soft, their situation more or less loose."[59] Finally, there are certain faculties which depend completely on the physiological state of the nerves. The discussion of all of these factors is designed to suggest that, if a complete understanding of brain physiology were possible, then the relationship between sensation and mental processes would be knowable.

This emphasis on the effect of the individual nerve on the sensation itself led La Mettrie to deviate from Locke, making Locke's tentative connections between mind and matter definitive; that is, the qualities of the soul become qualities specific to the organism that are determined and controlled by that organism and form the basis of La Mettrie's concept of the individual. Just as particular faculties depend on the organs, so too are differences between individuals the direct result of the diverse configuration of their organic constitutions. The notion that rational faculties depend on the organs themselves leads to both an extreme skepticism about what our sensations tell us of external reality and an irreducible individuality based on physiology. Though these points define La Mettrie's epistemology and distinguish it from Locke's, they were not completely foreign to more orthodox Lockeans. Locke himself raised the question of how much the variation in the perceptive and rational abilities of different individuals depended on differences in physical constitution but refused to speculate.[60]

In *L'Histoire naturelle de l'âme*, La Mettrie proceeded from those physiological and mental processes where the physiological connections are more easily demonstrated to those more difficult to substantiate. He assumed that his analysis was legitimate and would be persuasive even where the connections are less readily apparent and believed that all that could not be predicted or prescribed according to his analysis was due to the unique character of each nerve and the internal self-modifications of some physiological processes. The hope for greater knowledge thus rested on more thorough correlations to be drawn through empirical investigations.

He therefore began to define mental phenomena in physiological terms, first discussing those "faculties of bodies which are related to the sensitive soul." La Mettrie expanded his notion beyond the scope of the Aristotelian sensitive soul to include, in keeping with Lockean sensationalism, "the habitual modification of these same movements which necessarily recall the same sensations. These modifications, so many times repeated, form the memory, imagination, and the passions."[61]

A comparison of their discussions of memory will make clear

some of the differences and similarities of La Mettrie's and Locke's epistemology. For Locke, to remember is to retain an idea either by keeping it in view or by reviving it. In either case, it is an activity of mind. La Mettrie, who will not allow active powers of mind that he fears can easily be transformed into faculties or souls, is much vaguer on where the activity takes place and what kind of activity it is, and instead emphasizes passive tracings on the different parts of the brain. For Locke the random or unpredictable nature of memory is explained by the manner in which the sensations occurred, for example, in youth, with great impact, or with pleasure or pain. La Mettrie, however, posits a physiological explanation for the problematic character of memory by referring to the way physiological traces on the brain are connected to each other.[62] Locke merely raises the issue that La Mettrie considers fundamental: "I shall not enquire, though it may seem probable, that the constitution of the body does sometimes influence the memory."[63] This is the connection La Mettrie is determined to substantiate through case studies and the perspective from which he understands the issues of Locke's epistemology. If, for example, the connection between sensation and memory is conceded, and if it is acknowledged that this connection can be established by accounts of human behavior—which is just the case Locke consistently makes in the *Essay*—then La Mettrie contends that if certain brain injuries disrupt the connection between sensation and memory, Lockean epistemology supports materialism. La Mettrie constructed an hypothesis as to how this process works: "The cause of memory is entirely mechanical, like [the memory] itself; it appears to depend on which physical impressions on the brain follow it or are neighboring."[64] Thus an idea is able to evoke a similar tracing on the brain and take it out of sequence or call forth the entire sequence, as in the case where hearing a single word evokes an entire poem. If the physiological basis of memory is conceded, then, according to La Mettrie, it must also be acknowledged that memory and all the intellectual activities that depend on it are material and the result of brain function.

La Mettrie also invoked Locke to define the passions. Locke claimed that "pleasure and pain are the hinges on which our passions turn"[65] and that the desire to procure pleasure and avoid pain is at the root of all the emotions. La Mettrie repeats Locke's definitions and points to the physiological effect of strong love or hate.

"Our entire [animal] economy is overturned by it and no longer knows the laws of reason; then this violent state is called passion, which draws us toward its object despite our soul."[66] But whereas Locke then defines a whole range of human emotions as specific dispositions of the mind—for example, "fear is an uneasiness of the mind, upon the thought of future evil likely to befall us"[67]—La Mettrie's concern is specifically with the physiological manifestations of the passions. Perhaps taking his cue from Locke's statement that "[t]he passions too have, most of them in most persons, operations on the Body . . . ,"[68] La Mettrie discussed in detail the physiological effects of the passions and as a physician sought to modify their sometimes deleterious effects. Locke, on the other hand, broke the connection between the passions and their physiological effects by insisting that the effects of the passions on bodies, "not always being sensible, do not make a necessary part of the idea of each passion."[69] La Mettrie was forced to argue from analogy ("although we do not know the passions by their causes, the light which the mechanism of the movements of bodies has cast in our day, permits us at least to explain them clearly by their effects")[70] the physiological connection is the most essential part of this discussion because the nerves obviously play a crucial role in the passions. He nonetheless considered that the physiology of the nerves played the most essential role in the passions.

For La Mettrie, the passions determined the will, which he defined as simply a desire to act on the pleasure attached to the sensation. (Locke has exactly this same notion of the will.)[71] According to La Mettrie, sometimes the affections of the soul are made with an interior sentiment, which he called "conscience" (meaning consciousness), and sometimes without it. Those cases made with conscience, that is, when the body obeys the will, are characterized by the following physiological processes: "To explain the effects of passion, it is sufficient to have recourse to some acceleration or slowing of the movement of nervous fluids, which appear to be produced by the nerves."[72] Those passions that are not guided by an interior sentiment and in which the body is not subject to the control of the will provoke a host of far more extensive physiological symptoms, which can be debilitating. Although La Mettrie described the will in Lockean terms, he emphasized the circumstances under which the will is to no avail whatsoever in order to suggest the general subservience of the will to physiological processes. He made particular note of the substances that affect the will, an argument he would extend to the entire mind in *L'Homme machine*. La Mettrie's disparagement of the will is part of his attack on vitalism; because the will is completely a product of sensation and a relatively negligible one at that, it cannot be the case, as Stahl maintained, that the will is the direct cause of all physical activity "producing everything itself, even hemorrhoids."[73]

La Mettrie claimed to have explained man's memory, passions, and will as "faculties of the soul which visibly depend on a simple disposition of the *sensorium commune*, which is nothing but a purely mechanical arrangement of the parts of the medulla of the brain." There is no basis for ascription of any faculty distinct from the physiology of sensation. This position is not merely an epistemological position, it is also pragmatic. Knowledge of the physiological effects of the passions in particular and a materialist-sensationalist physiology in general provide essential information for the physician "to know, explain, and cure the diverse afflictions of the brain."[74]

The importance of this materialist reworking of Lockean memory and the passions to the development of La Mettrie's philosophy cannot be overstated. La Mettrie has first of all repositioned these functions in the brain in accordance with the Aristotelian tradition. Deliberately opposed to Descartes's denigration of these corporeal faculties, La Mettrie not only grounded these activities of the mind/brain in concrete physiological processes but also used them as the foundation for rational faculties. As part of his rehabilitation of these functions from the scorn attached to them by the Christian and Scholastic understanding of Aristotle and more recently and more emphatically by Descartes, La Mettrie consistently claimed that man has overemphasized the role of rational faculties in his behavior.

To a large degree, La Mettrie suggested, human behavior could be more accurately discussed as motivated by the appetites and instincts we share with animals. In discussing inclination and appetites La Mettrie adamantly and successfully emphasized the material bases of his sensationalist analysis. For example, inclinations, as he defined them, are dispositions which depend solely on the particular structure of the senses, that is to say, the solidity or the softness of the nerves found in those organs and the degree of mobility of nervous fluid. Thus the inclinations we feel are the direct product of our particular constitution.[75] "It is to this state [physical constitution] that one owes the natural penchants or disgusts one has for the different objects which happen to hit the senses."[76] The appetites too depend on certain organs destined to give us sensations that make us desire the enjoyment of "those things useful to the conservation of our machine and the propagation of our species." Because appetites depend completely on the quality of the physical organism, they are the bases of La Mettrie's initial comparison of men with animals. Instinct too can be used to undermine those characteristics we consider distinctly human. For example, instinct is the source of the compassion animals often show towards each other and even towards man. But just as instinct gives animals traits we consider human, under its sway men act as animals do. "When our body is afflicted with some illness, so that it can function only with pain, it is, as any other animal, mechanically determined to seek the means to remedy itself even without knowing them." Thus the organism itself seeks its own good: not a moral good, but the well-being and self-preservation of the individual and the perpetuation of the species. In other words, instinct, as a purely physical phenomenon, reveals not only man's fundamental comparability with animals but also the organic nature of human behavior. Furthermore, the preserve of instinct effectively curtails what La Mettrie called "the monarchy of the soul."[77]

La Mettrie also emphasized that certain ways of behaving are inherent to matter itself. Invoking the authority of Maupertuis, he contended that there is something other than simple mechanism in living bodies; "a certain force, which belongs to the smallest parts of which the animal is formed, characterizes not only each species of animal, but each animal of the same species, each of which moves and feels diversely according to its manner." According to La Mettrie, this innate force very clearly applies to man and is to be found "in each fibrous element, in each vascular element, and always essentially different in itself from that which one calls elasticity, since elasticity is destroyed and the other persists even after death."[78] This discussion of a force innate to each fiber of the body foreshadows the role that irritability will play in La Mettrie's philosophy of man and nature. As the quotation indicates, he distinguished this force from a simply mechanical force. Haller's findings on irritability gave La Mettrie the decisive empirical evidence to support the active force of matter which he so effectively used in *L'Homme machine*.

Continuing to argue the comparability of men and animals, La Mettrie claimed that, just as animals feel in the same way that we do, they also express those sensations, including emotions (which are by his definition only like or dislike provoked by a sensation), in the same way.[79] Although he conceded that animals have fewer ideas and therefore fewer expressions of those ideas than we, they nonetheless perceive and remember secondary qualities of size, shape, and so on and use the same affective language. The fact that parrots can repeat words without ever attaching any significance to them does not prove that they have no ideas since they are able to distinguish between people. So what is the difference between their discourse and ours? According to La Mettrie, theirs is pantomime and ours is verbal, but their signs are understandable to members of the same species. La Mettrie quotes the argument of a French physiologist, using Descartes's language test against him. "I know as certainly, says Lamy, that a parrot has understanding, just as I know that a foreigner does; the same signs used for the one, are used for the other; it is necessary to have less good sense than the animals to refuse to grant understanding to them."[80] Thus only our larger brain size has enabled us to develop a language that *seems* to support a qualitative break between our expressive abilities and those of animals. And if the sounds animals make seem arbitrary (though La Mettrie suggests they are not), human language was no doubt equally arbitrary at the beginning. The comparability of men and animals was a theme La Mettrie addressed in much greater detail in *L'Homme machine*.

Ultimately, for La Mettrie, sensation controls the human condition; happiness depends completely on the sensations the soul receives.[81] The lack of control that the individual has over how he feels, or senses, is a subject La Mettrie will pursue in his works on morality. Here he was provoked to begin his attack on traditional notions of happiness, which are based on metaphysics rather than on an understanding of the workings of the human body.

The Physiology of Mental Processes

La Mettrie had to reconcile man's rational abilities with both his sensationalist epistemology and its materialist implications by making all rational processes comprehensible under sensationalism. Intent on demystifying these processes, he linked them to physiological speculations, which he set forth with a great deal of confidence even though he was venturing into realms where the connections he drew were less than conclusive. He was less concerned to describe mental processes in any kind of complexity than to reduce them so far as possible to the processes he had already described in completely physiological terms. To this end he made as many comparisons between the intellectual activities of man and animals as possible, since presumably few would want to assert a rational soul for animals.

He emphasized the active nature of the physiological process and, since he had tied memory to physiology, made memory the root of all intellectual processes. "Because the soul can only contemplate one idea at a time, if I were to try to compare one idea with another without memory, I would no longer find the first idea. Therefore without memory, no judgment, no speech, no knowledge, no internal sense of our own existence could exist."[82] Perceptions could discover the connections between the sensations the soul had before, but these intellectual perceptions were not qualitatively different from other sensations; they required greater attention, but attention too has a physiological explanation. "When the fibers of the brain, being stretched taut, have put up a barrier that halts all commerce between the chosen object and the barrage of ideas which hasten to trouble it, then the clearest, most luminous perception is possible."[83]

In his materialist working through of Locke's epistemology, La Mettrie argued categorically against the ascription of any faculty to the brain or soul (at this point in his treatise he used the two terms interchangeably) that could not be adequately explained by his definition of matter coupled with this sensationalist epistemology. Thus reflection, which Locke considered to be an active faculty of the soul distinct from the faculty of sensation, required reworking. La Mettrie made it simply another way of perceiving or organizing sensations. However, if reflection is not for La Mettrie the active faculty of mind that it is for Locke, neither is it the simply passive process of Condillac's statue man. To begin with, La Mettrie made sensation a much more individualized and differentiated process, based on the qualities of fibers, nerves, and the brain itself, than Condillac's literal *tabula rasa*. But unlike Locke, for La Mettrie the force behind reflection is not generated by the mind but by the physiological imprint of the sensations themselves, "of the sort that the ideas that affect the soul, the sensation which occupies it at the present moment, brings it little by little, as if by the hand, to all the other ideas to which it has a connection."[84] This association or thread through the labyrinth of our sensations is not a completely mechanical or predictable process, for it does not always take the most direct route, but neither can it be differentiated from sensation.

Judgment, the most complex of the rational processes, La Mettrie defined as simply a serious application to the examination of ideas, and he substantiated his definition through physiological analogies and medical case studies. Judgment is not the active faculty of mind Locke claims or the determination of an active will Descartes describes. It is passive, because "when the soul perceives an object clearly and distinctly, it is forced by the very evidence of the sensations to consent to the truths that hit it so vividly."[85] To the degree to which it is active, the activity is impelled by the force of sensations. Though La Mettrie conceded that we cannot know exactly what takes place in the body, nonetheless he insisted that it is these physical processes that enable the soul to judge, reason, and feel. But he was not averse to somewhat nebulous speculation on those physical processes. "The brain changes its state continuously, the *esprits* make new traces there that necessarily produce new ideas and give rise to a continual and rapid succession of diverse operations in the soul."[86] La Mettrie also made judgment depend on the state of the brain by referring extensively to case studies which revealed that injuries to the brain produced some dysfunction of the memory.

In using Lockean epistemology as the basis for his materialism, La Mettrie treated Locke as a serious medical writer who was concerned with physiological questions. La Mettrie took Locke's descriptions of specific mental processes and considered them as physiological phenomena. He discussed mental processes explicitly according to a Boerhaavian medical analysis. He accepted as a given a correlation between mental processes and physiological events and suggested that what cannot be known about mental processes through physiological events is irrelevant, the only exception being some kinds of analogies drawn from physiological examples.

The Empirical Basis of a Physiologically
Grounded Lockeanism

Just as medicine must define epistemology, offering its approach and evidence to the committed physician, so too the case study must be recognized as the most decisive kind of evidence. Even though he initially restricted himself to metaphysical issues, La Mettrie felt that his positions would be most forcefully sustained by case studies; having defined a new method of philosophy, he wanted to demonstrate what could be gained or known through its use. The particular cases he used are quite familiar to anyone who studies the eighteenth century and presumably were to La Mettrie's readers as well. Perhaps he meant to capitalize on the familiarity of these cases to show that these bits of common knowledge inevitably support a Lockean epistemology with the materialist implications La Mettrie developed; that is, he exploited these cases, which were part of a common fund of knowledge, for their materialist potential.

The first case study substantiates La Mettrie's refutation of Descartes by demonstrating that religious ideas, especially the idea of God, are not innate but only acquired through contact with society. Thus, a deaf-mute who had faithfully attended Mass and the sacraments revealed, when he suddenly regained his hearing, that he understood nothing of God, the soul, or religious ritual. Having dismissed the notion of innate religious ideas, La Mettrie used the famous example of Saunderson's blind man, who upon regaining his sight could not distinguish between a globe and a cube,[87] to demonstrate that geometrical ideas, which Descartes claimed were, if not innate, so clear and distinct that they could not be questioned, are also acquired through education. La Mettrie also used Amman's[88] method of teaching the deaf to speak to illustrate the way in which the senses interact to produce ideas. He found Amman's method particularly intriguing, because if it could be used to teach animals to speak and if animals could convey their feelings through speech, the *bête machine* hypothesis would be completely destroyed.[89] He cited other famous cases as even more indicative of our close relationship to the animals, for example, the boy raised by bears who was a great deal more like a bear than a man and the accounts of Pliny, St. Jerome, and Tulpius of Amsterdam about discoveries of creatures who spoke in a rudimentary fashion.[90]

La Mettrie was not so much convinced by these accounts as fascinated with the possibilities they suggested, and he considered them to be a more decisive kind of evidence than metaphysical speculation. For example, since these creatures were reputed to speak in the husky tones characteristic of those men who had been raised by animals, La Mettrie supposed that it would be easier to teach them to speak than the deaf. And since we do not deny humanity to the deaf, there would be no grounds at all for denying it to creatures who could speak.[91] La Mettrie's argument hinged on language because if, as he felt he had done, one disproved the existence of an immortal soul, the only remaining distinction between men and animals was language. La Mettrie argued throughout his philosophical works that animals could be educated to speak. If this distinction could be broken down, we could not consider ourselves qualitatively different from animals. We, like them, have no immortal soul but simply the veneer of education.

La Mettrie claimed that all the information he had provided was meant to lead to these conclusions:

> Point de sens, point d'idées,
> Moins on a de sens, moins on a d'idées
> Peu d'éducation, peu d'idées
> Point de sensations reçues, point d'idées.[92]

In *L'Histoire naturelle de l'âme*, La Mettrie used his reworking of Aristotle and Locke to develop an alternative, physiologically grounded epistemology. It is possible that this was of more use to later materialists than the static, orthodox sensationalism of Condillac for defining an epistemological position from which to approach the study of nature and social and political issues.

Condillac and La Mettrie recognized, as did their contemporaries, that Descartes's dualist schism between the mind and external reality forced a reappraisal of the nature of human knowledge, and therefore they focused on epistemological issues such as the source of our ideas, the nature of mind, and the relationship between the mind and external reality. Both Condillac and La Mettrie found Locke's epistemology a convenient starting point for their own explorations of these questions. They shared an epistemological modesty, a sense that the nature of metaphysics must be changed, and a desire to apply philosophy to a wider array of issues.

But their positions and premises were almost entirely different. Condillac intended to be the Newton of philosophy, to establish philosophical premises on the certainty of mathematics. He was interested in reforming philosophy so that it might offer an analysis of language and a clarification of concepts; but La Mettrie intended to use philosophy to investigate nature, especially the human condition. Whereas Condillac tried to systematize Locke's descriptive accounts, La Mettrie sought to amplify Locke's physiological descriptions. La Mettrie was much more antimetaphysical, deeming a quest for certainty as misguided and considering attempts to apply the standards of mathematics to the study of nature a grievous distortion. Furthermore, though both La Mettrie and Condillac are considered proponents of naturalism, their notion of what that entailed are widely divergent. When Condillac looked to nature as the model for his philosophy, he was impressed by its order, simplicity, and universality; nature could easily be compared to mathematics. La Mettrie saw nature as complex and irregular; his naturalism glorified the diversity of nature and thus found the baffling manifestation of disease in the individual the appropriate (if difficult to apply) model for philosophy. Relying on medicine rather than mathematics as an ideal meant that La Mettrie advanced lower expectations for certainty and that he had a much less abstract notion of nature, human nature, and morality, a lack of rigidity which might have attracted the eighteenth-century reader.

While Condillac was orthodox and acceptable, he also distorted Locke to accord with his fundamental rationalism. When he ran into difficulties or inconsistencies between empirical findings and his rationalist premises he took refuge in metaphysical speculation. La Mettrie, unconstrained by a rationalist position, was less disturbed by inconsistencies; he would suggest a reasonable or probable explanation, and he was comfortable simply acknowledging what was as yet unknown. As a result, La Mettrie's philosophy was quite different from that of Condillac. While Condillac's philosophy could be adopted by radicals, conservatives, or even the pious, La Mettrie's philosophy was more consistent in its call for empiricism; it was not wedded to an underlying rationalism or to a role for God in nature. But La Mettrie's materialist thesis made his argument polemically stronger and more consistent than Condillac's texts. For example, he did not resort, as Condillac so frequently did, to what Isabel Knight has aptly called "jarring flights into the super-natural."[93] And La Mettrie's consistent and forceful exposition of materialism might have exerted a greater influence on eighteenth-century thinkers than is generally acknowledged, especially on the eighteenth-century understanding of Locke—a force perhaps most clearly indicated by the vociferous complaints of religious critics and philosophical opponents. As Knight has noted, Condillac's "position was one of popularity rather than influence, suggesting that his books had more the familiarity that confirms than the import that converts."[94] La Mettrie provoked no such moderate responses, and as his texts had the widely recognized ability to provoke outrage, they also quite likely promoted "conversion." But even if that were the case, La Mettrie could be claimed by no one as a source because of the very radical implications of this treatise. He spelled out those implications in his other philosophical works, which develop his views of nature, man, and society from his sensationalist-materialist epistemology.

Neither the style nor the method of *L'Histoire naturelle de l'âme* can be found in any other of La Mettrie's works. Yet this text was crucial to the development of his philosophy. In it he developed his theory of matter, his epistemology, and his method and raised crucial questions to be addressed in more detail in his later philosophical works: What is the origin of life? How does the faculty of sensation develop (*Système d'Épicure*)? Is there anything which distinguishes us from animals? What does it mean to be human (*L'Homme machine*)? What is a better basis for discussions about happiness than metaphysics (*Discours sur le bonheur*)?

Even more important, this treatise seems to play a significant role in the development of a distinctively Enlightenment epistemology. La Mettrie continued the attack on theology and metaphysics not by using the skeptical or logical criticisms of seventeenth-century thinkers but by arguing instead on empirical grounds. While this treatise seems wedded to the methodology of seventeenth-century metaphysical texts in terms of the issues addressed and the exposition of arguments, La Mettrie also felt free to use that tradition against itself by employing the playful but devastatingly effective polemical style of eighteenth-century philosophes. By criticizing theology and metaphysics with the tools of a polemicist and by suggesting a different standard for knowledge, La Mettrie, like most later philosophes, could refocus the grounds for philosophical discussion on empirical evidence and ultimately on the question of what kinds of knowledge are useful to man. For La Mettrie's philosophical work, the notion of what is useful is rooted in the medical sciences; but by suggesting empiricism and utility as the two standards for knowledge, La Mettrie opened the way—though he did not follow it himself in any well-developed fashion—to the social sciences. Although it is a puzzling and difficult text, *L'Histoire naturelle de l'âme* is important both to the development of La Mettrie's philosophy and to the epistemological stance of the Enlightenment.

7

La Mettrie's New Philosophy Applied

The Medicalization of Nature

All that which is not immersed in the very breast of nature, all that which is not phenomena, causes, effects, the science of things, in a word, has nothing to do with philosophy and comes from another source that is completely foreign to philosophy.[1]

Having explored as thoroughly as possible the metaphysics of materialism in *L'Histoire naturelle de l'âme*, La Mettrie looked to medicine and physiology (the eighteenth-century embryonic form of biology) for the most conclusive evidence available for his materialism. As La Mettrie himself argued, metaphysics could not lead to certainty, and therefore even if reason inevitably lent the highest degree of credibility to materialism that was not sufficient grounds on which to espouse it; without empirical evidence the reasonableness of materialism made it useful as a means to critique established authorities but ultimately no more tenable than any other system of thought. Thus La Mettrie's three fundamental works on the philosophy of nature, *L'Homme machine*, *L'Homme plante*, and *Le Système d'Épicure*, and his ironic refutation of *L'Homme machine*, *Les Animaux plus que machines*, were intended to provide an empirical base for materialism and to examine the physical world in materialistic terms.[2] Just as medical concerns could be applied to metaphysics to reveal its shortcomings as a way to knowledge, so too the evidence of medicine and its more open, flexible, and empirically valid standards could be applied to discussions of nature, especially human nature.

La Mettrie provoked vehement opposition when he broadened his investigation to address the implications of materialism for our understanding of human nature. He specifically attempted to refute the notion that human beings were unique in nature and to argue that they could not be considered exempt from the fundamental precept that there is naught but matter and motion. In *L'Histoire naturelle de l'âme*, he applied this principle to his discussion of human mental processes and claimed that a Lockean epistemology lent no credence to the existence of an immaterial soul and rationality did not separate humans from the material world. In *L'Homme machine*, he turned his attention to human beings as physical creatures to demonstrate as convincingly as possible just how completely they belonged to nature. Without the impediment to research and understanding that the notion of the immortal soul posed, there was hope that one could come to a more realistic assessment of human nature by studying all available physical and scientific data. From this point on in his writings, La Mettrie took virtually all the evidence he used from scientific theories and experiments, especially medical and physiological findings. In fact, scientists and physicians were usually cited at the expense of metaphysicians.[3] Without distinctive supernatural facets human beings could not be separated from the animal kingdom, and La Mettrie could then integrate them into nature by comparing them with plants in *L'Homme plante*. From this interconnectedness of nature, La Mettrie could then argue the plausibility of evolution in *Système d'Épicure*. In other words, once he had firmly placed man in the sphere of the natural, he could investigate more thoroughly what that implied.

L'Homme machine: Questions of Interpretations

L'Homme machine is La Mettrie's best-known work and the source of both his contemporary notoriety and his present reputation.[4] His medical satires had incited the medical community against him, but *L'Homme machine* swept La Mettrie to general prominence or, more accurately, infamy, which led to his exile even from the generally tolerant Netherlands. As Frederick the Great noted, Calvinists, Catholics, and Lutherans temporarily forgot their theological differences to unite in persecuting La Mettrie.[5] Although *L'Homme machine* became a contemporary *cause célèbre* that provoked both scientific discussion and religious polemics, religious critics were able to gain control of the debate and establish La Mettrie's reputation as a godless atheist. They rightly understood *L'Homme machine* as an attack on the authority of the theologian and attempted to discredit La Mettrie by making effective use of his most inflammatory statements in their polemics. Religious polemicists were galvanized because La Mettrie admitted no possibility of an immortal soul, robbed theologians of authority on scientific questions or indeed any questions about nature, and explicitly addressed both deism and atheism. The efficacy of these polemics allowed La Mettrie's religious critics not only to set the terms for the discussion of this text in particular, and La Mettrie and his brand of materialism in general,[6] but also to relegate the text and its author to a position beyond the pale of acceptability. Religious critics thus made La Mettrie and *L'Homme machine* a powerful symbol of the dangers of Enlightenment.

But an understanding of this text has not simply been thwarted by eighteenth- and nineteenth-century religious writers; a more significant contemporary obstacle to appreciating the text is the independent status of "l'homme machine" as a term that has taken on a life and a history of its own.[7] Historians have investigated the roots of the man-machine theory in part because it has become such a powerfully evocative image in the computer age; the distinctions between human intelligence and the capacities of machines have become blurred in discussions of artificial intelligence, and mechanical analogies for physiological processes have infiltrated common parlance.

The concept of man-machine has been traced back to Greek scientists. Democritus and the early atomists, for example, saw the universe as composed of matter and motion, put man into nature, and eliminated occult qualities. These attitudes, fundamental to the possibility of a man-machine view, found new currency in the seventeenth-century revival of atomism. The scientific revolution not only revived atomism but also combined it with seventeenth-century technological innovations to produce a view of nature in which machines functioned as analogic descriptions for certain body parts and physiological processes. Descartes, as La Mettrie recognized, took this process a step further by considering animals as mere machines because they had no rational soul.

But La Mettrie has not been particularly well served by the associations drawn between the early intimations of a man-machine theory and his text; they have been used to deny him originality or to cast him in the context of the seventeenth-century revival of atomism and thus diminish his importance to the eighteenth century and the development of the Enlightenment.[8] Having been reduced to a throwback to Lucretius or Gassendi, La Mettrie has not been considered crucial to defining a new ideology of the Enlightenment. Furthermore, by placing La Mettrie in the context of seventeenth-century mechanism, scholarly attention has focused almost entirely on the text of *L'Homme machine* and even more narrowly on its title. Such a narrow focus has provoked fundamental misconceptions about La Mettrie's view of nature, and his medical writings especially have been neglected as a fundamental source of his view of human physiological processes. Some historians, recognizing that La Mettrie's mechanism is not completely comparable to seventeenth-century versions, have suggested that La Mettrie added a dynamic quality to "dead" mechanism.[9] But even this distinction does not sufficiently recognize the organic nature of La Mettrie's physiology or adequately consider the insightful criticisms of mechanism developed in his medical writings. Treating La Mettrie in the context of the development of the computer has heightened modern interest in his text, but while La Mettrie himself was clearly intrigued by Vaucausson's automata, his text was not designed to further the mechanization of human nature, human physiology, or human intelligence. Thus the analogy of the robot or even the computer, frequently associated with La Mettrie's *L'Homme machine*, is quite foreign to the spirit of the text itself. In sum, the evolution of the concept of man-machine may be a better way to assess La Mettrie's subsequent influence than to discuss his text itself.

There are two particularly influential interpretations of La Mettrie's relationship to Descartes. Keith Gunderson, in his book *Mentality and Machines*, attempts to explicate the role of "l'homme machine" in the development of arguments about artificial intelligence. Gunderson understands Descartes in terms of his metaphysics and sees La Mettrie's text as a serious attempt to deal with the metaphysical issues Descartes raised. Vartanian, in *Diderot and Descartes*, asserts the fundamental influence of Descartes understood not as a metaphysician but rather as reflected in the mirror of "Cartesianism" as it developed throughout the seventeenth and eighteenth centuries. Both of these interpretations take seriously La Mettrie's acknowledgment in his subsequent philosophical works of Descartes's influence on him and see it as fundamental to *L'Homme machine*, although their understanding and appreciation of that influence is quite different. However, I would like to suggest that La Mettrie's medicine and his consistent and persistent criticisms of Descartes raise fundamental questions that require modifications of both of these interpretations.

Gunderson, in a chapter entitled "Descartes, La Mettrie, Language and Machines," recognizes some of the problems implicit in connecting La Mettrie's *l'homme machine* with Descartes's *bête machine*. As Gunderson acknowledges, La Mettrie criticizes Descartes's understanding of animals in *L'Histoire naturelle de l'âme*, but in *L'Homme machine* he credits Descartes with the discovery that animals are pure machines. Has La Mettrie changed his mind about Descartes? Gunderson considers a fundamental change in allegiance to be unlikely, because immediately after crediting Descartes in the text La Mettrie discusses animals as sentient beings, an opinion at odds with Descartes's *bêtes*. Perhaps, Gunderson suggests, La Mettrie was indulging in hyperbole in crediting Descartes, but he discounts that opinion as unlikely because La Mettrie also praised his own amplification of Descartes in a later text, *Les Animaux plus que machines*.

Before Descartes no philosopher had regarded animals as machines. Since this famous man only a single and most courageous modern has dared to revive an opinion which seemed condemned to oblivion and even to perpetual scorn; not in order to avenge his compatriot, but carrying temerity to the highest point, in order to apply to man, without any evasion, that which had been said of animals, in order to degrade him, to lower him to that which is most vile; thus to show no distinction between the master and his subjects.[10]

This quotation is the most frequently cited indication of the integral relationship between Descartes and La Mettrie. But what light does it shed on La Mettrie's discussion of Descartes? Does it decisively refute the notion that there is something disingenuous or at least hyperbolic about La Mettrie's attribution of credit to Descartes? Note that what is in fact being praised here is not so much the *bête machine* hypothesis as its utility in arguing the comparability of man and animals, a comparison explicitly based on the degradation of man to the level of an animal and a position entirely at odds with the thrust of Cartesian metaphysics. At the very least, it must be acknowledged that La Mettrie's use of Descartes to compare men and animals does not necessarily entail an application of the *bête machine* to humans.

Gunderson, rather than questioning La Mettrie's acknowledgment of the influence of Decartes, concludes that La Mettrie is sincerely praising Descartes and applying his own less than pure notion of machines to animals and men. In other words, La Mettrie muddled Descartes's notion of machine. Gunderson supports this claim by saying that if in fact La Mettrie had accepted Descartes's notion that animals were pure machines and tried to apply it to man, he would inevitably be claiming that nothing thinks or feels. Or, as Gunderson put it, La Mettrie would be suggesting that, in essence, Descartes had said nothing in his metaphysics.

Inadvertently, Gunderson has uncovered the implication of La Mettrie's crediting of Descartes. If La Mettrie first completely undermined fundamental tenets of Cartesian metaphysics and then redefined Cartesian positions in accord with his own refutation of Descartes, it seems naive to assume, especially given La Mettrie's well-developed polemical skills and adroit manipulation of the philosophical tradition, that he was confused about the implications. But instead of recognizing La Mettrie's effective polemical refutation of Descartes, Gunderson continues to portray La Mettrie as an inept Cartesian. According to Gunderson, by showing that there is no essential difference between animals and human beings, La Mettrie intends to argue that animals share our intelligence to some degree and that we share to every degree their "machineness." The assumption that La Mettrie is doing both of these things has led to much of the confusion about this text. The first argument is well supported by the text, but the second can be maintained only if one accepts the title as signaling the intent of the text and the protestations of indebtedness to Descartes as sincere. The second argument neglects the criticism of Cartesian physiology implicit in La Mettrie's description of physiological processes that do not correspond to the notions of animals, machines, or human physiological processes Descartes developed in his *Traité de l'homme*.[11] Concerning the first argument, Gunderson recognizes that La Mettrie appreciates the "language test," as Gunderson calls it, as a critical point of division between men and animals for Descartes and that La Mettrie does indeed attempt to establish that animals might speak. Since this application of the Cartesian claim that animals are machines to support a mechanistic view of man makes no sense in Cartesian terms (because there would be no *thing* which thought or felt), Gunderson concludes that La Mettrie did not understand Descartes's "pure machines."[12] This reading of La Mettrie has proven to be particularly influential in the philosophical community, but it resolves the problems inherent in the text by assuming that La Mettrie was naive and incompetent rather than by questioning his purpose in citing Descartes. Gunderson's reading seriously underestimates La Mettrie's abilities, particularly his deft manipulation of the philosophical tradition against itself and his habitual use of authorities on any subject to develop and sustain controversial positions. Furthermore, it does not take cognizance of La Mettrie's specific and thorough refutation of Cartesian metaphysics contained in the work, recognize the irreverent treatment accorded philosophers by the philosophes generally, or acknowledge the character of La Mettrie's treatment of the philosophical tradition and the malicious sense of fun that permeates his writings. In essence, Gunderson has not been sufficiently wary of the pitfalls of eighteenth-century philosophical writing.

Aram Vartanian is much more sensitive to its nuances. But he is also intent on crediting Descartes as the crucial influence in the development of eighteenth-century naturalism. To develop this argument he must contend with the fact that, with the notable exception of La Mettrie, there are very few favorable or even explicit acknowledgments of Descartes in the writings of the philosophes. Vartanian warns of the dangers of taking attributions of philosophical influence at face value (virtually all such attributions disparage Descartes and praise Locke and Newton). But Vartanian forgets his own warning and takes the clear allusion of La Mettrie's title and his acknowledgment of Descartes in the text too seriously. If Gunderson, writing as a philosopher, is inclined to consider Descartes principally in terms of his metaphysics, particularly the *Meditations*, which has been the focus of most recent scholarly discussion of

Descartes,[13] Vartanian, acutely aware of the permutations of Cartesianism in the eighteenth century, considers Descartes's metaphysics irrelevant to his eighteenth-century reputation and uses the *Discourse on Method* as the fundamental text. As a result, he emphasizes the reformist nature of Cartesianism, its pragmatic approach to knowledge, and the diminished role of metaphysics, perhaps not adequately taking into account the limitations of this popularized text as a vehicle for discussing the influence of Descartes. But a more serious problem is that, in order to trace the Cartesian influence on Enlightenment naturalism, Vartanian deems it necessary to discount not only Descartes's metaphysics but also his mathematization of the universe and natural processes and thus dismisses both of these aspects of Cartesian thought.[14] Vartanian also redefines "Cartesianism" as all positions taken in response to Descartes, whether favorable or negative. As a result, it is virtually impossible for any eighteenth-century thinker to be an anti-Cartesian. Even more problematic, Vartanian claims that those aspects of Cartesianism which can be connected to the development of materialism reflect Descartes's own real concerns, as opposed to more orthodox uses of Descartes, that is to say, the positions taken by those who followed him and took seriously his metaphysical or mathematical concerns. For Vartanian, then, those religious opponents of Descartes who raised the possibility that Descartes would be used to support materialism contribute to materialism just as much as those who genuinely argue or subvert Descartes as a materialist, and he defines both positions as Cartesian. Whether in favor of Descartes or opposed to him, these interpreters, insofar as they further a materialist or naturalistic reading of Descartes, are both the transmitters of Descartes to the Enlightenment and the genuine Cartesians. By working back from the Enlightenment to Descartes, through the Cartesian and anti-Cartesian debates, Vartanian has effectively undercut the argument that sees Enlightenment philosophy as a series of commentaries on Locke. However, the "Cartesianism" that emerges could as easily be called the critique of Cartesianism, and very little of what emerges as "Cartesianism redefined" can be directly correlated to Descartes.

In Vartanian's tracing of the evolution from Descartes to Diderot, La Mettrie is the key figure who makes the Cartesianism-materialism connection explicit. Yet his originality as a materialist philosopher is diminished because, according to Vartanian, La Mettrie simply articulated a well-established and generally accepted materialist understanding of Descartes. Most of Vartanian's examples of the obvious connection between *bête machine* and *l'homme machine* postdate La Mettrie, however, and thus suggest that the materialist reading of Descartes in fact owed a great deal to La Mettrie's text.[15] La Mettrie's lengthy critique of Cartesian metaphysics, based on a frequently cited reading of the *Meditations*, makes it improbable that La Mettrie considered metaphysics irrelevant to Descartes's philosophical endeavor. And La Mettrie's general treatment of Descartes as a benighted iatromechanist, better acquainted with mathematical theorems than with physiological functions, suggests that La Mettrie's appreciation of the naturalism Vartanian claims is implicit in Descartes's science was, to say the least, muted.

Critic of Descartes

In fact it is useful, although unorthodox, to read La Mettrie as an anti-Cartesian. Although La Mettrie's title seems to emphasize an indebtedness to Descartes almost to the exclusion of other points, *L'Homme machine* nonetheless provides a critical commentary on Descartes's *Meditations* and deliberately attempts to overturn the fundamental tenets of Cartesian metaphysics. La Mettrie was not subtle in his treatment of Descartes; he singled him out as one of the "fine geniuses" who produced "useless works" and "profound meditations" that have not benefited anyone. He was intent on demonstrating by numerous examples that there is no independent Cartesian soul, asserting instead that "the diverse states of the soul are always correlative with those of the body."[16] The authority for making any claims about the soul does not rest, as Descartes would have it, on our internal ideas but rather on physiological studies. To further support this connection, La Mettrie posited as probable a physical location of the soul within the brain, possibly, he suggests, the corpus callosum. Just as studies in comparative anatomy between men and animals reveal that our physiological structures are analogous to those of animals, so too, La Mettrie suggested, our reason is comparable to animal instinct, which even Descartes placed in physical organs. This assertion both challenged dualism with physiological evidence and set forth physiological investigations as a more fruitful way to truth than "internal truths."

Having connected soul to brain and men to animals, La Mettrie drew out the anti-Cartesian implications. First, reason is a function of the softness or hardness of brain matter (this invokes the authority of Boerhaavian physiology), and accordingly one finds little sign of reason in children, puppies, or birds, all of whom have soft brain matter.[17] Because language supports the distinction that Descartes drew between men and animals, La Mettrie must argue that the fact that men speak and animals do not is not a sign that only the former have a soul. La Mettrie claimed against Descartes that animals also used affective language, showing, for example, signs of remorse just as in humans.

To refute Descartes, La Mettrie argued the essential similarity between man and ape from two sides of the issue. On the one hand, he claimed that it was plausible, given the extensive comparability between the brain structure of the ape and man, that apes could be taught to speak. Perhaps, he suggested, they had not developed a language to date simply because of some defect in or insufficient development of their vocal cords. He refused to accept that language represented a qualitative leap in learning. With a deliberate slight aimed at Descartes, "géomètre par excellence," La Mettrie noted that "a geometrician has learned to perform the most difficult demonstration and calculations, just as a monkey has learned to take his little hat off and on."[18] On the other hand, La Mettrie assumes that humans did not always speak. Much in the way that animals try to express their feelings (directed at Descartes, whose animals have none), the earliest men began to speak to try to convey their feelings. (It is important to note that La Mettrie's comparisons go from animals to man rather than vice versa.) But language is possible only after the "soul" examines what has been imprinted on the brain through sensation. This stage of human experience is primitive, or as La Mettrie put it, "at a time when the universe was almost dumb, the soul's attitude towards all objects was that of a man without any idea of proportion toward a picture." Deliberately inverting the Cartesian sense of how knowledge is gained, La Mettrie claims that "men have used their feelings and instincts to gain intelligence and intelligence to gain knowledge."[19] Thus the independent, rational soul, which Descartes set forth as the defining characteristic of human beings, La Mettrie claimed had evolved from the sensations, which, with the development of language, allowed the further development of instinct and, finally, rationality.

The way in which knowledge is acquired also inverts Descartes's metaphysics. La Mettrie roots all intellectual abilities in the imagination and explicitly denies the importance of the will. In an aside which seems deliberately directed to Descartes, La Mettrie says, "In vain, you fall back on the power of the will, since for one order that the will gives, it bows a hundred times to the yoke." Furthermore, La Mettrie is intent on exposing the will, the soul, and anything that might be supposed to be a lofty human power as dependent on the senses and the body; for example, he claims that the will is exercised through the nerves. Finally, neither the will nor the soul can act except "with the permission of bodily condition,"[20] and those bodily conditions are prone to sickness, aging, and other infirmities, all of which have a clearly demonstrable effect on the will and the soul. Even such mundane considerations as diet can affect the power of the mind.

If the will is considered as bound to the body, how then does man reason? The key for La Mettrie is the imagination, a position which challenges Descartes's replacement of the imagination with reason as *the* significant faculty. Traditional psychology, from Aristotle through the Scholastics, considered the imagination as a physiological function of the brain. Thus, by making imagination central to all intellection, La Mettrie was asserting that reasoning must take place in the brain and must therefore be the result of physiological activity.[21] Even Descartes's geometric ideas must be understood, according to La Mettrie, as based on the representation of things by signs.[22]

But even if it is conceded that La Mettrie's text is intended to refute Cartesian metaphysics, the question remains: what did La Mettrie intend by making a deliberate reference to Descartes's *bête machine*? Can it be assumed that, even if La Mettrie rejected Cartesian metaphysics, he nonetheless relied on Cartesian science? Is Descartes's mechanism La Mettrie's way of understanding human physiology? Did La Mettrie simply apply Descartes's mechanism more widely than Descartes himself had by applying it to the human mind?

Because *L'Homme machine* is considered to be the ultimate evolution of the Cartesian *bête machine*, it is assumed that La Mettrie has simply and uncritically applied Descartes's mechanistic understanding of animal physiology to human beings. Scholars have more recently suggested that La Mettrie's medical concerns, especially his exposure to the teachings of Hermann Boerhaave, led him to mechanism. However, even Boerhaave was not a firm adherent to mechanism; although he thought a mechanical approach to human physiology was the approach most likely to be productive, his own treatment of the reigning medical ideologies was critical and pragmatic. And La Mettrie had criticized the shortcomings of mechanism as a way to understand human physiology much more stringently than Boerhaave largely because he feared that it would be applied as a new system. La Mettrie had also singled out Descartes for the harshest criticism, specifically for the rigidity of his mechanism, which made him unable to understand and describe physiological processes properly. Significantly, La Mettrie reiterated that criticism in one of his last works, *Ouvrage de Pénélope*, published three years after *L'Homme machine*.

While readers generally expect to be confronted by a text detailing mechanical physiology, replete with heart-furnaces, lung-bellows, gland-sieves, and so forth, the physiological perspective of La Mettrie's text, to the extent that *L'Homme machine* defines such a perspective, is eclectic, nondogmatic, and intent upon describing organic processes by examples supporting his polemical points. There are, however, four significant uses of the word "machine" in the text that have frequently been cited as examples of La Mettrie's fundamental adherence to mechanism. While these examples are striking, it is important to situate them in context, to see what arguments they are intended to support and what examples precede and succeed them. For example, La Mettrie claims that "man is so complicated a machine, that it is impossible to get a clear idea of the machine beforehand, and hence impossible to define it," not to emphasize man's machineness but rather to argue against a priori claims and in favor of a posteriori evidence. Similarly, La Mettrie notes that "the human body is a machine that winds its own springs. It is the living image of perpetual motion." His point is that the perpetual motion of the body is generated by food and drink, and the passage follows a discussion of the effects of wine. Another quotation, often cited as support for mechanism, notes that "we think we are, and in fact we are, good men only as we are gay or brave; everything depends on the way our machine is running." This point was also made in his discussion of the effects of particular substances on behavior, and it is followed by the acknowledgment that van Helmont was not far wrong in locating the soul in the stomach. As support for his anti-Cartesian argument that animals show intelligence and remorse just as we do, La Mettrie wondered, "Why is it absurd to think that [animals] almost as perfect machines as we, are, like us, made to understand and to feel nature." The term "machine" seems to function as the most obvious way to tie together the body and the soul when La Mettrie suggests that "since all the faculties of the soul depend to such a degree on the proper organization of the brain and of the whole body, that they are simply this, or, the soul is clearly an enlightened machine." Perhaps the most famous of these quotations is La Mettrie's concluding claim: "Let us boldly conclude that man is a machine and that there is nothing in the universe but one substance diversely modified." La Mettrie's emphasis is not on the mechanical nature of man but rather on his fundamental materialist premises that even the most complicated intellectual functions can be explained physiologically and, even more important, man is no exception to the uniformity of nature.[23]

What role then does mechanism actually play in *L'Homme machine*? In what sense can La Mettrie be understood as a mechanist? In *L'Homme machine*, La Mettrie did use mechanical analogies as part of his explanation of the functioning of the human body, but only as a small part of his overall discussion. In light of his critique of mechanism, the use of mechanical analogies is perhaps best considered as simply a reflection of the common descriptive language of the experimental tradition of the eighteenth century. La Mettrie can also be considered a mechanist in that he would not entertain occult explanations of physiological functions; as a result, physiological functions had to be automatic, that is, self-perpetuating and self-contained.[24]

But if La Mettrie's text is a criticism of Cartesian metaphysics, and if he is not fundamentally wedded to Cartesian mechanism as a physiological perspective, what purpose does his acknowledgment of Descartes serve? Perhaps La Mettrie was using Descartes in the ironic or distorted way he used other thinkers. Several considerations suggest that La Mettrie's attribution was ironic. By using a title that connected his work to Descartes, he was first of all drawing attention to his own work. Second, he was indicating, just as he had with Locke and Aristotle in *L'Histoire naturelle de l'âme*, just how easy it was to reconcile the works of other philosophers with materialism, in this case Descartes's. Putting himself within the tradition in order to criticize it, as he did with the Scholastics and to a limited degree Descartes in *L'Histoire naturelle de l'âme*, does not make La Mettrie a Cartesian or a Cartesian mechanist. This ironic use of the philosophers in general and of Descartes in particular is completely characteristic of La Mettrie's work. In fact, La Mettrie continued to use Descartes ironically in subsequent works. (For example, in *Discours sur le bonheur*, Descartes appears as a spokesman for Christianity.) And because La Mettrie took Descartes's metaphysics seriously enough to refute it at length, it seems likely that his acknowledgment of Descartes was ironic rather than genuine. In *L'Homme machine*, La Mettrie pointed out just how easily Descartes could be transformed into a materialist. He credited Descartes with the development of the *l'homme machine* hypothesis, for by arguing that animals were machines Descartes had opened the way for the contention that both men and animals were machines. But this credit seems ironic, especially at the point in La Mettrie's argument where it appears. He has just explicitly claimed that muscular irritability defeats Cartesian dualism and argued for the complete comparability of men and animals and for motion as inherent to matter, two fundamentally anti-Cartesian perspectives. It is also possible that La Mettrie capitalized on the outrage of critics who fulminated against his radicalization of Descartes, exacerbating their fury by claiming in his later work, *Les Animaux plus que machines*, his materialist reading as the only possible understanding of Descartes. But it is important to see this as a polemical response that La Mettrie chose to employ only after *L'Homme machine* had been tarred as Cartesian by his critics. Furthermore, and most indicative of the possible irony behind La Mettrie's remark, his *l'homme machine* does not resemble Descartes's *bête machine*, and none of the explicit physiological evidence La Mettrie provides to establish his conception of human nature is taken from Descartes, nor could the evidence he provides be used to describe Descartes's animals. La Mettrie has also extended Descartes's arguments about how we know anything about other human beings to animals. Rather than making Descartes's beasts men, La Mettrie has negated both parts of Descartes's dualist categories; La Mettrie's men resemble neither Descartes's beasts nor Descartes's men.

If making Descartes into a materialist was the point of his title, it seems to have served him ill by obscuring the principal point of his treatise: the complete comparability of man and animals, which La Mettrie considered to be the most decisive evidence of materialism. Since he compared men and plants with a similar purpose in *L'Homme plante*, it must be wondered whether, his joke on Descartes aside, a better title for his work might not have been *L'Homme bête*.

One of the unfortunate ramifications of the view of La Mettrie as a Cartesian is the belief that there must have been a dramatic break between *L'Histoire naturelle de l'âme* and *L'Homme machine*, that La Mettrie had completely altered his philosophical allegiances, away from Locke, the acknowledged inspiration behind *L'Histoire naturelle de l'âme*, to Descartes, and thus repudiated the materialism of that earlier work.[25] Vartanian bases his contention that a decisive shift occurred not only on the presumed Cartesianism of *L'Homme machine* but also on the self-critical letter which La Mettrie attached to the 1747 edition of the *L'Histoire naturelle de l'âme*.[26] In that letter La Mettrie made fun of his need to resuscitate substantial forms. However, the letter to Mme. de Châtelet must be recognized as the ironic and problematic piece it is; it cannot reasonably be considered simply as a rejection of his earlier work. While he was particularly vehement in denouncing substantial forms, he also, with blatant irony, claimed that *faith* alone had kept him from acknowledging a distinctly human soul, the soul as the source of human character, and God as a principle of human activity.[27] First of all, it is scarcely credible that faith should keep one from these perfectly orthodox positions, and, second, these are positions that La Mettrie specifically rejected in *L'Histoire naturelle de l'âme* and continued to reject in *L'Homme machine*; the irony of much of his letter to Mme. de Châtelet is blatant.

Admittedly La Mettrie was much more comfortable with the kind of physiological basis for materialism that muscular irritability seemed to provide. However, the argument that a decisive break occurred in La Mettrie's philosophy completely neglects the many indications that La Mettrie himself considered the work essential to his corpus (he both criticized and praised himself as the author of *L'Histoire naturelle de l'âme* in subsequent writings)[28] and that self-criticism was a constant feature of his work.

Perhaps the most conclusive evidence of continuity is the fact that La Mettrie's later works on natural philosophy addressed the same issues he raised in *L'Histoire naturelle de l'âme*: a critique of metaphysics; the question of language; the relationship between men and animals; the question of the relationship between the way sensations are organized (the imagination) and that which senses (the physical constitution); and the constraints of the individual physical constitution and the degree to which it can be modified by education. La Mettrie even used the same case studies he added to *L'Histoire naturelle de l'âme* to argue his points in *L'Homme machine*.

If the traditional interpretation of La Mettrie as a Cartesian mechanist cannot be sustained in light of his explicit criticism of Descartes and his qualms about mechanism, how is *L'Homme machine* to be understood? If La Mettrie has not fundamentally altered his philosophical allegiances from Locke to Descartes, what is he about in this treatise?

Despite the moderate and engaging tenor of the work, which has led some interpreters to suggest that La Mettrie's adherence to materialism was not firm, *L'Homme machine* must be understood as a work which furthered his materialist agenda. With materialism as his basic philosophical position and Locke providing the most probable epistemology, La Mettrie expanded on the issues he had defined in *L'Histoire naturelle de l'âme* to deal specifically with critiques of materialism, especially from the natural law tradition, to examine the physiological and anthropological evidence for materialism, and, most important, to develop a notion of the physiological mechanism of muscular irritability, which he saw as providing an effective explanation of the self-moving powers of living creatures. He reworked issues raised in his earlier works and began to treat questions that would receive more attention in later works. Thus *L'Histoire naturelle de l'âme* was an important philosophical exercise for La Mettrie because it defined the essential position from which he never veered. Though he abandoned forever the metaphysical style of that work, he never rejected his materialism, reiterating throughout his works that to think philosophically was to think as a materialist.[29]

L'Homme machine continues La Mettrie's quest to understand the nature of man with arguments that are daring to the point of being deliberately inflammatory. His departure from the constraints of convention in both opinion and style is more than adequately announced by the dramatic change in form from *L'Histoire naturelle de l'âme*. Having denounced the format of metaphysical treatises and traditional questions about the nature of the soul that cluttered them, La Mettrie no longer felt constrained to argue within the confines of that tradition or to show respect for the stylistic conventions under which philosophical tracts were written.

La Mettrie wrote *L'Homme machine* with the zeal of a crusader. He took neither time nor care to construct a tightly woven and logical treatise. Instead he aimed at persuasion. If in elucidating an idea his attention was caught by another, stronger case, he would go on to it even if he never returned to his original point. As a result his style is frequently convoluted and confusing and seems to reflect a dialogue of the author with an enlightened reader who is conversant with the anecdote, the innuendo, the contemporary controversy. Vartanian has said of La Mettrie's style that "the text of *L'Homme machine* pours itself out with the garrulous ease of an improvised monologue unconstrained by any plan of exposition."[30] Another critic, less kind and more bemused, has suggested that La Mettrie must have been drunk or insane when he wrote many of his later works.[31] Though the bemusement deserves sympathy, the assessment is implausible; given the number of revised editions of his works that La Mettrie personally supervised, it seems improbable that La Mettrie would have been selectively drunk or insane during the repetition of murky passages. Furthermore, La Mettrie's style closely resembles that of eighteenth-century medical tracts, which deliberately eschew metaphysical subtleties and instead rely on the persuasive qualities of vivid case studies and are driven by polemical and reformist zeal. The medical character of La Mettrie's philosophy must be continuously reemphasized. In fact, one of the fundamental points of *L'Homme machine* is to argue the authority of the physician over the metaphysician and the theologian. As a physician, La Mettrie naturally considered case studies to be the most conclusive kind of evidence. He was less concerned with logic or the structure of his argument because truth was a matter of empirical demonstration. Even the authorities he invoked were medical rather than philosophical. In *L'Histoire naturelle de l'âme*, La Mettrie drew examples from his medical works to support the philosophical arguments he made. In *L'Homme machine*, the weight of medical evidence defined the arguments he made. In terms of structure, argument, and evidence, *L'Homme machine* seems to be an eighteenth-century medical text. La Mettrie used materialism as a means to bring to bear on the question of human nature the standards of evidence and the issues of contemporary medicine. In *L'Homme machine*, he specifically began to work toward a redefinition of the philosopher and to demonstrate the methodology and the concerns of the *médecin-philosophe*.

The Physiology of Human Nature

Although scholarly efforts to fit La Mettrie within the particular schema of the man-machine theory have distorted the understanding of this text, La Mettrie himself was quite forceful in laying out his initial premises. He explicitly utilized the criticism of the philosophical tradition which he had developed in *L'Histoire naturelle de l'âme*. He reasserted the failure of metaphysics as a way to knowledge and reiterated his chastisement of Locke, Leibniz, and Descartes for failing to adopt materialism. But in *L'Homme machine* his stance became combative, and he was more inclined to challenge overtly traditional philosophical positions, especially those of Christian theology.

La Mettrie's initial appeal to the authority of empirical evidence was deliberately inflammatory. He set traditional arguments about the relationship between reason and revelation within a materialist context. For example, he used a traditional topos of scientific reformers of the sixteenth and seventeenth centuries, the two-book theory of knowledge. This argument, asserted by Paracelsus, Bacon, and others who wished to turn education away from established texts and toward the observation of nature, contended that the Bible and nature were complementary sources of divine revelation. Science could then be considered as an attempt to understand God by a means more accessible to the layman. La Mettrie, who was neither hypocritical nor cautious, used the argument to support materialism, noting that "to distrust the knowledge we gain about bodies is to regard nature and revelation as contraries which destroy each other and to support the absurdity that God contradicts Himself in his diverse work with the intent to deceive us." Of course, his purpose was not to use nature to support theological contentions but to argue the primacy of the observable over the theological by claiming that the evidence of nature was our only hope for knowledge and that evidence could not logically be refuted by revelation, since both were presumably God's handiwork. In fact, he contended that nature must be used to understand revelation, for "by nature alone, one can discover the sense of the words of the Evangelist, of which experience alone is the true interpreter." Others, church fathers and contemporary theologians in particular, "have only muddled the truth." Furthermore, theologians produce works completely without merit; they argue endlessly about the soul, which they cannot know. La Mettrie wondered, "Isn't it ridiculous to let them decide without embarrassment on a subject [the soul] that they are not at all on the verge of knowing?" The teachings of the theologians could only be called prejudice, since they were not based on any attempt to understand the workings of the body; the theologians had turned their prejudices into fanatical systems.[32]

Having stripped the theologian of intellectual authority to interpret nature or even revelation, La Mettrie bestowed it on the physician's quest for truth.

Experience and observation would be our only guides. They are to be found in countless numbers in the records of physicians who have been philosophers and not in those of philosophers who have not been physicians. Those [the physician-philosophers] have run through and enlightened the labyrinth of man; they alone have revealed to us so many marvels. They alone tranquilly contemplate our soul. They have a thousand times surprised it in its grandeur and its misery without scorning it in one state or admiring it in the other. Once more it is only the physicians who have the right to speak here.[33]

This is perhaps La Mettrie's most radical statement about the extent and purpose of medical inquiry. In his satires and his own medical works, he argued for empiricism, repudiated medical systems, and completely denied the existence of occult qualities. His satires also attempted to establish a standard for medical education and practice that made it possible to see the enlightened physician as the most competent scientist and one whose results would be of immediate social utility. Such a model physician was the seeker of truth, the essence of the philosopher.

According to La Mettrie, the reason that the efforts of ancient and modern philosophers were of so little use in understanding the nature of man was that they employed an invalid method. "Man is a machine so composed that it is impossible to have a clear ideal at the outset and consequently to define it. That is why all the research that the greatest philosophers have done *a priori*, that is to say, by wishing to use wings of the spirit, has been in vain. Thus it is only *a posteriori*, that is, by trying to disentangle the soul in the organs of bodies that one can, I don't say discover the very nature of man, but attain the greatest degree of probability possible on this subject with this evidence."[34] This is essentially La Mettrie's philosophical manifesto. A priori investigations could only lead to idle speculation and never to useful knowledge. Empirical investigations, on the other hand, by their very nature provide men with information upon which they can act. La Mettrie claimed as his purpose to "start out to discover not what has been thought, but what must be thought for the sake of repose in life,"[35] a mission in keeping with the iconoclasm of his age and the new movement for Enlightenment, which explicitly redefined the appropriate area of human inquiry into narrower but more useful bounds.

La Mettrie pointed to another failure of metaphysics: since it was constructed on the basis of a priori arguments, metaphysics could not adequately come to terms with the diversity of human nature. La Mettrie had tried to redress this problem in *L'Histoire naturelle de l'âme* by emphasizing the importance of organization, physical constitution, and that which senses; his preoccupation with this issue grew out of his medical practice and reflected his indebtedness to Hippocratic medicine. "It is true that Melancholy, Bile, Phlegm, Blood, etc., according to the nature, abundance, and diverse combinations of these humors in each man, make a different man,"[36] he claimed, emphasizing the variation, the individual character of each human body. This crucial preoccupation decisively militates against La Mettrie's easily being considered as simply or even primarily a mechanist. In these initial pages, where he essentially defined the principles of his philosophical argument, La Mettrie emphasized this point. "There are as many different minds, different characters, and different customs, as there are different temperaments."[37]

In *L'Homme machine,* La Mettrie canvassed all the scientific issues of his day for empirical, and *eo ipso* legitimate, evidence for materialism. Evidence of this kind was not meant to define human nature or even to enable one to make predictions about human nature (La Mettrie's sense of the primacy of the individual would have precluded such predictions) but rather to establish that these physical characteristics had a decisive effect on human behavior and to demonstrate that all his evidence yielded no sign of an immortal soul.

La Mettrie then launched into an elaborate discussion of the physical basis of human behavior. He meant to demonstrate that the effects of the body on the soul are so striking that one cannot reasonably assume that a soul controls the body; thus one must ultimately conclude that the soul, if the term has any meaning, must be considered part of the body. He cited the many effects of disease on temperament, intelligence, and even normal demeanor because "in illness the soul is so eclipsed it gives no sign of itself." He described in vivid detail the effects of disease on the imagination, citing as an example those who imagine themselves to be vampires. Similarly, mental states like violent passions had disruptive effects on the body. He meant to drive home the inextricable relationship between the body and any characteristic or any kind of behavior one might consider indicative of a soul. Because there is no empirical evidence to the contrary, those characteristics must be material and mortal. For example, the soul and body fall asleep together, indicating, as La Mettrie put it, "the mechanical relationship between the relaxation of the soul and a slowing of the circulation."[38] The soul is also quite obviously affected by drugs and intoxication. Food seems to nourish both the body and the soul, or at least, "without food, the soul pines away, goes mad and dies exhausted." Food can also affect the disposition so far as to unseat moral notions. Englishmen, he notes, are particularly violent because they consume so much red meat.

This remark brings to the fore the way in which physiological conditions affect the ability of the individual to act in accord with moral prescriptions. According to La Mettrie, hunger could clearly carry one to cruel excess, and "pregnancy also produced depraved tastes; it sometimes makes the soul execute the most horrifying conspiracies, effects of a subtle mania which extinguishes everything, even natural law."[39] These physiological effects on moral behavior were ample evidence for La Mettrie to conclude that men could behave virtuously only when their bodies were working properly. He also brought to bear his notion of the temperaments, based loosely on Hippocratic temperaments and reinforced by Boerhaavian physiology (thus dependent on the interplay of solids and liquids). For example, women, because they have more liquids than men, have a more delicate temperament and are thus much more prone to disturbances of the passions, and so less educable. (Presumably liquids are less easy to control.) Men, on the other hand, because their brains and nerves are more solid than those of women, have more vigorous minds.[40] La Mettrie also pointed out the environmental factors which affect behavior. For example, "one nation is of heavy and stupid wit, and another quick, light and penetrating. Whence comes this difference, if not in part from the difference in foods and in inheritance?" Climate, too, affects behavior, as do the immediate circumstances in which one finds oneself; for example, stimulating companions will heighten one's own intellectual abilities.[41]

The interesting thing about this smorgasbord of explanations of human conduct is its nonmechanistic tenor. In his discussion of the physical roots of mental behavior, La Mettrie occasionally uses a mechanical analogy, referring to the springs of the soul, for example. But mechanics does not by any means provide the only, a sufficient, or even the most useful explanation of the functions of the human body. La Mettrie offered a great many physical factors that could help to explain human behavior. His explanation was mechanistic only insofar as it suggested that if X then Y—if certain conditions exist then certain physiological functions are likely to occur. For example, he referred to the mechanical relationship between relaxation and the slowing of the circulation. By "mechanical" he seems to have generally meant "automatic" or "habitual," that is, a predictable correlation. More crucial to his argument is the claim that all factors involved in human behavior are physical. Inherent to this discussion of human behavior is an implicit determinism, a position he developed much more clearly in his later works.

La Mettrie relied on comparative anatomy for the most conclusive evidence of the complete dependence of the soul on the body and the effects of this relationship. Specifically, he concluded from Willis's work in brain physiology that human brains and quadruped brains have the same form and functions. Though Willis himself did not draw materialist implications from his study of the human brain (he was instead concerned to determine the cerebral location of intelligence, sensation, motor, and emotive functions), he did lay the foundation for a comparative anatomy of the central nervous system. Thus he provided La Mettrie with fundamental evidence of man's essential similarity to animals and examples of the effects of physical states on mental states, specifically the way in which the condition of the brain affects behavior. From Willis's findings La Mettrie drew several conclusions about the correlation between the brain and behavior: that the fiercer the animal, the less brain matter it has; that the gentler the animal, the larger its brain is; and that the more intelligent the animal, the less instinct it has. This information about brain size and behavior had a possible practical use, for it might one day lead to an understanding and treatment of aberrant human behavior. La Mettrie suggested, for example, that insanity might be the result of diseased brain matter, that is, "offending viscera, lacking by virtue of a bad consistency, too soft, for example." Studies like Willis's on the structure of the brain and the different states of brain matter represented the best hope for ultimately understanding and treating these problems.[42]

The similarity between the size and structure of human and quadruped brains led La Mettrie to blur the one remaining crucial distinction between men and animals: speech. Language was, of course, a preoccupation of Enlightenment thinkers, but it was crucial to La Mettrie because it was the grounds on which Descartes had denied sensation to animals. As La Mettrie suggested, perhaps the ape might overcome this barrier to thoughtful communication if he were instructed in the sign language Joseph Amman had used successfully in teaching the deaf. In other words, if the physiological limitations of the vocal cords of animals could be circumvented, perhaps some animals could be educated to communicate meaningfully. La Mettrie wanted to impress on the reader that neither language, nor reason, nor any other ability traditionally considered distinctly human set man apart from the animals. "From animals to man the transition is not violent, the true philosophers concur. What was man before the invention of words and the understanding of language? An animal of his species who had much less natural instinct than other species of whom man did not believe himself to be king because he was distinguished from them only as the ape is now; I mean to say by a physiognomy which announced more discernment."[43] La Mettrie thus denigrated the acquisition of language as simply a mechanical or automatic correlation between the brain and the vocal cords that did not herald a vast intellectual accomplishment and certainly did not suggest a definitive break between man and animals. He described the production of language as relatively simple: "as a violin string or harpsichord key vibrates and gives forth sound, so the cerebral fibers, struck by waves of sound, are stimulated to render or repeat the words that strike them."[44] To those who might suggest that educability separates man from the animals, La Mettrie, instead of considering education as a great intellectual accomplishment, described it as comparable to mimicry. "Nothing is so simple, as one sees, as the mechanism of our education. Everything is reduced to the sounds or the words which pass from the mouth of one to the ear of the other in the brain which receives, at the same time through the eyes, the figure of the body of which these words are the arbitrary signs."[45] Thus the weight of the evidence La Mettrie presented substantiated the complete interdependence of mind and body, and he used that relationship to claim that there was no evidence of any forces at work in human beings beyond those attributable to matter and motion. In other words, thought could be attributed to matter.

Furthermore, La Mettrie argued that there was no philosophical reason to suppose that matter was not self-moving. In *L'Homme machine*, he provided a veritable catalog of scientific experiments which demonstrated that matter was able to move without any perceptible intervention of the soul. Such small detached bits of matter carried out this movement that it would be impossible to posit a location of a soul. For example, he noted that the flesh of all animals palpitated after death, separate muscles retracted when pricked, and the intestines exhibited peristaltic motion for a long time after being removed from the body. According to Cowper's experiments, an injection of cold water would reanimate the heart muscle. Bacon showed that the human heart continued to beat long after there was no other sign of life. Boyle and Stenon's experiments showed that even pieces of the heart continued to beat. La Mettrie himself saw that parts of spiders continued to move in hot water, and chickens continued to run after their heads were cut off. Last but perhaps most important to his natural philosophy, La Mettrie noted the case of Trembley's amazing regenerative polyp. Trembley's polyp reinforced the close link between plants and animals and was the crucial piece of evidence for the development of materialist theories of epigenesis by both La Mettrie and Diderot. However, the polyp played a central role in defining the problematic implications of scientific findings for orthodox belief, implications that concerned Trembley himself, Haller, and Bonnet, and that were all too gleefully exploited by La Mettrie. His *L'Homme machine* was the most obvious example of the way scientific findings could be used to erode conventional religious beliefs.[46]

Trembley's experiments were meant to provide the clinching argument to convince the reader in an incontestable manner that each small fiber or even each part of a fiber moved by a force that was proper to it and did not depend, as voluntary motion did, on nerve impulses or, as La Mettrie put it, the circulation of spirits.[47] Muscular irritability, then, was a completely physical phenomenon that provided evidence that life consisted of matter and motion. In these fibers that continued to move La Mettrie found no evidence of a soul.

La Mettrie was intent on incorporating the functioning of the brain into his description of the purely physical phenomena of living matter. He suggested that just as the leg had muscles, so it might reasonably be supposed that the brain did too. Though he admitted that he had no evidence for his conjecture, he said he found Borelli's biological experiments on muscular injection to be a much more satisfactory explanation of the reciprocity of mental and physical states than Leibniz's preestablished harmony or any other metaphysical account.[48] It was the physician, according to La Mettrie, who was best able to investigate questions like the mind/body problem; his evidence and experiments carried more weight than all the arguments of metaphysicians.

Furthermore, the physician alone, La Mettrie claimed, could attempt to give to man greater peace through his understanding of the interrelation of the mind and body. For example, if each element of the body was an oscillating fiber, then the purpose of medicine was to give force to fibers which were weakened or to prescribe a temperate regime to keep the fibers in harmony. Thus hopes for reform lay in the hands of the physician, who might alleviate the physical ills of patients. But La Mettrie suggested an even more important role for physicians when he said, "all ethics is fruitless for one who lacks his share of temperance."[49] Just as the physician might cure the intemperate by diets or regimens designed to give greater peace to the afflicted, so too might his understanding of human physiology make it possible for some individuals to live an ethical life because the reformer-physician could suggest ethical standards human beings could reasonably hope to attain despite their physical limitations. La Mettrie focused on the role of the physician in moral issues in his later treatises.

One aspect of La Mettrie's work which made his conclusions particularly influential was his assumption that physiological research applied *equally* to man and other animals. Because he staunchly maintained that man was as much a machine as any animal (or as little, given La Mettrie's notion of a machine), he claimed that muscular irritability could be applied to man. If man's "springs," as he put it, were slightly stronger, that was no reason to consider him essentially different or to assert the existence of an immaterial soul. Perhaps, he suggested, some purely physical part of the brain acted as its main spring. But in any case, La Mettrie maintained that the forces of life should be discussed in purely physiological terms. For example, nutrition provided a particularly useful analogy for understanding life processes. (It should be noted that La Mettrie had pointed out that mechanism was particularly inadequate for discussing the process of nutrition, despite the fact that he here indicates its importance by invoking analogies that are at least loosely mechanical.) The body was but a watch whose maker was new chyle (food). This new chyle provoked a fever that "produced a great filtration of spirits that mechanically animate the muscles and the heart, as if they had been sent these by order of the will."[50] While he would not speculate on the requisite balance of solids to fluids for good health, La Mettrie nonetheless asserted that this balance assured health and ultimately life itself. While he could not explain how the brain controlled this process, he was intent on refuting Stahl's contention that an immaterial soul, active through the will, directed all movement by facetiously suggesting that Stahl was unique, not constituted in the same way as ordinary mortals.

More seriously, he noted the contortions into which Boerhaave was forced because he did not recognize the existence of irritability and again remarked on his own difficulties in resorting to substantial forms in *L'Histoire naturelle de l'âme*. He chided Willis and Perrault[51] for having supposed that the human soul extended over the entire body; any attempt to insert a soul into physiology simply made physiology needlessly convoluted.

This type of discussion is quite indicative of La Mettrie's method. Although discussing human motivation in entirely physiological terms, he did not assume that he had arrived at the definitive understanding or that sufficient information was in fact available. Instead he indicated the sorts of possibilities that were open if one dismissed the soul. His speculations were neither well developed nor presented as definitive arguments. Instead they were meant to refute established opinion, and, to that end, other possibilities needed only to be suggested, not substantiated.

Muscular irritability, then, was particularly attractive to La Mettrie as the most conclusive evidence to be marshalled against those who refused to admit that matter was capable of self-movement, in particular the Cartesians, Malebranchists, and Stahlians; for La Mettrie, irritability decisively demonstrated self-movement. With the same kind of equivocation which allowed him to conflate metaphysical terms in order to discount them, La Mettrie was able to build an argument based on irritability. He suggested that it is a form of sensation or feeling, that the step from sensation to reason is a short one, and that reason is simply a particular, developed form of feeling.[52] The conflation of these terms was legitimate in La Mettrie's opinion because the feeling soul was clearly physical, and the dependence of the thinking soul on the feeling soul could be demonstrated by physiological evidence such as the fact that in apoplexy, lethargy, and other disorders the soul ceased to think. But despite the probability and the utility of the evidence provided by physiology, La Mettrie did not make it the basis for claims to certainty. "As to the development of feeling and motion, it is absurd to waste time seeking for its mechanism. The nature of motion is as unknown to us as that of matter. How can we discover how it is produced unless, like the author of the History of the Soul [La Mettrie himself] we resuscitate the old and unintelligible doctrine of substantial forms?"[53]

The basic argument of *L'Histoire naturelle de l'âme* stands, but La Mettrie changed his approach to it and the evidence needed to support it. Because muscular irritability provided evidence for the argument that motion was inherent to matter, La Mettrie claimed that metaphysical arguments for materialism had been made obsolete by biological and physiological evidence. That evidence convinced him that organic matter was endowed with a principle of motion that alone differentiated it from inorganic matter, and man was simply a particularly complex configuration of matter.

La Mettrie had carried out the agenda he set for himself. Instead of arguing against other metaphysicians to support materialism, as he had in *L'Histoire naturelle de l'âme*, he presented physiological and medical evidence for materialism. He did not develop a systematic philosophy of nature or argue a coherent metaphysical position. Interested in challenging conventional ways of thinking and the claims that metaphysicians and theologians have made to truth, his task was one of destruction rather than construction. As a result the method and logic of his argument were far less important than the effect. La Mettrie quite deliberately took evidence from anywhere—case studies, isolated bits of scientific information, personal testimony, and experiments. His most compelling evidence was case studies that were either vested with the authority of the physician or familiar to his readers. Both kinds of examples were invoked in order to expose the radical challenges to established authority implicit in familiar scientific findings and cases. (This radical use of the familiar or the nearly conventional might help to explain the vehemence with which this work was received.)

L'Homme machine is freewheeling in style, organization, and argument, in part because La Mettrie was writing in a style quite common to eighteenth-century medical texts. He based his argument on case studies of patients because, for La Mettrie, the aberrant or the sick were the most revealing examples to use in discussing the normal and the well. The best evidence for materialism came from comparative anatomy, which was also the most reliable evidence for the physician. La Mettrie was willing to set forth his arguments according to the standard of eighteenth-century medicine, that is, a welter of case studies, suggesting but not confirming, tantalizing but never conclusive, and ultimately content with the possibilities offered rather than insisting on metaphysical certainty.

La Mettrie then turned his attention to one of the key areas where the authority of the metaphysician or the theologian had traditionally prevailed over that of the physician: ethics.

Working toward Moral Arguments

Although La Mettrie's philosophical works are most often considered as disparate and unconnected works, he often raised questions in one work which he later treated more thoroughly. His investigations into the workings of nature broadened his attack on established authorities and provoked questions about the basis of our moral notions by claiming that moral notions, like mental activities, must also be correlated to physiology. According to La Mettrie, the activities and abilities of the individual, especially his moral propensities, were largely dependent on the state of his physical "machine." To consider these moral qualities as constitutionally determined rather than acquired by human endeavor did not, according to La Mettrie, disparage them but rather made them analogous to qualities like physical beauty; "gifts of nature we do not scorn, but neither should we give undue credit to the individual who possesses these qualities."[54]

La Mettrie also refuted arguments that could be made against his treatment of man as the prototypic animal. He realized that the most substantial opposition would come from those arguing within the natural law tradition, a tradition whose principal tenet he took to be that "there is, one says, in man a natural law, a knowledge of good and evil, which has not been engraved in the hearts of animals." La Mettrie scrutinized this commonly held idea, querying, "Is there any way of knowing that only man has been enlightened by this gift? If we deny this enlightenment to animals on the basis that we do not know what goes on inside of them, can we make any better claim to understand other men?"[55] La Mettrie also ironically inverted Descartes's argument on the nature of remorse, using it as an attack on a distinctively human sense of natural law. "We know what we think and that we have remorse, a sentiment which compels us too much to deny it, but to judge the remorse of another, this sentiment which is in us is sufficient; that is why it is necessary to believe their word on the basis of the sensible and exterior signs we have noticed in ourselves, when we experience the same stricken conscience and torments."[56]

La Mettrie used the very argument Descartes had to extend feelings to other humans (although Descartes, of course, did not and would not extend the argument to animals) to claim that we are as able to determine that animals feel remorse as other humans do. In other words, all we have in either case is outward manifestations of remorse. Thus, since animals showed signs of remorse upon offending a master, the emotion could not be denied to animals. To the possible objection that animals were violent and therefore could not be compared to humans in moral terms, La Mettrie pointed to the role of warfare in human history as a more than adequate indication of the human propensity to violence. Nor was human violence confined to group actions. La Mettrie noted the cases of human cannibalism committed without remorse. Humans, like animals, were unequal in their ability to discern good and evil; nature and environment were the determining factors for both animals and men for how ferocious the one was or how well the other could distinguish between good and evil. Because nature distributed this quality unequally, La Mettrie suggested that this sensitivity could be completely eroded by such environmental factors as bad companions and that, in general, "custom dulls, blunts, and perhaps extinguishes remorse." Thus, La Mettrie insisted, even moral notions support his argument that men and animals are completely comparable, or, as he put it, "nature has employed one and the same dough of which she has only varied the yeast."[57] This variety of yeasts occasionally produced human beings and animals who felt absolutely no remorse despite having committed unspeakable atrocities—a characteristic which unfortunately could be inherited. Because of the physiological basis of moral behavior, La Mettrie argued for tolerance and a reassessment of the stringency of the penal code. "I realize all that the interests of society demand. But it is no doubt to be wished that there would only be as judges excellent physicians. They alone could distinguish the innocent criminal from the guilty one. If reason is the slave of a sense which is depraved or in fury, how can one control it?"[58]

La Mettrie also questioned how his understanding of the operations of nature affected belief in God, by claiming at the outset that there could never be conclusive evidence on the question of whether or not God exists. His own description of human nature, with his extensive comparison between men and animals and his denial of the existence of the immortal soul, did not refute the existence of a supreme being. But even though he recognized that the question was unresolvable and though he found Diderot's deistic arguments in the *Pensées philosophiques*[59] to be very strong, he nonetheless had several reasons to favor atheism. First, he found no evidence that a belief in God contributed to virtue in men. In fact, he personally believed atheists were more likely to be virtuous. Second, he saw no reason to claim that the design in nature required a supreme being who created and orchestrated this design. He suggested nature itself as responsible for design much in the same way Diderot later suggested in *D'Alembert's Dream*.[60] Finally, he claimed that the findings of naturalists could be considered self-evident arguments for the existence of God only for the convinced antipyrrhonist. Those same findings were more likely, according to La Mettrie, to "suggest that the motion that keeps the world going could have created it, that each body has taken the place assigned to it by its own nature."[61]

La Mettrie found no evidence that there was a God who had endowed his creatures with a natural law or that any God-given attribute separated man from animals. Nevertheless, he maintained that even if man could be demonstrated to have an innate characteristic like natural law, that would not call into question his argument that man was a machine. "A few more wheels, a few more springs than the most perfect animals, the brain proportionally nearer the heart and for this reason receiving more blood—any one of a number of unknown causes might always produce this delicate conscience so easily wounded."[62] Thus, according to La Mettrie, it was not necessary to conceive of anything beyond the principle of motion to explain all human actions or attributes "in the physical realm, or the moral realm which depends upon it."[63] Such forthright expressions of atheism, unfiltered by fictitious forms, were not common in the eighteenth century, and religious opinion, especially in German clerical circles, was mobilized against La Mettrie.[64]

La Mettrie's application of medicine to philosophy enabled him to endow the physician with a moral role. Just as metaphysics must give way to science, so the physician must replace the philosopher as the seeker of truth, since he looks to nature as the source of knowledge. The physician might also play a crucial role in society. Because the behavior of the individual is largely dependent on his physical constitution, he might be able to prescribe diets or regimens which would rectify physiological imbalances. He might also be able to identify and excise diseased brain matter, an operation that would presumably eliminate or ameliorate aberrant behavior. Perhaps physicians should serve as judges, La Mettrie suggested, since they might be able to determine to what degree the criminal committed his crime because of a defective constitution. Since human beings are completely physical, the physician must assume a role as a crucial agent of social reform.

Though La Mettrie shifted the ground of his philosophical position from the metaphysical argument of L'Histoire naturelle de l'âme to the scientific evidence of L'Homme machine, he continued to provide evidence for materialism. Having argued this position by comparing l'homme and bête, he then extended his materialism to all creatures and compared man to the lowest forms of life in L'Homme plante. Having used medicine and physiology to put man in nature, he then explored nature itself. But it is important to note that La Mettrie's investigation of nature is not sentimental or romanticized; it is instead directed to challenging the conventional.

The Great Chain of Being

La Mettrie challenged the traditional understanding of nature as a great chain of being and the most prominent figure associated with the argument, Blaise Pascal. La Mettrie used the concept to connect man to nature. He set man and plants at opposite ends of a spectrum through which to examine the workings of nature. Since the same degree of difference separates all the creatures on this plane, a dramatic break in the spectrum is inconceivable; or, as La Mettrie adamantly declared, "rien n'y tranche." The continuity of the great chain of being specifically precluded the possibility of a break which would allow the infusion or addition of a human soul separating man from his fellow creatures. La Mettrie ruled out any such distinction, saying that "man believes himself to be a God on earth but he is made of mud like all the others." But despite his comparability with animals, man is filled with amour-propre, an attitude which provoked La Mettrie's astonishment. "There is no animal so puny, so vile in appearance, the sight of which diminishes the self-esteem of a philosopher." If mere chance, according to La Mettrie, placed man at the head of the spectrum, man must keep in mind that a little less brain matter would precipitate him down the scale![65]

La Mettrie's reworking of the concept of the great chain of being was typical of the eighteenth-century formulation in that he placed man at the apogee instead of the middle of the chain, whereas in earlier formulations of the chain man was as far from God as from the simplest creatures. La Mettrie explicitly used the chain to reduce man's sense of his own self-importance. (As Lovejoy points out, the continuity of the chain implies that the other links [creatures] were not made to serve one [man].)[66] But La Mettrie's depiction of the chain was also more radical because he was intent on reducing the length of the chain, claiming that the distance between man and the lowest creatures was only a reflection of degrees of organization and that the distance between man and the animal next to him on the chain was minimal.

La Mettrie developed the radical implications of his recasting of the chain. In keeping with the ironic way he used other thinkers (for example, Aristotle and Descartes), La Mettrie took his notion of man's place on the chain and cast it in Pascal's terms in order to subvert Pascal's moral dilemma and the Christian view of man. For Pascal and many other seventeenth-century thinkers, man's place on the chain of being, midway between God and the lowest creature, was the source of man's greatest glory and misery. It made man an anxious creature, an uncomfortable muddle of soul and body. La Mettrie, however, concluded that man's place at the summit simply entailed a greater degree of complexity tied to greater needs and more animal spirits. Using Pascal's very words, he claimed that this position was the source of our "greatest misery and our greatest happiness."[67] Instead of casting the dilemma forced by his position in moral or religious terms, as Pascal had, La Mettrie saw it simply as a burden imposed by our greater organization. Furthermore, La Mettrie tied the soul to the constitution and made it simply the name given to our ability to satisfy our needs. "Certainly if our needs, as one can not doubt, are a necessary consequence of the structure of our organs, it is no less evident that our soul depends immediately on our needs, which it is so alert to satisfy and to anticipate so that nothing comes before them."[68]

Thus, according to La Mettrie, man's soul is an empty term by which we explain man's ability to fulfill needs occasioned by his greater brain matter. This merely quantitative difference in the amount of brain matter produces the greater degree of organization men exhibit. But because this need-fulfilling soul is the result of a purely quantitative distinction, La Mettrie claims that comparisons between man and animals are completely legitimate. For example, comparative anatomy has shown us that the monkeys resemble us, but even the "most spiritual" among monkeys is not skilled in self-instruction as man is. Even though animals never attain the "preeminence of our soul," they are certainly, La Mettrie contended, "de la même pâte et la même fabrique."[69]

To draw together the links of the chain, La Mettrie also articulated some of his fundamental perspectives on nature itself, particularly how nature ought to be investigated. First of all, La Mettrie was unconstrained in his investigations of nature. His use of the man-plant analogy was fruitful because he used it in an uninhibited manner; he was willing to entertain comparisons between human beings and other creatures which bordered on the outrageous and were not flattering to humans. He was neither averse to applying what he learned about man to creatures further down the chain of being nor unwilling to apply to man what he learned from a rather perfunctory observation of nature. For example, in likening the sexual functions of human beings to those of plants, La Mettrie meant to bring all aspects of human behavior into the realm of scientific discussion and experimentation.[70] Specifically, he suggested that since the sperm from men who are very young or very thin are not fertile, it might be useful to study sperm as a good reflection of the health of the man.[71]

According to La Mettrie, the analogies he drew and the whole notion of the great chain of being underscored the similarities between men and animals. He was not unaware of the differences but claimed that these are simply particular, specific details which did not interest him, as he was concerned to investigate nature or the general. This purpose, which dominates La Mettrie's biological or scientific work, has much to say both about his methodology and the scholarly neglect of any scientific import his work might have had. He characterized detailed studies of the scientific differences between man and animals this way. "They overburden us without increasing our knowledge, and besides these facts are to be found in the books of indefatigable observers."[72] La Mettrie claimed to find it incomprehensible that one could spend one's life studying insects; particulars were of interest to him only if they led to general hypotheses that would provide useful information. La Mettrie was clearly out of sympathy with the prominent naturalists of the eighteenth century like Réaumur and Linnaeus—a distaste also reflected in his scorn for medical nosology.[73] However, he acknowledged that this kind of general investigation is problematic and limited, inserting his characteristically skeptical caveat: one must exercise caution, using analogy only insofar as nature herself does; one must base all of one's conclusions on what is clearly observable and not flatter oneself that all is known because nature reveals a pattern. After all, La Mettrie warned, nature sometimes deviates (*s'écarte*) from her favorite laws.[74]

This occasional capriciousness of nature suggests much about La Mettrie's view of nature. He was, first of all, not a complete skeptic. There was for him a clear purpose in observation, experimentation, and other scientific methods. But underlying his arguments for empiricism was the sense that any certainty that men claim may well be completely illusory. First causes are unknowable; the senses provide us with the only knowledge that is possible, but it is only probable; ultimately even our notions of causation may be merely conventional. Even more than Hume, La Mettrie recognized those limits of human knowledge, yet he accepted them gracefully, contending forcefully that one must nonetheless avidly pursue the only possible avenue to knowledge, experimentation. This modest appraisal of what we can claim to know seems to color La Mettrie's sense of nature as well. Observation and experimentation may lead to as complete an understanding of nature as is possible, or our extrapolations of patterns and so forth from experiments may have some basis in fact. But despite these positive possibilities, nature may deviate from her favorite laws.

Further complicating this problematic view of nature is the personification of nature that La Mettrie is willing to accept when it fits his argument; at times he accepts as a given that nature is reasonable, rationally ordered, purposeful, and acts with economy and a sense of the appropriate. At certain points in his philosophical works, he even seems to subscribe to his own version of the classic argument from design, the design reflecting nature rather than God. For example, he employed a secular argument from design to explain the principle behind the variety of organizations of matter. Because nature is meet, just, and well ordered, the more organized a body is, the more needs it has, and the more means nature has given to that body to satisfy them. "The fewer necessities an organized body has, the easier it is to nourish and raise this body, the more its share of intelligence is slight." This intelligence, called instinct in animals and soul in man, has been, according to La Mettrie, wisely apportioned by nature according to the need her creatures have of it. This apportionment has occurred with some justice. For example, plants have no capacity for joy, but neither do they suffer.[75] Nonetheless, since this fundamental order can be disrupted by nature's whim, system building, claims to certainty, and even the incautious or inclusive use of analogy must be resisted.

The Possibility of Transformism

In *Le Système d'Épicure*, an intriguing and suggestive work, La Mettrie argued that transformism was completely probable, a probability he based on his own investigations and hypotheses about the workings of nature. This work is rarely considered important in the history of the development of evolutionary theory, even in discussions of eighteenth-century contributions, in part because the impact of La Mettrie's theory is diminished by his own treatment of the issues he raised. Aram Vartanian has been in the forefront in arguing La Mettrie's critical importance to the development of transformism.[76] But his interpretation has provoked a great deal of opposition. There are those like Bentley Glass[77] who argue that Maupertuis must be given greater credit. However, Vartanian argues in response that only the 1751 edition of Maupertuis's *Vénus physique*, not the 1745 edition, is transformist, and thus Maupertuis must have been strongly influenced by works on this theme written between 1747 and 1750, the most striking examples of which were La Mettrie's.[78] Others, most notably Jacques Roger,[79] deny any significance to La Mettrie by claiming that his work is simply a rehash of Épicureanism. Lester Crocker[80] also denies La Mettrie a role in the development of evolutionary theory. He points out that there are only inklings of transformism in *Le Système d'Épicure* (which was much more developed by Diderot in his *Pensées sur l'interprétation de la nature*[81] four years later). There are clearly legitimate arguments on both sides of the question of La Mettrie's contribution to evolution, especially insofar as the quest is for the roots of Darwinism. But perhaps a more relevant question for discussing this text is: what was La Mettrie's reason for raising the possibility of transformism? In other words, how did it serve his philosophical, medical, and reformist concerns? And what use was he making of this idea?

In his previous philosophical works, La Mettrie had argued against metaphysical systems as major stumbling blocks in the way of accepting a more naturalistic and materialistic assessment of the operations of nature and the nature of man. Out of his conviction of the uniformity and interconnectedness of nature La Mettrie developed a notion that transformism was indeed probable. In *Le Système d'Épicure*, he investigated the implications of his understanding of the workings of nature and human nature at the extremes of the natural spectrum, in the original elemental mud and in human reason.

La Mettrie warned his reader that he was venturing into subjects that could be addressed only speculatively. But even if epistemological modesty can be seen as a characteristic response in the post-Lockean world of the eighteenth century, La Mettrie's epistemological modesty seems far more thoroughgoing than was typical. His skepticism extends beyond first causes to our notions of causation, to whether we can possibly have an understanding of the workings of things that is any more than probable. He thus cast into doubt both the certainty of scientific inquiry and the utility of the social and political reforms of philosophes that were predicated on an understanding of man produced by science. Ultimately he cast doubt on the possibility of a foundational scientific principle that could then be applied to society. Furthermore, he claimed, even if certainty were possible, it would make men neither better nor happier.

Having made these daunting remarks as a preface, La Mettrie nonetheless did not hesitate to speculate. He had, after all, investigated some analogies which he found very persuasive, analogies that, despite his usual diatribes against system makers, convinced him of the essential uniformity and simplicity of nature, at least for the purposes of argument. Although in his other works La Mettrie certainly emphasized the discontinuities and the complexities, here he presumes a uniformity in order to radicalize naturalism. The presumed simplicity of nature leads him to assert blithely, "A bit of mud, a drop of mucus forms man and insect; the most infinitesimally small portion of movement would have sufficed to set the machine of the world in motion." Taking as a given this presumed simplicity and uniformity, La Mettrie goes on to speculate about the origins of the world. But in keeping with both his fundamental skepticism and his fervent desire to convince his reader of the plausibility of transformism, the tone of his remarks wavers between tentative suggestion and dogmatic assertion. Admitting that it is impossible to explain the origin of the world, and conceding therefore that any theory must be acknowledged as simply "une conjecture aussi hardie," La Mettrie expresses a thorough conviction that the world has evolved. He regards as extremely naïve and unthinking those who think that the world had always been as it was. "Indeed! to believe that they came into the world large, as fathers and mothers, and ready to create offspring." He instead found it much more reasonable to suppose that "men have not always existed, at least not as we see them today."[82]

Lester Crocker has isolated four philosophical positions which served to inhibit the development of evolutionary theories in the eighteenth century: the sense of man as distinct from nature, the dualist theory of mind and matter as two different sorts of things, the preeminence of the Newtonian world view, which tended to view nature as geometric, and the preeminence of the argument from design, which saw every creature as aptly created to fill some niche established by God. (A corollary of this theory was that all other creatures were created to serve man.)[83] La Mettrie was a significant figure in undermining these conventional ways of thinking even if he did not construct a new, full-blown theory of evolution. In *L'Histoire naturelle de l'âme* he claimed that mind was simply a particular organization of matter, and in *L'Homme machine* he emphasized man's integration into nature. His view of nature was if anything anti-Newtonian; in his medical works he contended that attempts to apply Newtonian geometry to nature were at best counterproductive and at worst completely frivolous. His own investigations into the nature of matter favored a dynamic, organic theory of matter. La Mettrie's speculations were completely unfettered by theological considerations, and he consciously sought to disassociate them from the argument from design (although, as previously noted, on occasion he invoked a *secular* argument from design). Thus completely uninhibited by any of these philosophical impediments, La Mettrie argued the probability of transformism. The notion of scientific method he developed in *L'Homme machine* also seems particularly conducive to transformism. He saw nature as generally rational yet occasionally idiosyncratic, and he was inclined to advance speculations that were loosely grounded in biology or physiology in his quest to understand nature at the general level.

These methodological considerations, which also characterize the work of other eighteenth-century figures such as Diderot and Maupertuis, has impeded recognition of their roles as precursors of Darwinian evolution; they simply do not seem guided by the same standards of scientific method as Darwin. Their method also inhibited a complete development of the theory of evolution. For example, although La Mettrie suggested the transformation of species and the notion that species develop and degenerate, he did not articulate a mechanism of evolution, nor did he have a definition of species. There are also key differences between the method and tone of this work and Darwin's. La Mettrie suffered no qualms of conscience about how his theory would affect belief in the biblical creation account. He also had no interest whatsoever in the collection and analysis of minutiae; in other words, he had not at all the character of the natural scientist. However, being virtually unconcerned with specific data, he was much more willing than Darwin to speculate on the origins of the universe. These characteristics give La Mettrie's work the aspect of a free-flowing speculation rather than that of a well-constructed biological theory.

La Mettrie deliberately challenged the notion of the original perfection of the universe and instead posited an initial development of all creatures from some sort of elemental mud. With that underlying assumption, he proposed that the relationship of nature to its creatures might well provide the key to recognizing a relationship that prevailed throughout nature and that might then explain transformism. To wit, he suggested that the earth nourished its creatures in the same way that the sexual organs of men and women cultivate "les germes humaines."[84] Since he assumed that men were not always as they are now, he considered it most probable that the earth itself acted as the uterus for human seeds which would have contained in themselves the seeds of man's evolution into the creature at the apogee of creation. In keeping with his elaborate plant-man comparison, La Mettrie thought that because nature had acted as host to so many plants there was no reason to suppose that it would not also nourish man. The fact that nature no longer performed that function for man, he suggested, was due to the age of the earth (menopausal) and the tendency of nature to evolve towards greater perfection, which would entail at the very least the ability of creatures to self-perpetuate.

La Mettrie postulated an account that he said was taken from Benoît de Maillet's *Telliamed*[85] and is close to that of Lucretius.[86] The earth was once covered with water, in which all existing creatures floated; the sea was eventually evaporated by the sun and absorbed by the earth; the human egg which floated in the sea was deposited on a bank where the incubation of the sun hatched it. Although it was likely in his view that these early creatures were much less perfect than we, these differences were not enough to deny our relationship to them or to disbar man from the evolutionary process.

La Mettrie further claimed that it is not inconceivable that this human fetus hatched on the bank of a river could have survived. It could perhaps have nourished itself from the earth, as the works of ancient historians and naturalists suggest. He also subscribed to the view, later popularized by Rousseau, that the physical capabilities of modern man had degenerated, "enervated by infinite succession of soft and delicate generations."[87] So our own lack of ability to survive adverse conditions cannot be taken as indicative of the adaptability of these first humans. Although La Mettrie did not develop this idea, it seems to suggest the notion of degeneration of species. He also claimed that these initial creatures, being more like animals than we are, probably had much more highly developed instincts. He therefore considered it possible that other animals might well have raised, protected, and even nursed these primitive humans. (He cited as perfectly credible the case of bears in Poland raising an infant.) Though he recognized the great difficulties involved in surviving under such adverse conditions, he also noted that the continuation of the development of the human species would have taken only the survival of two of these primitive humans. Thus the process of transformism was very slow, impeded by the large numbers of imperfect creatures who lacked the organs necessary to survive and reproduce. La Mettrie cited contemporary case studies of men and women with malformed genitalia who were therefore unable to reproduce. These he saw as throwbacks to earlier generations, to a remote time when "the generations were uncertain, difficult, and ill-established, and were more attempts than the works of masters."[88] Thus, according to La Mettrie, the most important evolutionary adaptation was that which endowed some creatures with the capacity to reproduce themselves.

This series of remarks about the possible manner of evolution is sometimes used to deny that La Mettrie advanced a theory of transformism and to suggest instead that La Mettrie was simply trying to resolve the problem of monsters, which preoccupied so many eighteenth-century naturalists.[89]

There is some basis for this interpretation in that La Mettrie was not explicit on certain points (though that is in part simply the product of the aphoristic style in which *Le Système d'Épicure* was written). However, this argument neglects what would seem to be the crucial link to transformism. La Mettrie tied man's evolution through an infinity of combinations of matter to the equally long, drawn-out series of fortuitous combinations that were necessary to establish a perfection of generations. La Mettrie was not simply concerned with the eventual production of the "perfect" individual or man developed to his present state, a restricted notion of "evolution" that might indeed simply involve the trial-and-error method of production, where the efforts of nature could be compared to the throw of the dice. But La Mettrie also noted that, even after human beings had acquired the ability to reproduce, an infinity of combinations occurred before man came into being in his present state. Thus, man's development across many generations was analogous to the long chain of combinations necessary for the development of the eye from a bit of light-sensitive tissue or the ear from a bit of sound-sensitive tissue.

What is clear is that La Mettrie was using these brief but suggestive remarks not to develop an evolutionary theory but rather to challenge the way men thought about themselves by using the

information at his disposal to point out and overcome the prejudices that kept man from acknowledging that he too is part of
nature, of its processes and transformations. First of all, according
to La Mettrie, man must change his attitude toward nature. He
must strip it of occult overtones and mysticism. He must not rever-
entially back away from a close examination of the unfolding of
God's plan but instead simply recognize that "things make themselves, as sight or hearing are lost and recovered, as some bodies
come to reflect light or sound. More artifice was not required in the
construction of the eye or ear than in the making of an echo."[90] If we
are able to think of nature's creatures as analogs to machines or as
random composites of elemental mud, we will be able both to
banish metaphysical and religious considerations from our science
and to deal more realistically with the complexity of nature. We
might then, La Mettrie suggests, be able to conduct more fruitful
scientific research.

La Mettrie also considered it absurd to postulate a special creation or unique process for the creation of intellectual ability. Reason, he claimed, was neither more remarkable than any number of
other natural creations, nor did it qualitatively separate man from
animals. Reason only helped man to compensate for his lack of
other important instincts for survival. In fact, a comparison between animals and men raised by animals revealed that "he [the
man] is more stupid than any animal but most fortunately organized so as to have memory and to be educable. Without the cultivation of this faculty, man would be an animal like any other."[91] La
Mettrie deflated pride in human reason as unwarranted; he noted
that man is a creature so feeble in strength that he can be destroyed
by a great many creatures. Although he purports to be an intelligent
creature, he is still often ruled by superstition. Furthermore, intelligence can easily be undermined, by drink or fever, for example. In
fact, La Mettrie argued that reason is no more and no less than
another spring in the machinery. "It is a spring that breaks down
like any other, even more easily." Thus La Mettrie argued that only
"nos seuls usages," or our customary ways of thinking, prevent us
from recognizing the plausibility of transformism. In keeping with
the spirit of the Enlightenment, La Mettrie clearly contended that
conventional ideas are meant to be challenged.

Le Système d'Épicure indeed challenged the way men thought

about themselves. Having stripped away some of the basic premises on which man constructed his sense of his special place in creation—his immortal soul, his rationality, and so forth—La Mettrie contested the creation account. Man became simply a part of natural processes, developing like all other natural creatures from an elemental mud. If La Mettrie's remarks on the nature of this process are often considered too speculative, too detached from observation, and too deliberately inflammatory—in a word, too unscientific to be considered essential to the development of evolutionary theory—they nonetheless combined several concepts that were crucial to its emergence: matter endowed with self-determining powers; the great chain of being, implying continuity in nature; and transformism. Thus, as part of his critical appraisal of conventional ways of thinking about human beings, La Mettrie also refuted crucial ideas impeding the development of a theory of evolution.

La Mettrie's three works on nature reveal his concerted efforts to find empirical evidence for materialism. He supported his sensationalist account of mental processes with the findings of contemporary physiological experiments. With his materialist theory of man substantiated by physiological experiments, La Mettrie was then able to compare man to animals, despite the damage that comparison would do to man's *amour-propre* and conventional notions of man's place in the universe. Man could be fruitfully compared to the lowest creatures and placed in the context of the unfolding of matter and motion in an evolutionary process. His materialist notion of man and his place in nature were the foundation for his subsequent philosophical works, which examine the implications of materialism for moral systems and for the individual in society.

As for the question of understanding La Mettrie's works, especially *L'Homme machine*, it is important to recognize what La Mettrie did not do. He did not endorse a mechanistic philosophy or present a mechanical explanation of the body or of life processes. He did, however, undercut conventional ideas such as the great chain of being, and he used thinkers like Lucretius in particularly subversive ways. Moreover, La Mettrie invoked the evidence of physiology to refute the notion that man occupied a privileged position in nature by virtue of his soul and his reason. La Mettrie's works investigating nature transferred authority from interested, partial, prejudiced theologians and metaphysicians to physicians, who are assumed to be disinterested, public-spirited, and nonprejudiced. His empowerment of the physician, whose physiological understanding of human beings was the most sound and the most likely to yield productive results, was supported, as far as La Mettrie was concerned, by the close connection he drew between the physical and the mental. He also produced a new understanding of knowledge as nonsystematic, noncautious, and unconstrained by standards of orthodoxy, bound instead by empirical standards. He then explored the connection between the physical and the moral.

8

Moral Theory in Medical Terms

Dissolute, impudent, a buffoon, a flatterer; made for life at court and the favor of nobles. He [La Mettrie] died as he should have, victim of his own intemperance and his folly. He killed himself by ignorance of the art he professed.
> —Denis Diderot, "Essai sur le règne de Claude et Néron"[1]

La Mettrie undermined the distinctiveness of human beings and questioned whether any aspect of human behavior could reasonably be assumed to be distinct from physiology by consistently emphasizing the physiological sources and causes of complex human behavior and by reenforcing the correlations between human behavior and the actions of animals. Because he considered man to be a slightly more complicated animal (but also one whose instinct had declined as his intelligence increased), and because he considered human behavior to be largely dependent on the nature of the individual constitution, La Mettrie raised serious questions about moral systems, questions he explored in detail and without concessions to orthodox sensibilities. As a result he was denounced by enemies and even by those, like Diderot, who were indebted to him. La Mettrie has generally been known as a purveyor of scandalous ideas.[2] The philosophes denounced him because, in addition to provoking their fears of repression by civil and ecclesiastical authorities, he exposed some of the pitfalls of their reform programs and some of the perils of constructing a secular morality. La Mettrie has also served as a useful scapegoat at the hands of certain modern historians for the demise of classical and Christian moral values. Their arguments presume that the mere criticism of those traditions inevitably produced the horrors of the modern age.[3]

Because his contemporaries, both philosophe and antiphilosophe,[4] bandied about the most outrageous statements contained in the *Discours sur le bonheur*,[5] La Mettrie has been considered amoral, antisocial and depraved, and denounced as a hard-core voluptuary, a grim pessimist, and a dogmatic atheist. (La Mettrie himself added fuel to this fire by consistently using the most provocative statements to make his points.) A closer examination of his moral philosophy makes it evident that, while many of La Mettrie's points are certainly disturbing, they are made rather tentatively, and that his moral position is more complex than has been acknowledged. His underlying purpose was to derive a fundamental understanding of the constitutional constraints on the individual. Thus his investigation of moral issues was a crucial part of the humanitarian crusade of the physician concerned with the sick, or in the case of moral behavior, with the deviant.

To assess more accurately La Mettrie's moral position, the *Discours* must be discussed in its entirety, not in terms of the inflammatory statements that are drawn from it to condemn La Mettrie as beyond the pale of respectability. It must also be placed within the context of La Mettrie's philosophical corpus and his philosophical and medical agenda.

There are stylistic indications that La Mettrie considered this work to be part of a larger whole; the *Discours* carries over arguments and peculiarities of style from earlier works. In it he employs a system of internal cross-references and ironic asides that refer to his earlier works, and he seems to take it for granted that his reader is conversant with his entire corpus and will easily pick out and follow the threads of argument. He continues to wage the battles fought in earlier works, specifically against the notion of an immortal soul and a unique, distinctly human nature.

Ironically, La Mettrie came to write his most controversial work because Maupertuis gave him a copy of Seneca to read to keep him out of trouble.[6] But even if the specific inspiration of the work was accidental, La Mettrie was clearly working toward the argument of the *Discours* in his other philosophical works. His earlier works dealt with moral issues, especially *L'Homme machine*, in which he treated some of the implications for morality (especially the natural law theory) of his notion of the essential unity of nature, a unity that did not support or allow a chasm between animal and man. In the

Discours La Mettrie came to focus on the moral ramifications of those positions.

But most crucial to an understanding of this text is that it is the outgrowth of his medical humanitarianism and his crusade for medical reform. The *Discours* underscores a fundamental tension between medical humanism and the social implications of materialism, a tension that creates, at certain points, an internal inconsistency. For example, although La Mettrie would like to discredit the moral position of the Stoics and the Enlightenment idealization of the man of letters as unrealistic, those positions are too personally appealing for him to entirely dismiss them. Despite his reputation for provoking outrage, La Mettrie's arguments seem to be less forceful; he seems to pull his punches, because although he wishes to present the most radical conclusions he also wants to disassociate himself from any hint of depravity.[7] But the most fundamental tension in this work is the conflict produced by La Mettrie's desire both to present the strongest conclusions of his materialism and to argue for social reform based on a humane treatment of individuals.

La Mettrie's moral philosophy must also be reassessed in the context of eighteenth-century thought rather than in light of twentieth-century political dilemmas. Such an examination can illuminate the moral philosophy of La Mettrie and his particular brand of materialism and increase our understanding of the Enlightenment. Many of the positions La Mettrie took in the 1740s became commonplace in the later Enlightenment. For example, his notion that physical pleasure is an important consideration in discussing human motivation became a common theme of later moral treatises.[8] Though La Mettrie was vehemently denounced by the materialists themselves, he articulated many points that they later discussed. He was also a much more cautious, complex, and subtle thinker on moral questions than some of the other materialists, d'Holbach and Helvétius, for example. In fact, when Diderot raised serious questions about the dogmatically sensationalist moral position taken by Helvétius in *De l'homme*, he used many of the arguments made by La Mettrie, especially about the importance of the individual constitution.[9] La Mettrie wrote early enough to be a danger to the burgeoning philosophical movement and yet before most of the philosophes who would later espouse materialism had come to embrace it. Nonetheless, La Mettrie's kinship with the radical Enlightenment and his influence on it cannot be denied. Despite the opprobrium attached to La Mettrie's moral position, he raised important moral issues that continued to be addressed throughout the century.

Virtue, Remorse, and Determinism: The Limits of Human Action

Like most Enlightenment thinkers, La Mettrie looked to nature as the foundation of morality. But his view of nature was not Newtonian or deistic, and he did not conclude that human nature was governed by a soul or reason. So while La Mettrie looked to nature, it was a nature, and especially a human nature, quite distinct from that held by most of the philosophes. Specifically, his medical and philosophical works offered a medical understanding of nature that he used as the basis for discussions of moral issues. Because he was convinced that virtue could not be produced by trying to attain an abstract goal foreign to our nature, La Mettrie tried to determine whether, given what we know of human nature, there is a realistic possibility of virtue and, if so, where it might be found. As a starting point, he looked to the state of nature and concluded that humans in their natural state cannot be distinguished from animals. Just as virtue and vice are not terms assigned to animals, neither can they be used to describe the actions of human beings in the state of nature. He concluded that our notions of virtue and vice can only be the outgrowth of social relationships. "The necessity of liaisons of life has thus been that of the establishment of virtues and vices, of which the political institution is consequently the origin; because without them, without this solid though imaginary foundation, the edifice cannot sustain itself and falls in ruin."[10]

It is interesting to compare La Mettrie and Rousseau on the question of how society is formed from the state of nature and how man differs after its formation. Both assume that some sort of necessity brought man into society, and for both of them this development had a detrimental effect on human beings. For both of them, human beings originally lived according to their nature, but that is essentially animal nature, and our ideas of vice and virtue would make no sense to man in such a state.

For Rousseau, society imposes a host of conventions which allow the strong to exploit the weak and the rich to exploit the poor, and so society, unless it should come to be governed by what he calls the social contract, is an abomination and an extreme distortion of the natural character of human beings. But for Rousseau there is a stage in human development between the state of nature and the development of society when human beings were *good*; and although it was perhaps only for the worse, man has evolved from a state of nature.[11]

La Mettrie's estimation of the role of society is both more modest and more problematic than Rousseau's. Admittedly, society has connived to deceive man by making him believe that its notions of virtue and vice are absolute, even though it has simply attached honor and glory to those things that serve its interests and attached scorn, fear, and ignominy to what undermines them. But although La Mettrie emphasized the absolutely arbitrary nature of vice and virtue, he did not castigate society in the way that Rousseau did. Instead, he simply wanted it recognized that this has been society's purpose, which is justified by society's need to preserve itself. But La Mettrie's position is more problematic for the philosophes because he did not rhapsodize about society at any golden age of human development. He would not brook the idea that the constraints that society places on man are, or have been at any time, anything but arbitrary: they neither correspond to man's "higher nature" nor are they the "good." Society does not have the right to use these ideas to remake man's nature or to suggest that the attainment of these ideals has anything to do with man's happiness beyond the fact that it might satisfy his *amour-propre*. Furthermore, it is not clear whether or to what degree the animal nature of man has been altered by socialization.

The fact that La Mettrie's conception of society is not developed—it is simply a given, a rather nebulous notion that human beings, like certain other animals but for unexplained reasons, live in societies—has been the source of many problematic interpretations. Denying society the right to define "the good" and yet cognizant of the necessity of preserving social order, La Mettrie has been understood as sanctioning any and all political regimes and requiring social conformism of the individual.[12] Interpretations such as these have been possible not only because twentieth-century totalitarianism has colored studies of the Enlightenment[13] but also because La Mettrie's notion of society is so nebulous that it can be interpreted in almost any fashion. However, his failure to develop a social or political philosophy can be partially understood in light of his purpose. He is, as in his discussion of the soul in *L'Histoire naturelle de l'âme*, intent on removing any metaphysical pretensions from our commonly held notions. Because society is not natural, its determination of the "good" cannot be natural either. What is natural, as he emphasized in *L'Homme machine*, is an understanding of human nature based on physiology, a view that emphasizes the comparability of men and animals, and the control exercised by the physiological constitution. Thus his initial discussion of society and morality expose them both as divorced from the nature of man. In other words, the very limitations of his conception of society are determined by the points he is trying to make: because society is not natural, and because human nature is both comparable to animal nature and dependent on a physiological constitution, socialization is simply a gloss over that basic nature. The question remains: what is to be done with that knowledge? While many philosophes would exalt the gloss provided by socialization as the source of human progress, La Mettrie vehemently insists that this gloss is at odds with man's nature. And thus the crux of the *Discours* is a discussion of the relationship between the individual and the process of socialization.

The absence of a well thought out social and political philosophy makes La Mettrie's philosophy considerably different from that of other philosophes. His philosophy takes as its starting point, much as a physician would, the concerns of the individual rather than those of society as a whole. It is not, as his critics have generally claimed, that he was antisocial, but rather that, unlike most of the philosophes, he was unconcerned with society, except in a peripheral way. He did not explore the relationship of the individual to his society or society's goals, nor did he examine the purpose, nature, or origin of society, because these things are not part of the study of nature and therefore not the proper subject of scientific, empirical investigations. He was instead concerned to carve out areas of individual freedom from societal repression based on his medical knowledge of man rather than to construct programs for broad-based social change. His approach to society was therefore completely pragmatic; his concerns were those of the physician and, against the predominant spirit of his age, he had little interest in the empirical study of human beings in society. According to La Mettrie, the proper study of man was man, but man understood as part of nature.

Instead of probing the individual's relationship to his society, La Mettrie simply accepted it as a given that human beings have formed societies and will continue to live in them. Society, to its credit, has civilized man. Though he bemoaned the heavy burden that socialization imposed on certain individuals, La Mettrie also recognized its positive aspects: the effect of socialization on the more complex organization of human beings has made, as he put it, "some animals *human*."[14] The brunt of La Mettrie's moral argument is the hope that society, recognizing that its notions of virtue and vice are relative and thus designed merely to further its interests and preserve its existence, will be persuaded to reward a greater array of human behavior. If social rewards corresponded better to human nature than in traditional moral systems, more individuals could aspire to social virtues. Society would be better served and the burden civilization places on some of its less civilized members would be reduced.

In addition to his generally limited sense of the possibility of social reform, La Mettrie's specific claim that virtue and vice are completely relative put him clearly at odds with the aspirations of other Enlightenment moralists writing within the natural law tradition. Those aspirations are perhaps best typified by a work such as Voltaire's *Essai sur les moeurs*,[15] which, though cognizant of the relativity of cultures, maintained that by tracing moral notions through various cultures one would be able to distill a kernel of truth, a notion of virtue that was common to all cultures because it was rooted in the nature of man. Montesquieu's definition of justice as an absolute relation, no matter what its subject, is a concise formulation of the natural law tradition. "Before there were any laws enacted just relations were possible. To say that there is nothing just or unjust, excepting that which positive laws command or forbid, is like saying that before one has drawn a circle all of its radii were not equal."[16]

The sense that positive laws did not correspond to natural law was a powerful impetus to reform. The philosophes meant to wipe away or dismiss from consideration the artificial moral constraints of society to uncover natural law. By means of this understanding of virtue, they intended to construct social and political systems based on man's innate sense of virtue, which would thereby produce good citizens. They aspired to be Newtons of the moral sphere.[17]

La Mettrie stands in clear opposition to this tradition. He was perfectly willing to grant society the right to try to make human beings good citizens, but he would not tolerate any assumption that the values instilled by society necessarily represent a higher value or that society can inculcate virtue. In fact, La Mettrie claimed, what citizens seek is not virtue but renown. "In fact, we are for the most part truly small masters of the practice of virtue; the favors virtue accords us are worth nothing unless they are heralded with a great deal of noise. Almost no one wishes to have a merit which is obscure and unknown; one does everything for glory."[18]

In addition to his claim that natural law could not be substantiated, La Mettrie went further and strongly contended that remorse was not an innate sentiment, a radical position because it denied man's innate goodness. La Mettrie argued staunchly for this point because it is both the logical outgrowth of his philosophy and the point at which even those who might have accepted his argument thus far would break with him. Indeed, his argument against remorse provoked outrage from many quarters. The most orthodox of his opponents argued for remorse as God's imprint on man's soul, or the knowledge of good and evil produced by Adam's fall from grace.[19] The philosophes, on the other hand, used remorse as a touchstone they could apply to a number of situations to determine what kinds of actions universally produce remorse. In other words, remorse could be taken as a negative proof of the existence of natural law, a punishment for violating it. At the very least, remorse was claimed to be *the* characteristic which distinguished man from animals and made man responsible for his actions.

La Mettrie willingly conceded that remorse does exist. But far from dignifying it as a principle of human virtue, he instead decreased its importance until it was simply a holdover from childhood. "Revert to our infancy and we will find that it is the epoch of remorse" (a notion Freud would develop later).[20] Remorse is such a strong sentiment simply because it was engraved on the brain at a very early age. In accord with La Mettrie's Lockean epistemology, the earliest, simplest, and strongest sensations or impressions are the most difficult to efface or blur through later sensations. However, in a way that is much more radical than the spirit of Locke's *Essay*, La Mettrie used Locke's epistemology as a cutting edge to whittle away at all of man's cherished beliefs about himself that encouraged the belief that he deserved a special place in the universe. Thus remorse was merely a sensation like any other, which La Mettrie defined as "only a simple sentiment, received without examination and without choice, and which was as strongly impressed on the brain as a seal on soft wax."[21] As simply a strong impression, remorse could have no moral force.[22]

The weakness of La Mettrie's argument is that, though he seems to consider remorse a universal human experience, he does not explain how or why it occurs so universally, or how the sentiment is related to the events that produce it. In fact, in *L'Homme machine*, published only a year earlier, La Mettrie maintained that remorse and hence natural law extended throughout the animal kingdom. The position he defined in *Discours sur le bonheur* might have been developed to respond to critics or to deal with other obvious problems of extending remorse to the animal kingdom. But this new formulation of the problem presents other difficulties. The fact that human beings will practice cannibalism rather than starve without feeling remorse proves to La Mettrie both that remorse is not innate and that there are no universal situations that produce it. But that example, the only one La Mettrie brings to bear, does not address the fact that this sentiment, dismissed as an infantile holdover, is apparently universal; despite his objections, one might want to argue that even the evidence La Mettrie provides suggests that it is innate to human beings.

But La Mettrie adamantly declared that the situations which produce remorse are completely relative; "autre religion, autres rémords: autres temps, autres moeurs."[23] An extreme example of the cultural relativity of remorse was the case of Lycurgus, who killed weak and malformed children and as a result was applauded for his wisdom. By pointing to the relativity of the situations which produce remorse, La Mettrie argued against its value as a means to virtue and suggested that a society which fosters guilt is not molding virtuous citizens. To those who argue that remorse is socially useful and thus ought to be cultivated, La Mettrie countered that guilt does not prevent crime because it occurs after the fact and rarely prevents a recurrence. Therefore remorse is, at the very least, useless to society. Fear of the laws, he suggested, would be a much more effective deterrent to crime than remorse. But he was quite concerned with those at the other end of the scale, those unfortunates who suffer the pangs of remorse for things they have not done. These individuals, he suggested, prove that remorse or guilt does not correspond to the degree of violation of a natural law but rather to one's constitutional predisposition towards feeling remorse, or reverting to infancy. Because remorse can be so exceedingly harmful to the individual, the pain it inflicts must be alleviated even if that means that some criminals will also be relieved of remorse, because "it [remorse] overloads machines already to be pitied that, badly regulated as they are, are swept along towards evil as the good are towards righteousness. . . . If I lighten the load of the burden of life, they will be less unhappy, not less punished. Will they be more wicked? I do not think so, because although remorse does not make them better, it is not dangerous for society to deliver them from it."[24]

Toleration is a solution to this problem. If society has a right to establish standards of behavior to ensure its preservation (and La Mettrie allows that right as long as it is not clouded with metaphysical pretensions) and if, as he has argued, virtue is arbitrary and we are constitutionally determined, then society has a responsibility to be as tolerant of the individual as its interest allows. Because remorse is neither innate nor socially useful (since it cannot make the individual virtuous or prevent crimes) and because it places a great burden on some individuals, society ought to do all it can to break down guilt rather than to foster this counterproductive and destructive sentiment. La Mettrie granted that if guilt is not fostered by society some scoundrels will live more tranquil lives, but for each scoundrel set free of remorse, he asked, "how many, wise and virtuous persons, inappropriately tormented while living sweetly innocent lives, will be able to have more beautiful days without clouds once they have shaken off the yoke of a too onerous education?"[25]

Because La Mettrie insists that the impact of remorse varies according to the particular determinants of an individual constitution, he seems to be arguing for a physiological determinism. But despite his conviction that behavior, including complex reactions like remorse, is the product of the configuration of the physiological constitution, La Mettrie nonetheless acknowledged that humans suppose they can be happy and act as if they were completely free. La Mettrie was not cynical about the optimism felt by his fellow man. Rather, he accepted that the individual must act and can have no other attitude toward his own existence. He was not arguing for determinism as a metaphysical position or recanting his disparagement of metaphysics as irrelevant to human concerns. He was arguing not for a metaphysical determinism but rather for a physiological determinism which limits, if not how happy man can be, at least the ways in which he will seek to be happy.

A belief in the ability of an individual to seek happiness persists even in those, like La Mettrie himself, who are convinced of a physiological determinism. This conflict between the physiological and the psychological makes La Mettrie's determinism intriguing rather than dry and despairing. His claim is that we are determined to a great extent by our physiology, and as we do not accept that determinism in our actions, some other factors must be brought to bear in discussing man in society. But our understanding of society must also be informed by our scientific knowledge of man's physiological determinism, an understanding that must inevitably produce tolerance for the individual. La Mettrie was not proselytizing for determinism. He recognized that even though there is no other scientifically supportable conclusion that human beings can come to about their own existence and capacities, it is not and cannot be a standard or principle by which human beings act. He then raised the question of the effect society can have on the individual, or the degree to which education can countervail physiological determinants.

Education and the Individual Constitution:
Determinism and Reform

In all of his medical works La Mettrie maintained that the nature of the individual constitution was the crucial factor in determining the appropriate prescription or regimen. In much the same way as the physician works within the parameters set by the individual constitution, La Mettrie sought to gauge the limits of the efficacy of the moral reformer. Just as the physician must acknowledge the effects of the individual constitution on health and disease, so too must the moral reformer recognize the limits that the individual constitution imposes on one's ability to behave in the ways society has defined as virtuous. The degree to which society can inculcate its values La Mettrie defined as education. Because they function as the crucial constraints on the moral reformer, La Mettrie weighed the relative strength of the fundamental influences on man, his constitution and his education. By emphasizing at every juncture the importance of the physical constitution, La Mettrie questioned the assumptions of classical political theorists and asserted the primacy of the physician over the metaphysician.

Like classical political theorists, La Mettrie took it as a given that human beings seek happiness. But his quest was to determine what that means in light of the constraints imposed by the individual constitution. His definition of happiness is the product of his sensationalism. "Happiness is a sensation that causes one to love life. If this sense of love of life lasts a short time, it is pleasure, if for a long time it is *volupté*, and if it lasts permanently, it is happiness."[26] He distinguished between two kinds of happiness, the internal and the external. The internal causes of happiness depend on man's individual constitution and the external on forces and circumstances outside man's physical being.

An internal constitutional cause of happiness which is specific to the individual is a very different notion from that of a human nature, and in this way La Mettrie radically changed the grounds for discussion of happiness. If one presupposes a rational soul, or a distinctly human nature, one can subsume all human beings under this rubric and determine one cause or combination of causes of happiness that can be taken as universal. But La Mettrie, unconstrained by an overarching metaphysical notion of human nature, was impressed by the diversity of human responses, and having discounted an immortal soul he contended that nothing could explain this diversity of responses except something about the physical organization of matter.

La Mettrie's observations convinced him of the constitutional basis of happiness, that is, some people seem to be more subject to "joy, to vanity, to anger, to remorse than others." This propensity can have no source other than the physical, and it will be reflected in particular kinds of behavior: "it is this disposition of our organs which produces mania, imbecility, vivacity, languor, tranquility, penetration, etc." He provided additional evidence from his medical practice, citing those "blessed ones" who have a constitution such that pains and misfortunes "slide over their soul so lightly that they make an impression only with great difficulty." These blessed ones who are predisposed to happiness are the beneficiaries of their physiology: "the same fortunate conjuncture, circulations, and interplay of solids which have produced the happy genius and the embittered narrow-minded man, also produce the *sentiment* that makes us happy or unhappy."[27] In other words, "the happiness that depends on our organization is the most constant and the most difficult to uproot; it has need of very little nourishment, it is the most beautiful present of nature. The unhappiness which comes from the same source is without remedy, or at best there are some very uncertain palliatives."[28]

The notion of a constitutional basis of human behavior is foreign to the systematic sensationalism of Condillac or Helvétius. Condillac assumed a predisposition toward goodness because he accepted as a given the infusion of an immortal soul. Helvétius considered complete malleability possible so that diversity of responses can only be the result of diversity of experience. Just as Diderot shared many of the scientific and physiological concerns of La Mettrie in the development of his philosophy, he also accepted, or at least entertained, many of La Mettrie's moral points, even if he considered them too dangerous to publish. In the dialogue *Rameau's Nephew*, Diderot has the character *Lui* discuss whether it is possible for a man to become good if his inheritance is that of Lui, in other words, depraved. "But if the molecule decides that he shall be a ne'er do well like his father, the pains I might take to make him an honest man would be very dangerous. Education would work continually at cross purposes with the natural bent of the molecule."[29]

However, in addition to these fundamental internal causes of happiness, there are external causes that leave some room for reform or the application of a philosophy of man to social issues. External causes of happiness "come from *volupté*, riches, science, honors, happiness, etc."[30] With the possible exception of *volupté*, all these sources of happiness are social virtues or rewards that most Enlightenment thinkers tried to link inextricably with happiness. The problem La Mettrie faced was to balance these two kinds of causes and determine how they relate to each other and how they contribute to human happiness. This problem plagued him throughout the treatise because he insisted on the primacy of the former but did not deny all influence to the latter.

This problem is also the source of the rift that develops within this treatise between the aspirations of the philosophes and what seems to be the much more pessimistic view of man and society held by La Mettrie. The philosophes quite clearly based their dreams for society on the notion that by appealing to or by attempting to provide some of these causes of happiness as rewards for virtuous behavior, men would be persuaded to behave virtuously or, as perhaps the more cynical of them might have put it, at least according to the needs of society. However, if an individual can be presumed to have a constitutional disposition, he must in some ways remain impervious to offers of social rewards.

According to La Mettrie, if society has convinced one to subscribe to its views of good and evil, that conviction can only be considered the effect of education on human nature, for "education alone can give us sentiments and a happiness contrary to what one would have had without it."[31] Although the practice of social virtues is essentially the result of the imprint of education on a malleable constitution, the effect of that education is by no means negligible or a simple veneer over the constitution that nature has given one. La Mettrie described that dramatic transformation: "The instructed soul no longer wishes nor does what it did before when it was guided only by itself. Enlightened by a thousand new sensations, the soul finds bad where it found good, it praises in others what it formerly blamed."[32]

Education, then, has fundamentally altered man, and La Mettrie does not disparage the change brought by education broadly construed, that is, socialization. For La Mettrie, as for the philosophes, the source of human happiness is to be found in society; as he put it, "a source of happiness that I cannot believe more pure, more noble, and more beautiful in the spirit of all men is that happiness which flows from the order of society."[33] The more distant man grew from the state of nature, the more horrible that state appeared to him and the more he sought to link socially useful behavior with rewards. "One has tied the idea of generosity, grandeur, humanity to the important actions of human commerce, . . . respect, honor, and glory to those actions which serve the country, . . . and by these goads a great many animals with a human shape have become heroes."[34]

The preceding quotations indicate some of the difficulties in this particular text. Although La Mettrie made adamant and radical statements about the unnatural state of social virtue, he included these laudatory statements about the virtues cultivated by society. A way to resolve the paradox is to recognize that although La Mettrie granted that social virtues are socially useful, he nonetheless insisted that they are unnatural, not easily acquired, and, for the most unfortunate members of society, impossible to acquire. Furthermore, the effect of education or socialization is not permanent, for the character of a man resembles a violin string which can be tightened to produce new sounds, or, in the case of man, to acquire new virtues. However, when the string is loosened, it produces its natural sound. Because the effects of education are impermanent, La Mettrie was not sanguine about what education can accomplish in society.[35] In the course of his argument, La Mettrie seems torn; he would like to advocate the orthodox sensationalist solution, that is, to find fault with man's education and thus argue, as Helvétius did, for reforms through legislation and education.[36] But as much as he might have been tempted to offer this palliative, La Mettrie could not escape the implications of his constitutional individualism which constrained him to emphasize nature at the expense of nurture and which absolutely precluded Helvétius's claim that human beings are only the product of their experiences.

Unlike those philosophes who had a sense that human beings are either innately good or neutral and that virtue could be inculcated, La Mettrie's view of human nature involved the possibility that an individual could have a constitutional predisposition to evil. Thus La Mettrie raised problems for philosophic schemes that aimed to ameliorate the human condition. "What if the disposition towards evil is such that it is easier for the good to become wicked than for the wicked to improve themselves? Please excuse this inhuman portrait of humanity."[37]

This sense of the impermanence of virtue and the difficulty with which the goals of society are assimilated (and the limits of that assimilation) La Mettrie defined as materialism. "This materialism merits consideration. It should be the source of indulgences, excuses, pardons, virtue being a sort of hors-d'oeuvre, a strange ornament always ready to fly."[38] Thus his materialism argued for a tolerant assessment of individual weakness because virtue must be admitted as being beyond the usual capacity of human beings; at the very least, it cannot be assumed to be universally attainable. La Mettrie used his philosophy of man and nature to develop a moral philosophy, and so clearly connected are these principles that they bear the same name of materialism.

However, he also recognized that the interests of society did not allow for complete tolerance. Society has and must have its own criteria for vice and virtue, vice being what is detrimental to the interests and continuation of society, virtue what furthers it. In fact, La Mettrie made the association between the goals of society and our understanding of the nature of virtue absolute. "One sees that the difference between the wicked and the good is that, for the one, particular interest is preferable to general interest, while the others sacrifice their well-being to that of a friend or the public."[39]

This quotation adds something to La Mettrie's notion of society as simply an aggregate of individuals. What people *do* in a society is act in the public interest. In other words, what society means to him is not a particular social order or regime but rather a more nebulous sense that a society by definition cultivates those virtues that make it possible to act in the public interest. Society not only defines virtues but, as a result, virtue must necessarily be in the public interest.[40] The weakness of this amplification is that La Mettrie nowhere explores in detail what public interest entails beyond a vague concern with good health and a commitment to enlightened science. But those values are not natural to man. As harshly as La Mettrie was criticized for the dangerous implications of his morality, he nowhere argued that it is illegitimate for society to set standards of virtue in the public interest. Since man does not act freely, he should not be blamed if his constitution does not enable him to acquire what society deems to be virtue. Nonetheless, society is forced to and must "tuer les chiens enragés."[41]

To Challenge Traditional Moral Values

Having laid the groundwork for a materialistic moral theory, La Mettrie evaluated traditional moral systems and theories of the good life under the dual perspective of whether they corresponded to his sense of human nature and whether they fostered qualities that were socially useful. In other words, he reappraised traditional moral systems in light of his medical understanding of human nature and his medical methodology of critical empiricism. His reappraisal was motivated by his sense that moral notions formed a part of the corrupt status quo that must be criticized because those moral notions, based on unfounded metaphysical assumptions, have proven to be inaccurate and because they have been used by privileged corporate social groups like politicians or priests to bolster their unwarranted positions. Instead moral notions must be reappraised by the standards of empirical evidence, evidence which acknowledges and reflects man's integral involvement in nature.

The Christian moral tradition was his first target, though his method of attack was idiosyncratic. Using the tools of the polemicist, La Mettrie examined it through Descartes, whom he portrayed as both the most recent spokesman of that tradition and as a closet atheist and materialist. The fact that La Mettrie was continuing his long polemic against Cartesian metaphysics with its dependence on God and independence of actual phenomena has not been recognized because this treatise contains the famous remark in which La Mettrie points to the easy step from Cartesian *bête machine* to his own *l'homme machine*, an evolution that has set the agenda of La Mettrie scholarship. "But one recognizes that he [Descartes] regarded animals as pure machines, well imagining that one day men would be considered in the same way by men who might be more mediocre thinkers but would be bolder, and who also said that one has no assurance of the immortality of the soul."[42]

But this remark, like so many of La Mettrie's, is ironic and a fine sort of vengeance to wreak on Descartes. If one finds Descartes's metaphysics entirely objectionable because it is predicated on God and requires God to sustain it at every point and because it has divorced man from nature in both his own nature and his quest for knowledge, and if one abhors the fact that Descartes tried to gain acceptance for his metaphysics from a university community dominated by Scholastics and thus melded questions of science and theology in a completely inappropriate manner (all positions La Mettrie had taken), what better way to destroy Descartes than to insist that he meant none of those things! Thus, everything about

Cartesian metaphysics which La Mettrie rejected had been inserted simply to avoid entanglements with Church authority. Rejoicing in Descartes's ability to deceive religious authority about his true intent, La Mettrie praised Descartes's philosophy because "the human spirit desires all the progress that experiments can bring about, and, hypothetical as it is, his philosophy has made us feel the necessity of experiments."[43] La Mettrie claimed that Descartes advanced his *bête machine* theory with the clear understanding that it would only be a matter of time before that theory would be expanded to include man, despite the absolute sense in which *l'homme machine* would completely discredit the notion of an immortal soul. This praise is ironic; La Mettrie is claiming that Descartes had so divorced metaphysics from experience that a refutation like his own was inevitable. In other words, La Mettrie has recast Descartes as an atheist and a materialist in the spirit of philosophical polemic.

But he also used Descartes to discredit Christianity. La Mettrie quite rightly recognized that Descartes's God plays a fundamental role in Cartesian metaphysics, but he might have also recognized that Descartes's God, for all Descartes's protestations of orthodoxy, is quite remote from Christian beliefs and values. By selecting Descartes as a spokesman for the Christian moral tradition, La Mettrie pointed to the weakness of Cartesian dualism as an anchor for the moral authority of Christianity. La Mettrie recognized that Descartes had been forced to leave the "sure and certain" foundations of morality in abeyance, arguing no better foundation for morality than custom.[44] La Mettrie effectively reduced the moral authority of Descartes's God to the expediency that underlies Descartes's discussion of morality. Furthermore, by claiming that Descartes's God is a ploy, La Mettrie meant to suggest that Christianity, especially the immortal soul and the authority of Christian morality, cannot be and is not seriously maintained by any modern thinker who has even the scientific knowledge of the seventeenth century, much less by an eighteenth-century physician with the physiological knowledge of his own day![45]

Thus, in a very short discussion connecting Descartes and Christianity, La Mettrie has been able to tar Descartes as a fellow materialist and atheist, yet at the same time point to the weak link between Descartes's God and Christian moral theory. These remarks would have been thoroughly inflammatory to an orthodox

Cartesian; La Mettrie had, in essence, taken the vehemence of the critical response directed against his own *L'Homme machine* and turned it back against Descartes with particular polemical dexterity. He also suggested that a metaphysical system anchored by God, such as Cartesian dualism, is fundamentally at odds with scientific investigation. By choosing Descartes as the defender of Christianity but one whose weaknesses are quite apparent, La Mettrie attempted to kill the two metaphysical birds of Descartes and the Christian moral tradition with one polemical stone. La Mettrie may in fact have used the most effective method possible to ensure that the taint of materialism adhered to Descartes in subsequent philosophical discussions.

But La Mettrie was not interested simply in using Christianity to impugn Descartes. He also cast aspersions on the immortal soul as an effective incentive to virtuous behavior, thereby questioning its social utility. Pointing to the difficulties of living in this world if one is continually weighing one's actions in this life against the possibility of rewards in the next, he claimed that one can make only one decision for his own good and that of society. "Finally, all things well considered, to restrict one's self to the present, which alone is in our power, is the choice worthy of the sage; no inconveniences, no disquietude about the future in this system. Uniquely occupied in filling well the narrow circle of life, one finds himself as happy as possible in that he lives not only for himself, but for his country, for his king; and in general, for humanity, which one makes himself glory in serving. He thus assures the happiness of society with his own."[46]

La Mettrie shared the concern of the philosophes that religion directed man away from this life, but this concern led him to attack not only the institutions or the canons of the church but also to deny the moral authority of the Christian tradition, a position not usually taken by the philosophes. For as Voltaire noted, "there is a great difference between combatting superstitions of man and breaking the ties of society and the chains of virtues."[47] In his attack on religion, La Mettrie focused on the immortal soul primarily because he saw it as a fundamental impediment to understanding human nature. The tone of his attack was less vehement than Voltaire's campaign to *écrasez l'infame*, but La Mettrie went further than most of the philosophes in undermining the moral authority of the church.

La Mettrie treated ancient moral philosophy as a more worthy adversary than Christianity. He took Seneca as the paradigm of the ancient tradition which claimed "the good" as equivalent with man's end and virtue as the only path to happiness. Perhaps Seneca and the Stoics were chosen because their restrictions on the concept of "the good" seemed to La Mettrie to be the harshest and thus the easiest to refute. Or perhaps they were selected because their scorn for the things of this life could easily be tied to the abnegation and the otherworldliness explicit in the Christian moral position. For whatever reason, armed with the notion of human nature he had developed in his other works, La Mettrie denounced the Stoics as fundamentally inhuman, for they maintained that to be happy was to live tranquilly, untroubled by ambition or desire, unaffected by wealth or its lack, impervious to emotions, disdaining pleasure, *volupté*, and even life itself. La Mettrie proudly proclaimed himself an anti-Stoic and set up a rigid dichotomy between the Stoic and those like himself. "These philosophers are severe, sad, and hard; we are soft, gay, and compliant. They make themselves inaccessible to pain and pleasure; we glory in feeling. They place themselves above events and therefore they cease to be human."[48]

Stoicism, like other moral systems, could not substantiate its claims to have identified "the good" primarily because abstract moral notions are not a meaningful way to talk about human morality; Stoicism is, according to La Mettrie, fundamentally misbegotten because it defined human nature abstractly rather than empirically. La Mettrie claimed that because the Stoics had such a distorted view of human nature, their moral system could not foster social virtue. "The more they distance themselves from nature, without which morality and virtue are equally foreign, the more they distance themselves from virtue."[49]

Stoicism was an attractive alternative to Christianity for many of the philosophes, and the fact that La Mettrie attacked Stoicism provoked Diderot's famous denunciation of him.[50] La Mettrie himself, despite his denunciations, acknowledged the writings of the Stoics as a great comfort that calmed his troubled soul and allowed him to face with equanimity the trials his work brought him and the pain of his exile from France.[51] Nonetheless, he vehemently berated the Stoics for advocating suicide, and ultimately he found their denial of the self and of life virtually incomprehensible. "What folly to prefer death to the most delicious, delightful course of life, to believe that those who cannot lead a solitary and philosophical life cannot be happy and should consequently leave life sooner than wear chains of flowers." As opposed to the abnegation and other-worldliness of the false philosophies of Stoicism and Christianity, true philosophy, La Mettrie insists, invokes carpe diem. "It spreads the roses and flowers in our path and teaches us to gather them."[52] La Mettrie, it might be suggested, is a foul-weather Stoic, finding Stoicism a comfort in difficult times but too rigid and self-denying under better conditions.

Another classical ideal of the good life that La Mettrie scrutinized was the life of the eighteenth-century man of letters. He himself had, of course, chosen this career and seemed somewhat at a loss to account for that choice. From his exile in Prussia, it can scarcely have appeared to have been a choice conducive to the quest for the happiness he expounded. La Mettrie seems so steeped in classical ideals that, as he noted, the decisions he made seem to be more in keeping with Seneca's philosophy than his own. "Let us go further and let us preach a doctrine which we have had the honor *not* to follow: it is not necessary to cultivate one's soul except to procure more conveniences for the body. Perhaps one should only write, as some authors do, to gain money from the booksellers . . . love of life and well-being are evidently rights more pressing than those of *amour-propre* and, just as pleasure is more important than honor for one who has good taste; bread is nourishment more solid than reputation."[53]

Unable to explain the appeal of the life of the man of letters to himself or others, specifically the crusading zeal of the philosophe with its attendant risks to personal safety, he wondered: "What is this trumpet, more powerful than that of Mars, which raises our courage and emboldens us in the face of dangers, calling us to combat with only the weapons of reason?" Though La Mettrie called it folly to sacrifice so much "to the chimerical honor of immortalizing the letters of the alphabet that compose our names," he acknowledged that "there is great delight in seeing one's ideas accepted by some contemporary connoisseurs." However, even that delight is promptly dampened by the recollection of the danger that philosophers face under most regimes, for "the glory which follows in the wake of the muses cannot compensate the loss of physical well-being." Since "chance has thrown us here," he concluded that it is more reasonable to suppose that we are here not to suffer the rigors of a quest for fame, but rather "to live tranquilly, content, and at ease, for to think of our bodies before our souls is to imitate the wisdom of nature which made the one before the other."[54]

La Mettrie looked to another classical ideal of the good life, the *vita contemplativa*, to see whether it produced happiness. While La Mettrie did not deny the pleasures of the intellectual life, he could not subscribe to any philosophy which touted the life of the mind as the only true pleasure for man or claimed that this sort of pleasure is natural to man. He acknowledged that for some the drive toward intellectual pleasures is akin to a sexual drive and that he himself would be bereft without books, ink, pen, and paper. (He himself experienced *volupté d'esprit* while writing *L'Homme machine*.) Nonetheless, the intellectual life can also be completely without pleasure, even for those who try desperately to attain it. The most convincing evidence for La Mettrie that happiness was not generally to be sought in intellectual pleasures were the "innumerable multitude of happy ignorant!" Even though his own life and that of the philosophes were at odds with his conclusion, La Mettrie supposed that nature intended us to seek happiness in the tranquility and ease of the body rather than in the pleasures of the mind. Thus, to place human happiness in study, according to La Mettrie, essentially misconstrued human nature. "To generally place happiness in the culture of letters, for the pleasure one gains from it, is to neglect the goods of the body and to mock nature. To attach happiness to the chariot of glory and fame is to put it, as a child might, in the noise that a trumpet makes."[55]

La Mettrie's argument that all men would not find happiness in the cultivation of reason undermined those Enlightenment reforms predicated on the assumption of an almost completely malleable human nature. Some of the philosophes supposed that all men would aspire to the ideal of the cultured, educated man. Others assumed that, at the very least, their fellow human beings could be constrained to be virtuous according to their talents through the perceptive identification of the interests of society by the philosophes and the application of suitable rewards for actions furthering those interests. Except for the Christian moral tradition, La Mettrie found these other theories of the good life somewhat persuasive. But despite their personal appeal, La Mettrie claimed that society had too narrowly interpreted human character. To be more successful at promoting socially useful behavior, society must recognize as "good," and therefore reward, behavior that better and more widely corresponds to the range and diversity of the human constitution.

For *Volupté*

In part, La Mettrie's adamant desire to discredit the classical moral tradition was based on his sense that nature has endowed human beings with so many means to be happy that happiness cannot be restricted to the life of a philosopher or scholar; because these states are attainable by so few, they cannot possibly be the happiness nature intended for us. This sense of nature as an egalitarian or perhaps only an arbitrary distributor of the capacity for happiness led La Mettrie to argue for *volupté*, or sensual pleasure, as a legitimate source of happiness, although he qualified the sense in which happiness can be said to be *volupté*. "It can be the refined sensual pleasures of love or it can be sensual pleasure moderated, made reasonable, governed not by the extravagant caprices of an irritated imagination, but only by the needs of nature; here, it is the sensual pleasure of the spirit engaged in research, or enchanted by the possession of truth; there, finally, is the contentment of the spirit, the motive, and the end of all our actions."[56]

Although La Mettrie is frequently portrayed as a hard-core voluptuary, his argument is moderate, defensive, and at times apologetic. Since *volupté* is much more accessible than science, and since it is empirically demonstrable that happiness is not parceled out to those with particular intellectual abilities, La Mettrie argued that *volupté* was probably the natural route to happiness. However, he made this argument in a tentative fashion. In addition to his own ties to Stoic philosophy, La Mettrie retained a great deal of respect for Seneca and the whole body of traditional moral philosophy. He tried to reconcile his argument with the objections Seneca had to *volupté* by claiming that Seneca's objections were based on the misconception that the voluptuous could not be good soldiers, or good citizens, or good friends. La Mettrie produced the French as a counterexample, a well-known nation of voluptuaries renowned for valor, patriotism, and loyalty![57]

La Mettrie's argument for *volupté* is in large measure the source of his unsavory reputation. The arguments for sensual pleasure are set forth more provocatively in the *cause de scandale*, his *L'Art de jouir*, also printed as *La Volupté*.[58] It seems ironic, at least from the perspective of this century, that his work would have caused such outrage. Much of it is spent evaluating other works on the subject in terms of whether they are obscene and dissolute or whether they convey a pure voluptuousness. La Mettrie's view of human sexuality in *L'Art de Jouir* is full of beauty and charm, expressed in pastoral imagery. He proclaimed in no uncertain terms his abhorrence of depravity and violence and noted that any picture of human sexuality which is not tinged with gentleness and delicacy is a misrepresentation. "*Volupté* is as different from debauchery as virtue is from crime." He cited *Manon Lescaut* and *La Princesse de Clèves* as examples of proper depictions in which "love, in a word, of the most voluptuous sort is most delicately portrayed."[59] It is also possible that as sexual mores changed at the end of the eighteenth century, La Mettrie's portrayal of female sexuality came to be seen as particularly perverse or that the very attempt to discuss human sexuality would have been taken amiss by his German pietist critics.

La Mettrie described at length his ideal of "la volupté plus épurée," the simple love of a shepherd and shepherdess, untainted by the corruptions of society—a love very similar to Rousseau's description of Émile's discovery of love. Although such sentimental descriptions dominate this work, La Mettrie also emphasized the physical pleasures of love, because sensual pleasure, like all other sensations, must be related to a physiological process. Sensual pleasure specifically depends on the tension and tickling of the nerves.

Much of the criticism of La Mettrie is predicated on the assumption that he was a proponent of complete license. Yet instead of exhortations to depravity, which the acerbity of the criticism heaped upon him leads one to expect, one finds arguments for sympathy or tolerance for those whose constitutions lead them to seek happiness in what society does not condone. Yet La Mettrie did not urge society to be permissive. In fact, in his opinion, the ability of society to affect the character of the individual is quite limited. In other words, for La Mettrie the possibility of reform or a more efficient working of society was not predicated on the ability to alter the character of man but rather on the recognition of the diverse ways nature leads him to seek happiness.

Modern critics of La Mettrie have been quick to connect his moral views with the ills of modern society. The basis of this argument is a comparison between La Mettrie and de Sade.[60] While it is true that for La Mettrie, like de Sade, virtue did not inevitably lead to happiness, and that La Mettrie also invoked a hedonistic ethic, he neither encouraged criminality as a way to happiness nor counseled war between the individual and society. Instead he pitied the individual whose machine was so ill-constructed that he sought happiness in what society condemned; and he asserted that the interests of society must prevail against the criminal. La Mettrie, unlike de Sade, did not point to the criminal as the human prototype, the example to which the weak or virtuous person should aspire. Instead, in his attitude toward sensual pleasure, La Mettrie reflects less the license of de Sade than the hedonism of the seventeenth-century *libertins*,[61] those savants who extolled the refined pleasures of sensuality. But once again he used thinkers of the seventeenth century to argue for an evolution toward reform through polemics and a scientific understanding of human nature. Unlike the *libertins*, he explicitly emphasized the physiological basis of sexual pleasure and its relationship to the imagination, a point he had earlier raised in *L'Histoire naturelle de l'âme*, for which he was condemned as a degenerate.[62]

Although this discussion of *L'Art de jouir* is meant to qualify the disrepute which hangs over La Mettrie, it must also be recognized that even if the terms "depraved" and "debauched" seem inappropriate, there are very real grounds for unease in La Mettrie's work. These grounds derive from the problematic implications of his philosophy that he did not shirk; he admitted that there are those who do not find happiness in moderation but rather seek it "in the breast of debauchery, madness, and disorder,"[63] and there are virtuous men who take no pleasure in virtue. Crucial to La Mettrie's moral philosophy and a direct outgrowth of his physiology is his sense that, though they may not be the norm, the depraved are not so monstrous as to be denied humanity. This notion develops from La Mettrie's use of the Hippocratic theory of the temperaments. For La Mettrie that theory highlights diversity to such a degree that it is simply a means of describing patients, of categorizing them only in the very loosest sense and emphasizing the great number of variables. Since he denied the existence of the immaterial soul or any occult forces, differences between individuals had to be explained only in physical terms. Presumably, then, those who are depraved have a slightly different balance of solids and liquids in some part of the body. But that difference is so slight in comparison to all the other physical conditions they share with members of their species that they cannot be excluded from the society of human beings. Thus, not only have proponents of traditional moral theories too narrowly considered where man might find happiness, but they have also argued too naively for either his complete malleability or his innate goodness. According to La Mettrie, the mere existence of the depraved or the individual with criminal tendencies is crucial empirical evidence that repudiates these naive assumptions. Furthermore, it cannot be assumed that any projects of the philosophes or any incentives to virtue or social conformity could modify or reform the individual who finds pleasure in debauchery.

What must have seemed particularly outrageous to the philosophes is that La Mettrie expanded upon their much-vaunted arguments for tolerance to argue on behalf of the depraved. He asked not only tolerance but also understanding, because the depraved act for the same motives we all do. "Do they not follow this instinct and this taste, by which each animal seeks its well-being? Have they not finally the only sort of felicity which is really within the range of their organs?"[64] The form of tolerance La Mettrie advocated for the depraved is that society not seek to burden them with remorse.

La Mettrie was torn between his concern to gain tolerance for the depraved individual and his intent to advance the interests of society through reform. But this argument, like his notion of reform through good medicine and empirical analysis, seems designed to sustain the interests of the individual. And perhaps because it was not usual to argue for the criminal or perhaps because his sense of what the interests of society were did not conform to those of traditional moralists or even of the philosophes, La Mettrie is best remembered for his outrageous defense of depravity. But an equally important part of his argument is his warning to the criminal that he must exercise care that his quest for happiness not transgress the interests of society because "politics is not as accommodating as my philosophy." This unfortunate must ultimately fear the hangman. If such an individual were bent on the destruction of society, one would have to hope for a man of virtue and courage to deliver society from such a creature, because he cannot be reformed. "To speak of temperance to one debauched is like speaking of humanity to a tyrant."[65] The philosophes, unlike La Mettrie, were willing to attempt both.

La Mettrie's defense of the depraved provoked such outrage that the more moderate points of his moral philosophy have been largely forgotten. Nonetheless, he accepted it as a given that nature was beneficent and made man for happiness (although he was equally inclined to emphasize the randomness and capriciousness of nature). He accepted the right of society to exist, although he did not develop a social or political philosophy. He suggested that the positive value of society is that it teaches those of us who are susceptible to education to favor public rather than private interests. Since our moral notions are determined by what society considers useful, La Mettrie argued that it would be beneficial to society and to the individual if society defined "the good" more broadly. If society rewarded a wider array of human behavior, more men would be able to serve its interests.

For the philosophes, the disquieting aspects of La Mettrie's moral philosophy were the limits he set on reform. He denied natural law and therefore considered any programs predicated on a belief in the innate goodness of man likely to be ineffectual. Furthermore, he contended that there were men who were constitutionally predisposed towards wickedness. Because he had little evidence that the individual character was malleable and no sense that it was perfectible, La Mettrie could advise toleration for the deviants only insofar as the interests of society allow, and for the depraved he ultimately could advocate only pity. La Mettrie recognized the problematic implications of his position but could not fail to proclaim what he saw as the truth. "I am angered to believe all that I say; but I do not repent to have said what I believe." He was aware that he had depicted human nature as much grimmer than the classical ideal to which he personally was attracted. He knew, too, that his conclusions had fundamentally undermined many of the hopes for social reform of his contemporaries. So in his conclusion he sought to explain his motives. He claimed to have described things as they are: "Je ne moralize, ni ne prêche, ni ne déclame, *j'explique*." He asserted that the recognition of facts in no way affects their existence; he was not proselytizing for depravity. His purpose was to discover the cause of certain kinds of human behavior. He concluded that a physiological determination could be overlaid with social values through education but only to a very limited degree. He had not made criminality more rampant or more difficult to control by discussing it. Nor, he claimed, could his advocacy of tolerance for the criminal be taken as approbation, for relief from remorse would create no greater inclination to crime. Furthermore, La Mettrie argued that his plea for the criminal could not be used to indict his own character. "I am honored to be a zealous citizen, but it is not with this character that I write. It is as a philosophe."[66] These are the general tenets of the moral philosophy that he brought to bear in defending his own philosophy and in proclaiming his adherence to the growing philosophical movement in the *Discours préliminaire*, his last philosophical work.

The *Discours* and Enlightenment Moral Theory

In the 1750s La Mettrie's moral position was a liability to the philosophes, a liability their enemies adeptly used against them. Though his views remained more radical than those of the philosophes, by 1770 many of his moral pronouncements had become acceptable enough to become part of a late Enlightenment tradition. The role of physical pleasure in motivating human behavior was a consideration the philosophes tried to incorporate into their plans for social reform. The question of determinism continued to plague them, but La Mettrie's solution, that even if one were completely determined by physiology it would not affect the way an individual conducted his life, was adopted by some of those who entertained it. La Mettrie's atheism or his complete rejection of theology and his agnostic refusal to allow the unknowable God into any discussion of nature or human nature also became a more acceptable position in the late Enlightenment. Materialism too became much more common, winning d'Holbach, Helvétius, and Diderot as principal adherents. And even more conservative philosophes like Voltaire made some concessions to a materialist understanding of human beings. Most of the philosophes also occasionally doubted the malleability of the human character, especially the educability of *le peuple*, on which so many of their social programs were based.

Nonetheless, La Mettrie's moral philosophy is at the heart of his problematic relationship to the Enlightenment. While his moral philosophy may not be as simplistic, dogmatic, nihilistic, or debauched as it is generally considered to be, it still raised crucial issues for the reformist hopes of the philosophes. He not only cast doubt on their programs by delineating the problems of the philosophic endeavor and limiting the efficacy of the philosophes themselves; he also attempted to connect his radical philosophy to the developing encyclopedic movement in his final work, the *Discours préliminaire*, in which he explicitly identified himself and his philosophy with the *mouvement philosophique*.

Even though La Mettrie and his moral views were subject to stringent criticisms from virtually every quarter within the philosophical party, the points he raised in the *Discours sur le bonheur* lurk in the background as direct influences or as troublesome considerations for subsequent moral discussions within the philosophe camp. For moderate philosophes such as Voltaire, La Mettrie indicated the dangers posed by any intimation of materialism. In fact, the *Discours* provoked Voltaire to write his poem on natural law, and his objections to d'Holbach's *Système de la nature* revivified his objections to La Mettrie's *Discours*. Perhaps Voltaire was so vociferous in attacking d'Holbach because he saw d'Holbach's position as lending a tinge of philosophic orthodoxy to the anathematized La Mettrie. And Voltaire's association of La Mettrie with d'Holbach was not unreasonable, for La Mettrie exerted a much more direct influence on materialist moral writings, particularly d'Holbach's *Système de la nature* and Diderot's *Réfutation de l'Homme*, than is generally acknowledged; even the extreme sensationalism of Helvétius in *De l'Homme* is also in part a response, albeit a negative one, to La Mettrie. Moral issues continued to be discussed throughout the Enlightenment according to the agenda set by La Mettrie.

Materialists recognized the dangers of being associated with La Mettrie and explicitly or implicitly distinguished their work from his. In *Système de la nature* d'Holbach was obviously concerned to respond to La Mettrie and differentiate their positions. He asserted his fundamental premise that "vice necessarily follows from unreasonable institutions" in opposition to those (and La Mettrie seems the most obvious example) "who see so little relationship between human goals and social institutions that they claim that society is foreign to human nature and that human beings are incurably ignorant." La Mettrie was more specifically the object of allusion when d'Holbach noted that "some say that the distinction between vice and virtue is only a matter of social convention" or conclude from crime that human nature is depraved. D'Holbach repeated Voltaire's charge against La Mettrie (without naming him) that "true philosophy is not misanthropy but rather philanthropy."[67] But d'Holbach most sharply deviated from La Mettrie in his adherence to the theory of natural law, which he claimed derived from the nature of man and not by virtue of his association in society. Despite his vehement criticism of existing institutions, d'Holbach insisted that natural law could not be broken in the social state and that civil law was simply natural law applied to a particular situation.

Despite his disclaimers, d'Holbach shared many conclusions with La Mettrie. He too believed that the passions are natural, that their object is happiness, and that their strength depends on the temperament, organization, and degree of imagination. He contended, as did La Mettrie, that a morality appropriate to man must be founded on human nature; "we will not err when we are able to establish a *science des moeurs* on our physical sensibility." Like La Mettrie, he wanted to discount other moral treatises and positions[68] because they were not in accord with human nature. But while La Mettrie emphasized the individual suffering produced by traditional moral systems because they had such a narrow view of human nature, d'Holbach simply suggested an alternative but equally monolithic view of human nature; his key to human nature was sociability. He claimed that society is useful and necessary to happiness; those who claim that the savage is happier than the civilized man are wrong because the savage is nothing but a strong child deprived of reason and experience.[69] According to d'Holbach, man has not degenerated from the state of nature; rather, his nature, which is sociability, has not been sufficiently cultivated. These points likely had Rousseau as their direct target, but La Mettrie, who contended that moral values are the arbitrary constructions of particular societies, was implicitly attacked.

D'Holbach was also intent on stripping the positions he shared with La Mettrie of any dangerous implications. For example, though he claimed that the passions are natural, he insisted that the bad use of them is unnatural. Thus all excess of passion, which he called crime, is contrary to the nature of man. D'Holbach's fundamental premise of man's sociability is a way to avoid the dilemmas posed by La Mettrie. For example, d'Holbach defines virtue as "nothing but the utility of men united in society," and for him the quest for happiness necessarily involves a quest for the happiness of others, that is, the individual's quest will invariably serve the interests of society.

D'Holbach also modified La Mettrie's emphasis on the organic and constitutional effect on morality by saying that though the passions depend on organization, whether the passions were directed to good or evil was not rooted in their organization but in the environment. For example, according to d'Holbach, if Newton had been raised by Tartars, he would have been a ferocious vagabond. Ultimately, for d'Holbach our conduct depends less on organization than on the ideas of true and false to which we have been exposed. He confidently expected that "if education, public opinion, government, and law give only true and sane ideas, it will become as rare to find a perverse man as it now is to find a virtuous one."[70]

La Mettrie would have deplored d'Holbach's positing of sociability as the basis for the ascription of a universal nature without taking into account the plethora of individual constitutions and behaviors, and he would have rejected d'Holbach's underlying premise that evil institutions created evil human beings. Ultimately, d'Holbach had posited a moral system based on an a priori concern for society.

Even those moral theorists who were most intent on denouncing La Mettrie's understanding of human nature as physiologically defined formulated their attacks in ways suggesting that they were responding in detail to his arguments. In De l'Homme, Helvétius took a staunchly sensationalist position which was designed to challenge most of La Mettrie's beliefs about human nature and its relationship to moral issues. He raised in a more consistent, dogmatic, and problematic fashion the environmental roots of evil and the qualities that make us distinctly human, qualities he identified as understanding, virtue, and genius. He determined that our aptitude for understanding was the product of our education, which he defined as the sum of all our experiences. The experiential must, according to Helvétius, be maintained over the interior or the physiological. If understanding were in any way dependent on physiological organization, then man would be determined by the nature of his organism, an understanding of man in general would be much less susceptible to empirical investigation, and the primacy of the individual would weigh heavily against prospects for social reform.

But although Helvétius vehemently denied La Mettrie's emphasis on the importance of the individual constitution, he employed the same kinds of criticisms of social standards of virtue and vice in claiming that notions of virtue depended on where and when we live. He suggested that every age has had different notions of virtue and that these notions have gradually evolved; for example, Old Testament standards of virtue would horrify modern sensibility. Helvétius concurred with La Mettrie that the terms "good," "interest," and "virtue" are arbitrarily employed according to the society in which they are used. But Helvétius saw a correspondence between society and its notion of virtue, not, as La Mettrie did, a fundamental dissonance between individual constitutions and the interests of society. And Helvétius was more optimistic about the civilizing potential of society's notions of virtue and vice.

But to criticize Helvétius's neglect of human physiology Diderot returned in *Réfutation de l'Homme* to many of the points of La Mettrie's treatise. For example, because physiology did not support the claim that men are uniform in ability or simply the product of their sensations, Diderot did not accept education as the means to altering the human character. "In a word, I would very much like to know how education will give warmth to a cold man, verve to a narrow mind, or imagination to him who has none." Even more problematic to Diderot was Helvétius's understanding of human motivation. If sex and power (the narrow sense in which Helvétius discussed the pursuit of pleasure) are the key to understanding human motivation, why did Leibniz spend twenty years in a solitary room working on a differential calculus? Against Helvétius's claim that human beings could be perfected under enlightened political regimes, Diderot pointed to virtuous human beings under the most repressive regimes and claimed that freer societies do not demonstrate widespread virtue, genius, or heroism. Diderot, of course, appreciated Helvétius's advocacy of education and political reform.

However, for him, as for La Mettrie, physiology underscored diversity, and a more reasonable conclusion than those suggested by Helvétius was that each man is led by his particular organization, character, and temperament to prefer to combine some ideas rather than others.[71]

La Mettrie's *Discours* was obviously the critical text for materialist moral theorists, whether they fundamentally agreed or disagreed with him. But although d'Holbach, Helvétius, and Diderot all dealt with moral issues along the lines laid out by La Mettrie, they were very careful to take some measure to set themselves somewhat at odds with him—for example, sociability as innate for d'Holbach, complete malleability for Helvétius, and an uneasy ambiguity between social and individual morality for Diderot. In taking these positions, French materialists both sought to avoid the extremism of La Mettrie and implicitly recognized how close their own views were to his. Ultimately, the unflinching adherence of these three thinkers to materialism was stronger than their desire to conciliate moderate opinion within the philosophic camp. Materialism became a wedge which split the philosophical party, a wedge whose shape can early be discerned in La Mettrie's *L'Homme machine* and *Discours sur le bonheur*.

9

From Philosopher to Philosophe

The Role of the Médecin-Philosophe

I propose to prove that Philosophy, completely contrary as it is to Morality and Religion, cannot destroy these two bonds of society, as one commonly believes, but can only tighten and fortify them more and more.
—La Mettrie, *Discours préliminaire*[1]

The intriguing paradox posed by this quotation, loaded as it is with implications for the nature of religion, morality, politics, and the role of the philosophe, is the fundamental thesis of La Mettrie's last philosophical work, *Le Discours préliminaire*. Written in 1750 as introduction to an edition of his philosophical works, it was also intended to define his philosophy and defend it from the charges of critics that it was pernicious. Thus one might assume that this work would resolve crucial questions of interpretation in La Mettrie's philosophy,[2] especially the fundamental issue of his relationship to the philosophes. However, one is foiled not only by the complexity and confusion typical of much of La Mettrie's work but also by the fundamental paradox he suggested.

One problem that comes to the fore in reading this text is the way in which twentieth-century historiography has dealt with the materialists in general and La Mettrie in particular. Because the materialists were singled out by Marx, they have been held accountable in this century for the practices of communist regimes. As historians have sought the roots of the ills of the twentieth century, especially the rise of totalitarian governments and the Holocaust, the Enlightenment, with its sometimes modern-sounding texts and unfettered attacks on tradition has seemed a good place to locate the beginnings of the modern world: for the good, as in Peter Gay's interpretation, or for ill, as in J. L. Talmon's work. But La Mettrie's moral philosophy, with its hedonism and its overt challenge to traditional moral systems, has been singled out by historians as responsible for the development of nihilism and its attendant political ills.[3] It is difficult to extricate La Mettrie's moral philosophy from these polemical and ideological analyses.

The reading of the *Discours préliminaire* is further complicated by the conventional understanding of La Mettrie's philosophy in general and in particular by the remarks made by the philosophes to distance themselves from the too-radical La Mettrie after his death in 1751. The conventional reading of the *Discours préliminaire* assumes that La Mettrie intended to conciliate political and religious authorities by arguing that philosophy could not undermine the religious or social order and that his specific purpose in writing the treatise was to persuade the French authorities to allow his return to France or, at the very least, to ensure the continued protection of Frederick the Great.[4] This interpretation is often used to deny La Mettrie the status of philosophe. If La Mettrie was sincere in taking this position, then he is taken to be an anti-philosophe. But if expediency motivated him, that is, if he wrote this treatise merely to influence friends in high places, then it is claimed that he was too craven to be a philosophe. Ultimately this latter interpretation reads La Mettrie out of the camp of the eighteenth-century philosophes, and because of his apparent appeal to the established authorities he is considered to more accurately mirror the intellectual attitudes of the seventeenth-century *libertin* tradition.[5]

There is some circumstantial evidence for this. La Mettrie might well have considered caution a wise course in 1750. The publication of *Le Discours sur le bonheur* had already provoked Frederick's disapproval.[6] A desire to appease him might well have led La Mettrie to write the final passage of the *Discours préliminaire*, which upheld Frederick as a model of the way rulers should treat philosophes, that is, offering them shelter and encouraging the free expression of ideas.[7] Scholars have accordingly assumed that the opposition of the philosophes to this work was provoked by the reactionary political position it articulated. La Mettrie's argument that philosophy has no influence is also taken to consign him to the ranks of armchair thinkers of the seventeenth century rather than the *philosophes engagés* of the eighteenth.

However, there are several serious problems with this interpretation. First, to deny La Mettrie any connection to the philosophes on this basis fails to note that many of his arguments were those used by the philosophes themselves. Second, La Mettrie's argument that philosophy could not undermine religion or society was not nearly conservative enough to garner support from eighteenth-century civil or religious authorities.[8] Third, to claim that the *Discours préliminaire* offers support for despotism or is a plea to civil authority mistakes a bit of self-protecting rhetoric attached to this work, almost as an afterthought, for its substance. Fourth and most important, this argument completely disregards the second half of the treatise, which is essentially a panegyric to the philosophe.

To resolve these problems, it is necessary at the outset to acknowledge the seriousness of La Mettrie's purpose, which militates against any argument that either part of the work is disingenuous and compels one to accept it as the *whole* La Mettrie evidently considered it to be. He wrote this treatise to justify his entire philosophical effort. Forthright and earnest in style, the entire treatise aims to be persuasive, and therefore it is also necessary to look to the response La Mettrie expected from his readers. He acknowledged that the work presented a paradox. But with a confidence in his readers that the reception seems to belie, he claimed that though his paradox appears difficult "at first glance, I do not believe, however, after all that has been said here, that profound reflections will be necessary to resolve it."[9] Perhaps La Mettrie's confidence in his readers ought to raise the question of just whom he was addressing and why he used the paradox.

By what audience might both parts of La Mettrie's paradox have been well received? To whom might La Mettrie have wanted to make his philosophy better known and acceptable? With what group might he have wanted to identify in 1750? The obvious answer, and one that might make it possible to reconcile both parts of La Mettrie's treatise, is the philosophes.[10] The reading of La Mettrie's treatise that I would like to develop here contends that in the first part of his treatise La Mettrie attempted to overcome the opposition of the philosophes to his more radical philosophy by using the arguments they frequently made to vindicate theirs, in particular, the argument that philosophy could not affect the masses. In the second part of the treatise, La Mettrie identified himself completely with the philosophic movement; as if, once he had persuaded the philosophes that his radical materialism, like their own works, could not affect the masses who might misconstrue them, he could freely proclaim himself a philosophe in exile. He thus addressed *en philosophie* issues of critical importance to the developing *mouvement philosophique*, such as the place of the philosophe in society, the most effective means for bringing about Enlightenment, and whether a program for Enlightenment was more effectively directed to the elites or the masses. As a philosophe he maintained that philosophy was the means to reform every art by scrutinizing it in light of reason. The philosophe was, in the terms of his materialist physiology, constitutionally predisposed to the exercise of reason and also a model of probity. The philosophe should therefore have the authority to reform institutions so that they might be more reasonable. As a philosophe in exile, La Mettrie thus defined his task as the encouragement of his beleaguered brothers in France.

Philosophy Poses No Danger

At the very outset of the first part of his argument, La Mettrie proclaimed the critical importance of philosophy as the scientific quest for truth and the application of reason, a definition of philosophy and its role that would have appealed to the philosophes. Philosophy, like "la vraie médecine," was completely grounded in natural phenomena. He also defined philosophy as inherently good and utilitarian. "What a frightful light would be that of philosophy if it only enlightened those who are such a small number by the destruction and ruin of the others who compose the entire universe."[11] Both these definitions seem to embody the philosophes' sense of themselves as carrying out a scientific method for the public good.

La Mettrie warned of the danger to society that the suppression of philosophy would entail: all of science would be without practical use. The "flambeau de physique" would be extinguished, and collections of "curieuses observations" would be rendered completely insignificant if philosophy were prevented from examining them with the light of reason. Such a proscription would also prohibit all discussion of human nature. "Can't one even try to guess and explain the enigma of man?"[12] he asked. Furthermore, to suppress philosophy was to deny entirely the importance of reason. Although he himself questioned the notion of grounding moral systems on the premise that all men were reasonable or sought happiness through reason,[13] La Mettrie did not disparage reason. In this treatise he, like many of the philosophes, made it the hope for man and society. The suppression of philosophy then was tantamount to a declaration that reason was a superfluous human appendage. The effect of such a suppression on society La Mettrie described in harsh terms. "To sustain this system is to wish to break and degrade humanity; to believe that truth is better left eternally entombed in the breast of nature than to be one day brought to light is to favor superstition and barbarism."[14]

La Mettrie has radically reappraised and redefined his notion of philosophy from his early medical works, where he saw the intervention of philosophical disputes into medicine as introducing irrelevant metaphysical concerns that served no practical purpose and fostered senseless factionalism. Indeed, the preceding passage points to philosophy as a benefit to humanity and as a weapon against superstition and barbarism, clear points of affinity with the development of the philosophical movement. This reappraisal seems to involve less a change of heart than the application to the concerns of the philosophes of his own redefinition of philosophy, which had been produced by his concern with medical issues. The medical controversies of the 1730s convinced him of the vanity of medical authorities and the importance of empiricism as an essential corrective to medical system-making. His own medical works impressed upon him the necessity of introducing reason into medical opinion and systems. His satires and his medical experience led him to describe an ideal medical practitioner, the *médecin-philosophe*, a man of learning, but even more important, a man of wide-ranging experience who sees medicine as the means to ameliorate some of the ills of mankind rather than to advance his social status. In fact, the physician had to be a philosophe, a model of probity and a practitioner of reason.

In his earlier philosophical works, La Mettrie indicated the results that could be attained by the work of such a philosophe. He himself had cleared the philosophical ground of metaphysical impediments to allow the unfettered investigation of nature. Without those impediments, man could be placed within nature and the implications for human society understood as part of nature could be freely explored. Thus, La Mettrie's definition of the "philosophe en médecine" is far removed from his earlier assessment of the value of philosophy; his notion of the philosopher has evolved into a repudiation of the seventeenth-century metaphysician and an appreciation of the new philosophy of the eighteenth-century philosophe. This new philosophy, instead of applying the arid "esprit de système" of the seventeenth-century metaphysician to arcane issues, uses reason in an "esprit systèmatique" to work for the amelioration of the human condition.[15] This new definition of philosophy, based on reason and science and directed towards utilitarian, practical ends, is well in accord with the understanding the philosophes had of themselves and their mission. By putting his own work into the context of the Enlightenment, La Mettrie was pointing out the crucial role his philosophy had played in laying the groundwork for subsequent philosophical investigation.

Thus the activist and reformist stance of his *philosophe engagé* decisively puts La Mettrie into the camp of the philosophe, in terms of both his own self-definition and his explicit agenda for reform. That is not to deny that his work is considerably influenced by seventeenth-century thinkers in general and the *libertin* tradition in particular. As Ann Thomson rightly points out, La Mettrie found some of the ideas held by *libertin* thinkers attractive. For example, he acknowledged *libertin* thinkers whose appreciation of refined sensual pleasures had influenced his own work, especially *La Volupté*, and he shared with the *libertins* a skeptical attitude toward religion and a rather pessimistic view of human nature.[16] But these acknowledged affinities do not make La Mettrie one of them. First of all, his aggressive materialism and forthright atheism were at odds with the deism of the *libertins*.[17] The character of his materialism also evinces a desire to proselytize and an activism completely foreign to the passive and resigned *libertin*. La Mettrie also criticized those who did not share his reformist concerns. For example, he disparagingly dismissed Fontenelle as a mere *bel esprit*, someone not sufficiently committed to reform.[18] Like other philosophes, La Mettrie's debts to the *libertin* tradition were extensive; he built on their skepticism and irreverence and turned it into an activist, reformist notion of philosophy. However, it seems particularly strange that the influence of the *libertins* has been thought to provide sufficient grounds on which to consign La Mettrie to the rank of a retrograde, armchair philosopher arguing for the status quo and advocating social conformism, when in this treatise he sounded an unequivocal battle cry for reform.[19]

La Mettrie would not allow his reader or any authority to be lulled into the false sense that the philosophy he extolled was a conservative one. For, as he maintained throughout his philosophical work, to think "en philosophe" invariably meant to be a materialist. And his argument that philosophy could not destroy religion, far from being reactionary or even conciliatory, was so radical that perhaps the only audience that would not have been completely outraged was the philosophes. Like many of them, La Mettrie assumed that religious beliefs were essentially myths constructed by priests and theologians, "la fruit arbitraire de la politique." These beliefs were perpetuated as the "received ideas" or prejudices passed from one generation to another. Thus they were completely relative and in no way relevant to the philosophical quest for truth in nature and through reason. That does not mean that because all political systems are divorced from truth the existing systems are thereby sanctioned, as Thomson suggests.[20] While philosophes will not, according to La Mettrie, look to political systems for truth, neither will they allow to go unchallenged any claims made by political or religious authorities to represent the truth. Specifically, philosophy as reason applied to nature will expose the groundless bases of theological dogma and challenge the claims to truth of the theologians and moral theorists.[21] So when La Mettrie argued that philosophy posed no threat to religion, it was because the two addressed different concerns (philosophy truth and theology myth), not because he endorsed the status quo and certainly not because he repudiated his fundamental materialist position. It seems inconceivable that any religious authority would have been deceived by this argument. In fact the response to this treatise was outraged and vociferous, and it was by no means placated by La Mettrie's protestations of innocence. The Faculty of Theology cited La Mettrie's *Discours préliminaire* in its condemnation of Helvétius's *De l'Esprit*, and the argument of the *Discours préliminaire* was explicitly cited in Pope Clement VII's decree of 1770 condemning La Mettrie.[22] The adamant declaration of materialism which runs through this treatise precludes any possibility that La Mettrie intended to be conciliatory.

But the philosophes would have recognized that La Mettrie was making overt some of their veiled anti-religious arguments. In fact, because La Mettrie frequently cites Voltaire's *Lettres philosophiques*, it is possible that he took Voltaire's claim in his letter on Locke as a model. As Voltaire put it, "we should never fear that any philosophical opinion could harm the religion of a country. Let our Mysteries be contrary to our demonstrations, they are no less revered for it by Christian philosophers, who know that matters of reason and matters of faith are different in nature."[23] The philosophes, however, concentrated their attack on the power of the church and some of the superstitions they saw as obstacles to Enlightenment. They were not as determined as La Mettrie to attack the notion of the soul as an impediment to understanding human nature, nor were they as inclined to challenge the moral authority of the church. Voltaire in particular wanted to preserve some of the traditional moral beliefs of the Catholic church in order to control the masses, claiming, for example, that "the common good of mankind requires that we believe the soul immortal; faith commands it; nothing is more necessary and the question is settled."[24]

La Mettrie also went further than virtually any other philosophe, claiming that moral values belonged to the category of arbitrary myths promulgated by theologians, which had only mistakenly come to be considered a part of philosophy. One of the principal aims of the *Discours préliminaire* was to establish this point so that "all the efforts one has made to reconcile philosophy with morality and theology will appear frivolous and impotent." (The philosophes were similarly intent on separating theology and philosophy, but not philosophy and morality.) La Mettrie argued the benefit to mankind of recognizing the break between philosophy and religion, for philosophy would certainly destroy the groundless belief in the soul. "I would dare to say that all the rays that flow from the breast of nature, fortified and as if reflected by the precious mirror of philosophy, destroy and turn to dust a dogma that is only founded on some pretended moral utility."[25] He placed this argument clearly within the context of his philosophy as a whole; he reaffirmed his definition of philosophy as reason applied to nature, argued for medicine as the epitome of this endeavor, and claimed that any attempt to consider man as anything but the most complexly organized animal could be dismissed as an appeal to the *amour-propre* of man.

La Mettrie also used the arguments of the philosophes to claim that philosophy did not and could not rupture the chains that bound men together in society. But he based them on convictions derived from his materialist philosophy, rather than on expediency, as most of the philosophes did. Because his arguments on this point are better developed and more earnest than those of the philosophes, it has generally been assumed that La Mettrie's bear no relationship to theirs and that he was arguing for the inefficacy of philosophy in a way that would have undermined the entire philosophic endeavor. Those scholars who have emphasized the antisocial nature of La Mettrie's moral philosophy have contended that he was not simply arguing that philosophy cannot harm society but rather that the position he took in the *Discours sur le bonheur* forced him to espouse complete social and political conformism in the *Discours préliminaire* as the only possibility for a philosophic public policy. But the text does not support such a conclusion. One must see instead, as La Mettrie did, that the work of the philosophe is difficult, that it is hampered in fundamental ways. The philosophe must recognize the fundamentally arbitrary nature of religion, social structures, and moral values. However, these social institutions should be scrutinized by philosophical inquiry (as he himself did in the *Discours sur le bonheur*), and reform, though limited, is possible (the case he will argue in *Discours préliminaire*).

Because his point was not to argue for social or political conformism but rather to make common cause with the philosophes, La Mettrie employed their very arguments to convince them that his philosophy, more radical than theirs by virtue of his willingness to draw out the implications, could be accepted as the fruit of scientific investigation without fear of the effect this philosophy might have on the people. In other words, even though the philosophes might find his philosophy objectionable, and many certainly did, they should not fear its effect on the people. He claimed that a philosophical position, no matter how radical, could have very little hope of influencing the ignorant masses. This argument is sometimes construed as reassurance to rulers that their realms will remain intact no matter what conclusion philosophers reach, but it also seems to reflect, in La Mettrie's case, a fundamental pessimism about the ability of any philosophy to modify general human behavior.

La Mettrie's use of Bayle highlights some of the problems inherent in his attempt to use the arguments of the philosophes.[26] Bayle serves him as the preeminent example of the virtuous atheist, one who espoused dangerous ideas but lived a virtuous life himself and did not proselytize or spread dissension among the people. Other philosophes likewise invoked the name of Bayle to make these points. But La Mettrie also used Bayle's arguments to contend that the radical philosophical stance of atheism produced model citizens.[27] Instead of leading to blind debauchery, atheism produced enlightened reflection. Atheists were in fact *more* likely to be virtuous citizens because, he staunchly maintained, the principles of probity were completely unrelated to those of religion. In fact, the practice of virtue could sink deeper roots in the heart of the atheist because his acceptance of the social standards was based on reason rather than on the more emotional, more suspect practices dictated by the "coeur dévot." Atheism was also beneficial to society; it did not lead to the contentiousness of Christendom because atheists did not presume to scrutinize and criticize the morals of others. Atheism was also beneficial to the individual, producing "the tranquility of a Virgil rather than the fears of hell of a monk."[28]

By taking the typical philosophical endorsement of Bayle's virtuous atheist and driving it to the more extreme position that atheists made better citizens, La Mettrie in effect exposed the dangers implicit in the arguments of the philosophes. For while the good citizenship of individual atheists might support the innocuousness of philosophy, the explicit argument that atheism produced better citizens than Christianity came too close to proselytizing for atheism and could only call into question more conservative arguments and less radical uses of Bayle's name.

La Mettrie used his own philosophy to demonstrate the irrelevance of philosophy to life. For example, he argued in *Discours sur le bonheur* that remorse was simply a prejudice engendered by education and that man was a machine imperiously determined.[29] He admitted that he might be wrong on these points, but he believed he was correct and went on to ask what difference it made. "All these questions can be put in the class of mathematical points, which exist only in the heads of geometers!"[30] His philosophical position would thus have no effect on the general populace or even on the conduct of his own life. Even if one regards materialism, or the determinism implicit in materialism, as a dangerous philosophy, it has too narrow an influence to do any harm. This argument is obviously meant to justify his philosophy: the moral position he articulated in the *Discours sur le bonheur* was not intended to injure the people or undermine society, nor was his argument for tolerance of the criminal intended to extol the crime.

La Mettrie sought for himself the same tolerance the philosophes accorded Bayle, the outstanding example of the man of proven probity but radical ideas, by comparing his own character to that of his detractors, most notably Albrecht Haller, "le vil Gazetier de Göttingen,"[31] and by urging the distinction between citizen and philosophe employed by many philosophes. He claimed that in the practice of philosophy one sought truth, but as a citizen one did not preach this truth to crowds because they, unprepared for it, would be likely to misconstrue it. Falsehood was the general nourishment of men in all ages, and La Mettrie saw it as the means appropriate "to conduct this vile troop of mortal imbeciles."[32] To speak philosophically to the multitude was to prostitute an august science by addressing those who had not been initiated and were thus incapable of understanding philosophy or applying it in their lives. For La Mettrie, as for Kant in *Was ist Aufklärung?*,[33] the proper means of disseminating philosophical ideas was through the written word, because written ideas would make their way into an illiterate population slowly, bringing philosophy "by degrees." La Mettrie also vehemently defended the character of the philosophe, as Diderot later did, as inherently virtuous. For example, Diderot claimed in "Les Sages" that the moral conscience of the philosophe is in perfect accord with the "morale universelle" because he is the physiologically perfect example of the human species.[34] Both Diderot and La Mettrie made the claim because they shared the same medical notion, derived from their physiological understanding of man, of the importance of the individual constitution. According to La Mettrie, although the philosophe shares the failings of others, he is less inclined to crime and disorder because even though he might espouse *volupté*, his passions, "constrained by the compass of wisdom," are better regulated than those of other men. The philosophe is a model of humanity and probity even while writing against natural law, as La Mettrie himself had done. "Let us not accuse the philosophe of disorder, of which he is incapable,"[35] La Mettrie advised.

But, according to La Mettrie, even if the philosophes were inclined to harangue crowds on the street, they would not have much influence. Although the people sometimes seem to accept the arguments of the philosophes, they usually take on only superficial mannerisms and gestures that would eventually be overcome by their stronger habits. (The stronger habits were those based on the constitution of the individual; the weaker, those acquired by education.) La Mettrie held out some limited hope of reform in suggesting that one must be prepared for enlightenment "by degrees," which left open the possibility that the more recently acquired "façon de penser" could eventually become the stronger.

But because of his sensationalist understanding of how we learn—that is, the strength of an idea was related to the strength of the sensation which produced it—La Mettrie considered this to be an improbable development. Only consistent and striking exposure to philosophical ideas could drag the masses out of the morass of ignorance. Both the common constitutional predisposition and the weight of received opinion fostered ignorance, so that it was doubly difficult to eliminate. In order to be effective, the philosopher would first have to overcome the prejudices of the people. Not even the eloquence of Cicero, La Mettrie contended, would be sufficient to sway the masses from received ideas. But the people rarely associated with philosophers or read their books, so it was difficult for them to acquire new habits of action or thought. Were they to come in contact with the works of philosophes, "either they would understand nothing or, if they understood something, they would not believe a word of it."[36] When Voltaire decided to come to the defense of Helvétius in the aftermath of the publication of *De l'Esprit*, he too proclaimed the innocuous character of the philosophe, saying that it seemed most unreasonable that a work containing "pauvre et inutile" philosophical truths that would be read only by the few should be suppressed when the works of all the philosophes would do less damage than one inflammatory placard.[37] Voltaire also claimed that philosophy would be unlikely to reach the masses: "Divide the human race into twenty parts. Nineteen of them are composed of those who work with their hands, and will never know if there is a Locke in the world or not. In the remaining twentieth part how few men do we find who read! And among those who read there are twenty who read novels for every one who studies philosophy."[38] La Mettrie postulated a radical difference between the character of the people and the philosopher, as if "one were low notes and the others high notes, one *basse-taille*, the other *haute couture*. These are two physiognomies which never resemble each other." While the philosophes are refined, the people are "crude, just as they left the hands of nature. Once the fold is made, it will remain; it is not easier for the one [the people] to raise himself than for the other to descend."[39]

Other philosophes also defined themselves as distinct from the masses.[40] For example, the author of the article entitled "Le Philosophe" in the *Encyclopédie* made this distinction: "The philosophe forms his principles on the basis of an infinite number of individual observations. The people adopts the principle without thinking about the observations which produced it: It believes that the maxim exists, as it were, by itself." He also noted that not all people were equally susceptible to Enlightenment. "Other men are driven by their passions, without reflection preceding their actions. These are men who walk in shadows. On the other hand, even in passionate moments, the philosophe acts only after reflection; he walks at night, but a torch precedes him."[41] Voltaire contended that "the people will always be composed of brutes" and "the people is between man and beast."[42]

La Mettrie, like other philosophes, was concerned to ascertain the proper means of disseminating the new philosophy, and like them he made distinctions in terms of receptivity between the educated elites and the masses. He saw the inability of the masses to be enlightened as a defense of his own philosophy; he denied that it could be dangerous or have a pernicious effect because it would not reach or influence the common man. He drew the same sharp distinction between the philosophes and the masses that other philosophes made. But the philosophes were less likely than La Mettrie to couch that distinction in terms of a constitutional proclivity or predetermination. The philosophes might well have been unwilling to suggest a gap between themselves and the people as inveterate as that suggested by two physiognomies.

La Mettrie also differed with the philosophes about the degree to which ignorance was responsible for the chasm between the philosophe and the people. The philosophes, unlike La Mettrie, were more inclined to consider ignorance, brutishness, and moral failings to be the result of one's condition rather than one's constitution. Since for the philosophes the people were not constitutionally confined to their lowly and depraved place, they were able to be enlightened to some degree. For example, Helvétius, one of the philosophes most optimistic about such prospects, confidently proclaimed, "Destroy ignorance and all the germs of moral evil will be destroyed."[43]

But La Mettrie had a rather different perspective on the relationship of the philosophe to the people; he did not recognize a degeneration produced by corrupt political systems but rather acknowledged the intrinsic limitations of the aberrant physiological constitution. Because of the inveterate nature of physiological predispositions, La Mettrie was neither naive nor optimistic about reform. By raising the questions provoked by the ill or the aberrant, La Mettrie crystallized the problematic relationship between physiology and the philosophic plans for reform. But despite the fact that La Mettrie identified himself as first and foremost a physician, he also proclaimed himself to be a man of letters. Like other philosophes, he had the sense that he was breaking new ground intellectually and that if his positions were unpopular posterity would nevertheless vindicate him. Despite his sense that progress would be difficult and limited, La Mettrie saw reason as the vehicle of progress, and he shared the philosophes' "passion for the public good." He advocated the implementation of empirical methods to study man and based his own understanding of man on scientific evidence.

La Mettrie and the philosophes differed on the issue of Christian morality. For the philosophes, as for La Mettrie, *le peuple* were hampered in their chances for enlightenment by the traditional myths to which they adhered. These, most notably the myths associated with Christianity, gave the people a moral code. Though the philosophes generally battled the strictures of that code and certainly challenged the right of any ecclesiastical authority to impose it, they nonetheless acknowledged the usefulness of these myths in maintaining social control. So while they were often willing to make and accept just the distinction La Mettrie here made between the writings of the philosophe and his life as a citizen, they were not generally willing to follow La Mettrie into the argument that all moral values were simply predicated on social utility. Though they did acknowledge in their historical accounts of the development of society that morality was based in part on the impositions of the powerful or the devious (a description most often assigned to the clergy), and though some of them accepted the cultural relativism of moral codes, nonetheless, for most of the philosophes, a prescriptive natural law or an innate sense of right and wrong was thought to underlie all moral notions.

Ultimately the arguments the philosophes made about the limited efficacy of philosophy were at least somewhat disingenuous, disguising their real hopes for Enlightenment and seeking, more earnestly than La Mettrie in his appeal to Frederick, to mollify established authorities. Their arguments then were designed at least in part to lull authorities into complacency so that the work of Enlightenment could proceed unimpeded. And while they expressed their exasperation with the receptivity of the people and the slow progress of Enlightenment, they believed more strongly than La Mettrie in people's educability and the feasibility of Enlightenment. La Mettrie, on the other hand, used the same sorts of arguments, but because he supported them with his materialism they could not have allayed the fears of any authority about the implications of Enlightenment. And with his sense of a predetermined constitutional proclivity and the propensity of the masses towards invincible ignorance, La Mettrie, while using the arguments of the philosophes, at the same time raised serious obstacles to Enlightenment and limited the possibility of reform.

Although La Mettrie did not persuade the philosophes, he couched his arguments in terms whose implications were immediately apparent to them and not at all congenial to his critics. And thus it cannot be assumed that La Mettrie's arguments are in essence responses, albeit ineffectual responses, to the horror expressed in the German periodical press.[44] Nor is it reasonable, given the nature of his self-defense, to assume that they were directed at either those critics or established authorities. But if the argument was directed to the philosophes, it was a notable failure; the philosophes not only did not embrace him, they vehemently repudiated him.

There are several possible explanations for the lack of success of La Mettrie's appeal to the philosophes. First of all, the fact that his philosophy, which most of the philosophes considered to be pernicious and a great danger to society, could be proclaimed as innocent by using the same arguments they launched to vindicate their own more moderate positions exposed a critical weakness in their defense. If La Mettrie could turn those arguments to his advantage, it would expose the entire philosophic movement to criticism. Secondly, because the philosophes made these arguments at least somewhat disingenuously, they would likely have found a perfectly serious presentation unconvincing and suspect. Furthermore, La Mettrie's formulation of the argument, especially in conjunction with his materialist notion of man, curtailed expectations of reform to a degree the philosophes would have found unacceptable. Ultimately, and perhaps most crucial, the philosophes simply did not believe that radical arguments about the relativity of vice and virtue and against remorse could be made without danger. They would have considered any attempt, like that of the *Discours préliminaire*, to connect their philosophy with La Mettrie's radical materialism dangerous to their cause, especially in those early years of the encyclopedic movement. But if the philosophes were not persuaded by La Mettrie's use of their own arguments, could they fail to respond to the second part of his treatise, a rousing exhortation directed to them?[45]

The Merits of Philosophy

La Mettrie explicitly identified his own philosophy with the developing philosophic movement by claiming that philosophy by its very nature bestowed benefits on society and by endorsing the philosophe as the architect of the reform of social institutions. He exhorted rulers to recognize the virtues of philosophy and proclaimed the authority of the philosophes to propose reforms. He praised the efforts of the philosophes and urged them to greater feats of daring.

La Mettrie defined the philosophe in terms of his materialist philosophy; the philosophe was one of the select few described in the *Discours sur le bonheur*, blessed by nature with a constitution inclined to reason. Since La Mettrie, like most of the philosophes, was perfectly willing to equate reason and progress, this reasonableness precluded any possibility that the philosophe could be a revolutionary, since philosophy equaled truth and *lumière*, forces that according to his definition could not work toward the destruction but only the amelioration of the human condition. (Presumably revolution is inherently destructive but reform inherently productive, and thus reform was the focus and the product of the activities of rational men.) In other words, the character of the philosophe, by which La Mettrie meant a physiological constitution, guaranteed that philosophy could not have a destructive effect on either religion or society. However, the limited efficacy of the philosopher had, as La Mettrie made more explicit in this part of his treatise, as much to do with his style as with the substance of his message. The philosophe, because he was reasonable, inevitably had to question theological absurdities. But as a model of probity, he would refute those absurdities without resorting to the contentious wrangling of the theologians. As far as the political sphere was concerned, La Mettrie, in this part of the treatise, modified his original assessment of the benign effect of the philosophe on the social order; this modification would have had the support of the philosophes. Though they could not by definition destroy, the philosophes, also by definition, would certainly work in accord with reason to improve social and political conditions. The interests of the philosophes were clearly not to be directed toward bolstering any particular regime but rather toward ascertaining and promoting the interests of society.

Though the philosophes would inevitably confront in their labors the intransigence of society and government as well as the almost insurmountable ignorance of the people, they were, La Mettrie claimed, the key to any hope for reform in the social and political order. The inherent reasonableness of the philosophe made him knowledgeable, indeed seemingly omniscient, in determining the need for reform. This acute perceptive faculty was the result of the philosophe's ability to reason, to think in a clear and orderly fashion. Reform would be motivated by a desire to modify political and social institutions so that they would be more in accord with reason. Reason was both the key to the virtuous character of the philosophe and the guarantor of the benefits to be derived from the crusade for reform. The license La Mettrie granted to the philosophe to act as social reformer was highly unlikely to win him approval from civil authorities. Nor would his simplistic sense of reform as productive and revolution as counterproductive have provided guidelines for concrete reform or allayed the fears of rulers who feared it.

Although he sanctioned the philosophe as the agent of political and social improvement, La Mettrie did not envisage sweeping reform. Never unaware of the effect of the individual constitution, he conceded that the number of individuals amenable to the influence of reason would be few. If social institutions were made more rational, then those who were constitutionally susceptible to the influence of reason would be able to modify their way of thinking. The gap between the irrational social instincts of the people and the reasonableness of the philosophe was a factor he quite clearly pointed out in the first part of his treatise. But he also defined the philosophes as the bridge between past and future, between the arbitrary social institutions of the present and the more reasonable social institutions of the future. Although he made no attempt to describe the abuses of the old order or project the improvements of the new, nonetheless, in the second part of his treatise, La Mettrie clearly argued the benefits of philosophy and sounded a rallying cry for the philosophes, maintaining that philosophy exerted a beneficial role in all aspects of life. "As it is she [philosophy] who treats the body in medicine, it is she also who treats the laws, the spirit, the heart and the soul, etc. It is she who directs the art of thinking, by the order she puts in our ideas. It is she who serves as the basis of the art of speaking, and involves herself usefully in jurisprudence, in morality, in metaphysics, in rhetoric, in religion, etc."[46]

Furthermore, philosophy, as the use of reason in the pursuit of truth, could serve as the critical test for determining where truth was to be found, for "it is sometimes possible to draw the truth from an impenetrable well in which it was formerly placed. Philosophy will show it to us." La Mettrie described this role of philosophy in chemical terms. "It is the touchstone of solid thoughts, of just reasoning, the crucible in which everything foreign to nature evaporates." Although philosophy might prove ineffectual in altering the habits of the masses, La Mettrie nonetheless endowed the philosophe with near omniscience in the ability to detect what was false, not simply in the abstract but also as applied to social institutions. He proclaimed that "it [philosophy] has a fixed point by which to judge sanely what is honest or dishonest, equitable or unjust, vicious or virtuous; it discovers the error and the injustice of laws and shelters the widow and the orphan from the traps of this Siren."[47] Thus philosophy alone provides the perspective from which to judge social institutions.

La Mettrie's political philosophy was clearly not an endorsement of the status quo or an argument for social conformity. To say that philosophy cannot harm society does not entail that the philosophe will therefore accept uncritically its conventions. And while the philosophe by his character, according to La Mettrie, is incapable of disorder, that character does not make him passive, complacent, or withdrawn from the concerns of society, but rather the appropriate agent of a philosophical examination of the social sphere. The activism implicit in this argument—that the philosophe cannot harm society but will certainly reform it—is a quality the philosophes would certainly have understood and supported, in part because the argument was one they were inclined to make on their own behalf. Instead of responding by retreating or being indifferent, the philosophe, La Mettrie insisted, accepts the fact that the laws are continually in need of reform, a need produced when the right of reason is undermined by the right of power. Who but the philosophe can reform the law? he asked. It is the task of the philosophe to guide the laws back to "le point fixe" which all social and institutional reforms must seek to reinstate.[48]

The notion of a "point fixe" seems to refute the relativity of moral notions that La Mettrie had so adamantly asserted. Although he denied the existence of a principle of natural law, he also seemed to acknowledge that, because social institutions were in need of reform, some must be "better" than others, which must also imply that those that were "better" must come closer to fulfilling some definition of the "good." However, La Mettrie continued to maintain that this was not a moral notion; instead, "the balance of wisdom and the interests of society is the fixed point from which the philosophe can distinguish just from unjust."[49]

Though the philosopher would seek to reform social institutions, La Mettrie insisted that he posed no threat to society, for the reforms he would suggest would necessarily be in the interest of society. "One may say of them [the laws] and all human actions that those which are just or equitable are those which favor society; that those alone which injure its interests are unjust."[50] This amorphous, nonspecific assessment of the philosophes' role is both an indication of La Mettrie's attempt to identify with the cause of the philosophes and the product of his own philosophy. The authority he confers on the philosophes and his confidence in their ability to discern the best interests of society reflect his idealized version of philosophy as reason and the character of the philosophe as the manifestation of the constitution predisposed toward the cultivation of reason. However, he developed no program of reform. He did not, as later philosophes did, describe an ideal legislator. Instead he simply suggested that, in much the same way that the physician can detect illness, the philosophes will detect injustice in the law and propose the remedy for it. Like his moral philosophy, La Mettrie's general philosophy here again seems quite remote from that of the philosophes because he developed no political philosophy. He did not discuss the role of the individual in society, and though the philosophes are proclaimed as agents of reform he did not investigate the role of particular institutions in society or propose any concrete ramifications of the philosophes' role as legislators. He did not offer any guidelines as to what "rational" institutions would be like or how they would differ from contemporary, presumably irrational institutions.

Despite this nebulous sense of what the application of philosophy to social and political institutions might entail, La Mettrie was wholehearted in his endorsement of philosophy because, by its very nature, it is always beneficial to the individual and society. "Fire does not dilate a body more than philosophy ennobles the spirit." Even the most outrageous, radical philosophy, like his materialism, produced a positive effect on the individual and society, for it "increased the public enlightenment and diffused *l'esprit* throughout the world." Even if he were to be proven wrong, exposure to his philosophy would be beneficial to his reader because, as he put it, "in making my reader think, in sharpening his penetration, I extended the limits of his genius, and for that reason alone I do not understand why I have been so ill-welcomed by *les bons esprits*."[51]

In addition to the manifest benefit to those individuals who were exposed to philosophy, the dissemination of philosophy would have a beneficial effect on society at large. La Mettrie took it as axiomatic that "the people will always be easier to lead as the human spirit acquires more force and enlightenment." This statement is sometimes used by scholars as evidence of La Mettrie's support for absolutism and, by extension, modern totalitarianism. But La Mettrie's sense of the philosophe as absolutely incapable of disorder entails that, if society as a whole enjoyed the benefits of the diffusion of reason, it would also become less prone to disorder, including political disorder. And a philosophic examination would, as he maintained in *Discours sur le bonheur*, bring greater understanding and tolerance.[52]

La Mettrie offered specific advice to the philosophes in their quest to reform social institutions. One effective means of reform was to enlighten the princes and their ministers, for the more enlightened they became "the more they would be able to understand the essential difference between their caprice, their tyranny, their laws, their religion, and truth, equity, and justice."[53] La Mettrie also directed an impassioned plea to rulers to acknowledge the benefits that philosophy would bring to their kingdoms by honoring the philosophes and giving them complete freedom. Although his ties to Frederick's court and his suggestion of this kind of philosophical program have branded him as a political reactionary, it must be acknowledged that La Mettrie recognized the urgency of enlightening rulers because he had experienced the danger of living under rulers who were not enlightened or who claimed to be enlightened but were not sufficiently so as to allow a philosopher unfettered freedom of expression. The notion that the philosophes might bring about enlightened social and political institutions by converting men of power and influence to their cause was also the approach Voltaire articulated in the early days of the philosophic movement.[54] La Mettrie seems in fact to define or at least reflect the political stance that most of the philosophes took in 1750, that is, to bring Enlightenment to society through society's rulers. Presumably, those rulers would then reform their social and political institutions and make them more reasonable and tolerant. Even if this is not the most progressive political argument developed in the course of the Enlightenment, it seems scarcely credible to suggest that this treatise was directed to civil authorities who wished to have their failings, their tyrannies, and their caprices pointed out to them!

As the philosophes became disillusioned with despots like Frederick, who pretended to be enlightened only to pursue despotic ends, they abandoned this program, and the political position La Mettrie represented became anathema to some. However, hopes for enlightened despots died hard. As late as 1770, Helvétius penned this panegyric to despots like Frederick: "The horizon of the North becomes every day more bright and effulgent as a Catherine II and a Frederick render themselves dear to humanity. Convinced in their own minds of the value of truth, they encourage the cultivation of it in others."[55]

Even though he suggested the conversion of the princes to the cause of Enlightenment as the political program of the philosophes, La Mettrie also recognized as early as 1750 the pitfalls of such an approach; he specifically noted the imprisonment of Diderot as an example of the risks one ran in assuming that *les grands* were friends of philosophy. Thus he sought to define those dangers and specify the proper relationship of the philosophes to *les grands* and the problem involved in such a relationship much in the way d'Alembert did in his *Essai sur les gens des lettres*.[56] But in his eagerness to protect the integrity of the philosophes against the lure of fame and position, La Mettrie was much more stringent in the restrictions he imposed on them. For example, he claimed that the philosophe must never dissemble, because he is fundamentally a seeker of truth "who does not believe anything imbecilic, anything which does not serve the reason of man." To support or even tacitly accept hypocrisy was, according to La Mettrie, completely unacceptable behavior for the philosophe. It made him "an actor in a comedy unworthy of man." The attraction of public office must also be warily appraised by the philosophe, for "whoever sacrifices the precious gifts of genius to political virtues, trivial and limited, as they all are, could well say that he corrupted his spirit in stupid instinct and his soul in sordid interest." If this refusal to accept prudent hypocrisy and this advice to avoid the perils of public office made life difficult for the philosophe, he could not look to La Mettrie for sympathy, for "the more the sea is covered with foam and notorious for storms, the more I would consider it wonderful to seek immortality across so many perils." La Mettrie ended his discourse with this rousing exhortation to the philosophes: "Let us be free in our writings, as in our actions; let us show there the proud independence of a republican. A timid and circumspect writer serves neither the sciences, nor the human spirit, nor his country."[57]

Though he may have seemed too conservative from the perspective of the 1770s, La Mettrie might have also seemed too outrageous and incautious in his calls for courage. And of course La Mettrie's philosophy itself posed dangers to the philosophes. But he was not completely oblivious to the dangers the philosophes faced; he advised them to "pensez tout haut, mais cachez vous,"[58] an injunction perhaps more difficult to fulfill in Paris than from the comparative safety of Frederick's court.

The philosophes did not eagerly embrace La Mettrie as one of them. His identification with their cause did not even have to be acknowledged because he died so soon after he wrote the treatise and the dangers he came to pose made it foolhardy to suggest a common crusade. Beginning to coalesce as a party around the *Encyclopédie*, the philosophes were acutely aware of the difficulties involved in making that venture acceptable to religious and civil authorities. La Mettrie's remarks were also used by the enemies of the philosophes to discredit them. As a result, the philosophes were so eager to distinguish their philosophy from La Mettrie's that they denounced him as vehemently as did the enemies of the philosophes.

Had the philosophes seriously responded to La Mettrie's attempt to identify with them, they might well have quarreled with his limited sense of the possibilities of reform. Despite the fact that he authorized reform at the hands of the philosophes, La Mettrie was too skeptical about its efficacy; philosophy was ultimately too weak a weapon against ignorance. Even more problematic for the philosophes, his reform would be more constrained by a physiological perspective than by the more typical quest to make laws and institutions reflect natural law.

Although the philosophes did not respond favorably to La Mettrie's attempt to ally with them, nonetheless the *Discours préliminaire* must be acknowledged as a fundamental and timely discussion of the nature and role of the philosophes. It can no longer be seen as an endorsement of the political status quo, and his wholehearted attempt to espouse and speak for the cause of the philosophes calls into question the traditional interpretation of him as an antiphilosophe.

The *Discours préliminaire* must be set in its temporal context; this particular text was composed in 1749 and published in 1750, when the philosophes had not yet organized themselves around the *Encyclopédie*. Most attempts to write La Mettrie out of the Enlightenment are based on attempts to compare his positions with much later, better-developed expressions of a more self-conscious and more coherently organized philosophical party. In this particular text, La Mettrie raised and addressed pivotal issues for the philosophes, advanced the discussions of the nature and purpose of philosophy, and also exposed some of the problems they were forced to confront in a more developed form in the 1770s. Just as La Mettrie set the critical agenda for the discussion of moral issues with his *Discours sur le bonheur*, so too did he raise difficult questions about the nature and purpose of the philosophe in the *Discours préliminaire*.

In justifying his philosophy, La Mettrie not only invoked arguments the philosophes themselves used to define their role and discuss their purposes; he also relied extensively, as did many of the other philosophes, on the definition of "Le Philosophe" which had circulated in an anonymous tract for twenty years before the emergence of the philosophic party.[59] That tract develops many themes that were essential to the philosophes' understanding of themselves and to the argument La Mettrie developed about their nature and concerns in the *Discours préliminaire*. For example, La Mettrie endorsed the notion that the philosophe was the model of probity, endowed with an "esprit de lumière." In almost the very words La Mettrie might have used to describe his own position, this tract claimed that "the philosophe was a machine like other men, but he acted knowing the causes of their movement," and that he recognized that thought, like the ability to see or hear, was completely dependent on the organic constitution. This pamphlet also developed the argument that adherence to religion was not necessary for a virtuous life and noted that the "honnête homme" who did not believe in the afterlife was more likely to behave virtuously than someone who did. The pamphlet also hinted at the abilities of philosophes to reform and to lead. Citing the Emperor Antonius, it noted: "People will be happy when kings are philosophes or when philosophers are kings."[60]

Although La Mettrie shared many of the fundamental points of

"Le Philosophe," he also radicalized others. For example, the text idealized the notion of "penser en philosophe," but La Mettrie explicitly claimed that to "penser en philosophe" was to be a materialist. Unlike the pamphlet, La Mettrie did not idealize human beings; he did not substitute "société civile" for a religious definition of community. The notion of the philosophe presented in the pamphlet was an outgrowth of the humanist tradition and was not explicitly connected to the scientific developments of the eighteenth century that La Mettrie's philosophy so thoroughly developed. "Le Philosophe" was also much more concerned than La Mettrie to use the notion of the philosophe as part of an antireligious polemic against the *dévot*s.

La Mettrie's *Discours préliminaire*, rather than looking backward to the seventeenth century, as is often charged, reworks the notion of the philosophe as defined in this early tract to reflect more specifically the concerns of the developing philosophic movement. Despite his differences with some philosophes over various issues, his endeavor to make common cause with them and to work within the definitions they were just beginning to develop should not be entirely surprising. Because he intended to identify with them, La Mettrie was particularly sensitive to the nuances of their arguments and singularly adept at molding his philosophy to reflect those concerns in the *Discours préliminaire*. (In other texts, where this was not his primary concern, it is much more obvious how La Mettrie differed from the philosophes.)

This text suggests a more positive assessment of the roles and activities of the philosophes in the social sphere, a notion of the philosophe that became more clearly articulated in the course of the 1750s.[61] In particular, La Mettrie's notion of the importance of the character of the philosophe as a model of probity and as a leader in the quest for a reform predicated on the assumptions of progress and toleration was characteristic of the later, activist philosophical party centered around the *Encyclopédie*. Like other adherents to the philosophical party, La Mettrie proclaimed the possibility of reform of social institutions by the philosophes. However, because his approach to these problems was so thoroughly medical, the program he defined was simply that the philosophe was constitutionally able to detect "le point fixe," the proper balance between wisdom and the interests of society. Like other philosophes, he saw toleration as a fundamental goal of reform, but he argued for tolerance towards socially unacceptable behavior rather than for dangerous ideas.

In 1750 La Mettrie, like the philosophical party itself, was poised at a point of transition from criticism to positive activism, from destruction to construction. And La Mettrie clearly understood the positive force that could arise from vehement criticism. Just as his medical satires with their grim denunciations of medical practitioners were intended to clear the way for a new sense of the reformist concerns of the enlightened *médecin-philosophe*, his pessimism about the constitutional proclivities of human beings has as counterpoise his exhortations to the philosophes to reform.

Conclusion

The Legacy of a Medical Enlightenment

Il est vrai que La Mettrie n'est pas philosophe, mais il a de l'esprit et cet esprit vaut bien la philosophie. Il ne vous donnera pas des saines idées, mais il vous guérir de vos vieux préjugés.

—Frederick the Great[1]

La Mettrie's attempts to align himself with the philosophes not only fell on deaf ears but also provoked a decidedly hostile repudiation. The protracted, concerted campaign against La Mettrie by German pietists[2] is perhaps not particularly surprising, although the vehemence of the attack, even in an era of religious polemics, is striking. But the philosophes, even those like Diderot and d'Holbach who shared many of La Mettrie's radical ideas or those who espoused them later or expressed them in unpublished writings, not only did not acknowledge a debt to La Mettrie but also heaped abuse on him.

In the nineteenth century criticisms of La Mettrie became even more vituperative because materialism was anathema, outside the constraints of acceptable discourse. Repudiations of materialism functioned as an effective element of anti-Revolutionary rhetoric in which materialism was opposed to truth and portrayed as the antithesis of natural theology or natural science; conservative politics was tied to conservative science. Because materialism had seemed to play a significant role in the new notions of science boldly set forth in the table of contents of the *Encyclopédie* under the faculty of reason, post-Revolutionary disparagements of materialism attempted to resuscitate the scientific pursuits relegated by Diderot and d'Alembert to the less significant realm of memory, that is, "histories of animals, vegetables, and minerals."[3] This return to earlier notions of science was not accidental. By placing materialism in a pejorative context, more moderate opinions could also be questioned. For example, if materialism was assumed to lead to atheism, then a spectrum of dangerous opinions could be posited with atheism at one end of the continuum, materialism in the middle, and anticlericalism as the starting point for the dangerous descent into error.[4]

Nineteenth-century critics of materialism were particularly vehement in denouncing La Mettrie's character. His posthumous reputation derives largely from his inauspicious manner of dying; contaminated pâté was thought to be the cause, leading his critics to charge him with gluttony. His critics characterized him as immoral or demented, denunciations derived from statements made by the philosophes but now wielded with greater polemical vehemence. They, unlike the philosophes, did not denounce La Mettrie to save themselves but rather to disparage the radical tendencies of the Enlightenment.

While contemporary historians are not generally sympathetic to the political agendas of nineteenth-century ideologues, contemporary assessments of La Mettrie nonetheless often parrot nineteenth-century invective, albeit with moderated vehemence. Historians have generally taken their cue from a long tradition of Enlightenment criticism that rescued some of the philosophes from the unsavoriness of La Mettrie. For example, Sainte-Beuve distinguished sharply between the mechanism of La Mettrie and the vitalism of Diderot, which, according to Sainte-Beuve, cloaked Diderot's latent religiosity.[5] Although more subtle in the distinctions they draw, recent historians have devoted attention to emphasizing slight differences of perspective which allow them to distinguish their subjects from the anathema La Mettrie represented.[6] For example, Vartanian distinguishes Diderot from La Mettrie as more vitalistic than mechanistic.[7] Historians have colluded with their eighteenth-century subjects by trying to substantiate their claims that they were indeed less relativistic, less radical, or even less depraved than La Mettrie. As a result, La Mettrie has been made to appear an antiphilosophe, an idiosyncratic figure completely outside the Enlightenment.

But it seems quite foreign to the spirit of the Enlightenment to look on conformity of opinion as a necessary criterion for influence on or inclusion in the philosophic movement. At times a thinker's self-identification as a proponent of the philosophic movement has been considered the best way to unify the group across such a welter of opinions.[8] After all, the philosophes made many statements that undermine the accepted commonplaces about their beliefs; for example, expressions of pessimism about human nature, denunciations of naive faith in reason, and expressions of intolerance can be found in the writings of Voltaire, Helvétius, and Condillac.[9] Furthermore, on political ideas philosophic opinion ranged from support for monarchy to anarchy, on religious ideas from orthodoxy to atheism, and in literary talent the philosophes ran the gamut from original thinkers to hacks. But despite the diversity of opinion within the philosophical movement, La Mettrie stands as perhaps the only example of someone who identified himself with the philosophes yet was repudiated loudly and repeatedly by those he claimed as confreres.

However, the reason for that rejection lies less in the content of La Mettrie's ideas than in his posthumous role within the Enlightenment, a role which defined and necessitated the thoroughgoing criticism of La Mettrie for the next thirty years. La Mettrie played two crucial roles in the subsequent history of the Enlightenment. By the critics of the philosophes, La Mettrie was portrayed as *the* representative of Enlightenment. As a result the philosophes had to avoid the appearance of resembling him in any respect, a problem which was particularly acute for the materialists, who could more obviously be tarred with the same brush. Even within the philosophic party La Mettrie could be cited as the author of dangerous and insupportable opinions. Moreover, he foreshadowed the danger of a schism between the materialists and the less radical philosophes, a danger which came to the fore in 1770 over the publication of d'Holbach's *Système de la nature*.[10] So throughout the Enlightenment, La Mettrie was a powerful force, always behind the philosophic scene but never acknowledged as a philosophe.

Although La Mettrie clearly identified with the cause of the philosophes, he was not a member of the "little flock" identified by Peter Gay,[11] nor could he be considered a member of "la partie philosophique" as it formed around the *Encyclopédie*. La Mettrie was already dead by 1751 and therefore not a part of the ongoing encyclopedic movement. Furthermore, it is not likely that he would have shared the kind of party loyalty Voltaire tried so hard to foster throughout the 1750s and 60s. La Mettrie never acknowledged in any of his writings that caution, deviousness, or even the expedient use of literary allusion to protect the movement (as well as oneself) might be advisable. (La Mettrie's allusions were either patently obvious or he himself exposed them.)[12] In fact, his recognition of the dangers faced by philosophes seemed only to embolden him. For example, when he faced increasing danger even at Frederick's court, he exhorted the philosophes to behave equally fearlessly in a work which argued that his dangerous philosophy was similar to their more moderate positions. The philosophes could reasonably conclude that with such an advocate they needed no enemies. Voltaire, who sought to forge party unity, to protect the philosophes, and to foster their interests throughout the period of the *Encyclopédie*, found La Mettrie's failure to protect himself or exercise any caution at all particularly exasperating and denounced him vehemently as *fou*.[13]

For the philosophes, La Mettrie's attempt to identify with the burgeoning movement produced horror and outrage in the face of what they perceived as growing political danger. La Mettrie was too incautious in his attacks on orthodoxy and too overt in disseminating radical ideas. Although the similarities between the ideas of Diderot and those of La Mettrie are often acknowledged, Diderot, unlike La Mettrie, was willing and eager to work in the interests of the growing philosophical movement,[14] and he did not publish his works of radical materialist philosophy. Of particular concern to the philosophes, La Mettrie's willingness to draw the radical conclusions from the arguments they used to make their works seem harmless negated their ability to deflect criticism. To both philosophe and antiphilosophe, La Mettrie was the perennial example of the hazards of philosophy. Not only did he expose the philosophes to the danger of persecution or suppression of their works, his own life was a glaring example of the dangers of incaution. La Mettrie's exhortation to courage, written from political exile in Prussia, must have seemed a chilling example of what the excesses of philosophical zeal could reap.

The stories of the reactions of the traditionalist critics and of the philosophes to La Mettrie unfolded together, and the reaction of the philosophes was largely conditioned by the vehemence of his critics. Specifically, the critics of the Enlightenment could argue that just as La Mettrie was the characteristic philosophe, so was irreligion the hallmark of the Enlightenment. In 1752 the connection between irreligion and the encyclopedic movement was substantiated, to the gleeful satisfaction of the philosophes' enemies, when censors determined that certain ideas in Abbé de Prades's thesis, condemned by the theology faculty of the Sorbonne, were discovered to have also appeared in de Prades's *Encyclopédie* article "Certitude." After the defeat of France in the Seven Years' War, the fact that La Mettrie and other philosophes had praised Frederick the Great as a model of the enlightened despot created the suspicion that the philosophes were disloyal to France. The attempt on the king's life by Damiens (1757) was attributed to the promulgation by the philosophes of republican ideas that had undermined respect for the king. This connection was spelled out in a royal edict that stated, "All those who shall be convicted of writing, of having written, or printing any writing intending to attack religion, to rouse opinion, to impair Our Authority and to trouble the order and tranquility of Our State shall be punished by death."[15]

In this particularly perilous time for the philosophes, and for the publishing venture of the *Encyclopédie*, Helvétius published *De l'Esprit*, a work considered subversive by the church and which further inflamed opinion against the philosophes. Initially, the philosophes concluded that discretion was the better part of valor. But late in the affair, Voltaire resolved to support Helvétius. He suggested the establishment of a colony of philosophes remote from public scorn and determined to uncover the plot against the philosophes, concluding that Helvétius must have had enemies in high places who had animated fanatics against him.[16] While this crisis galvanized Voltaire to become a spokesman for the philosophes, Helvétius and the *Encyclopédie* were nonetheless subject to increasingly vehement attacks. On 23 January 1759, the Attorney General harangued members of Parlement, claiming that in *De l'Esprit*, "you are seeing in fact, Messieurs, simply the principles and detestable consequences of many other books published earlier, especially the Encyclopedic Dictionary. The book of *De l'Esprit* is, as it were, the abridgement of this too famous work . . . which has become the book of error."[17]

As the attacks on the philosophes increased in intensity, La Mettrie was consistently invoked as the prototypic philosophe. For example, Guy de Saint-Cyr, in his scathing critique of the philosophes in *Catéchisme à l'usage des Cacouacs* (1758), used a long series of quotations culled from La Mettrie's works to indict the entire philosophic movement. In 1759, when the Faculty of Theology condemned Helvétius's *De l'Esprit*, its censors cited passages drawn from La Mettrie. While the philosophes could be moved to defend Helvétius, an admired if incautious friend, they had no reason to assert their connection or debt to a long-dead, politically dangerous thinker like La Mettrie. The playwright Palissot, in *Les Philosophes* (1762), explicitly claimed that the most outrageous remarks of La Mettrie were characteristic of the philosophes, an argument which provoked Voltaire to write to Palissot that La Mettrie had nothing to do with them. But his protests were to no avail, as critics of the philosophes such as Boncerf continued to attribute La Mettrie's positions to the philosophes in general in order to more effectively denounce them.[18]

But La Mettrie also played an important posthumous role *within* the philosophic party. In the 1770s the radical implications of his philosophy, combined with the role he had played up to this point as a bogeyman used to denounce the Enlightenment in general, made him a key figure in the falling-out among the philosophes over d'Holbach's *Système de la nature*. The philosophes essentially split into two factions over this text in which d'Holbach developed many of the positions taken by La Mettrie. The division within the movement thus made painfully obvious the dangerous ramifications of La Mettrie's philosophy for the philosophic movement.

The battle between the two philosophic factions had been taking form for some time. Ever since the publication of *L'Homme machine*, Voltaire had been monitoring the works of those who claimed to be philosophes but whose works showed signs of materialism. For example, he challenged the materialist and atheist implications of Diderot's *Pensées sur l'interprétation de la nature* and the *Lettres sur les aveugles* as dangers to society.[19] Voltaire's position hardened in response to La Mettrie's *Anti-Sénèque* in his *Poème sur la religion naturelle*, in which he argued that a natural religion was essential to guide human conduct. Ironically, while many of the materialists regarded Voltaire's "Letter on Locke" as a fundamental source of their materialism, Voltaire himself was horrified by the connection between materialism and atheism and invoked materialism only as a weapon to attack the authority of the church.

The philosophes also began to fall out over the question of the best strategy to pursue to gain acceptance for their ideas. Voltaire persisted in his quest to gain the adherence of *les grands*, a position which became progressively less persuasive to the more radical of the philosophes. By the 1760s both Voltaire and Diderot recognized the necessity of uniting the philosophes, but their notions of the tactics to pursue and the philosophy to promote were dramatically different. Voltaire still hoped that the philosophes would be persuaded to return to his leadership, but Diderot hoped to convert the patriarch of Ferney to materialism. The issue that irremediably split the two factions was the issue of whether religion is necessary to inculcate virtue in society. D'Holbach vehemently insisted in his *Système de la nature* that "Il n'y aura jamais qu'un pas du Théisme à la superstition."[20] The fact that La Mettrie had twenty years earlier cautiously endorsed a filiation with enlightened despotism would not have endeared him to his fellow materialists. And more conservative philosophes like Voltaire could not but notice that all of the positions they violently opposed seemed to originate with La Mettrie.

But beyond this role as scapegoat and backdrop to party disputes, what is La Mettrie's legacy to the philosophes and beyond? La Mettrie is a good indicator of the Enlightenment at mid-century, before it had become a self-conscious *partie philosophique*. He understood the positive value of criticism but had no sense that its exercise should be constrained by caution or expediency. His work, like so many eighteenth-century texts, is driven by a critical sensibility. It is in fact so critical of much of the inherited wisdom of the seventeenth century as to seem ungrateful, but one must remember that his thoroughgoing disparagement of the old was motivated by his zeal for the new. La Mettrie saw himself poised on the brink of a new movement defined by new methods, new approaches, and a different sense of the possibilities knowledge offered. He assumed, as did other philosophes, that the new philosophic method would produce great benefits for humanity. This belief, though consistently tempered by his knowledge that diseases can persist despite the best efforts of medical treatment, allowed him to develop a critical stance toward existing knowledge, especially systems of knowledge mired in the errors of metaphysics. But La Mettrie's use of criticism was typical of Enlightenment criticism that had not yet been structured by a party agenda and ideology; his arguments for Enlightenment are the cries of an exile, unstructured by the concerns of an emerging, self-defining group. Furthermore, his incautious use of criticism, his failure to tone down the radical moral and social ramifications of his materialism, and the simple fact that he published everything he wrote indicated to the philosophes a blatant disregard for safety and a failure to recognize the difficulties inherent to the pursuit of philosophy in France.

Despite this close connection to the critical spirit of the French Enlightenment, La Mettrie's position within the movement is problematic. It might be fruitful to regard the case of La Mettrie as analogous to that of Rousseau. La Mettrie, like Rousseau, proved to be in many respects an embarrassment and a sign of fragmentation within the movement. Denise Leduc Lafayette has suggested that La Mettrie's work disturbed the philosophes because of its extremism, because it tended, as she put it, towards a "désordre riche" as opposed to the more conventional "ordre banal,"[21] a characterization which seems to apply equally to Rousseau. Both thinkers also had dangerous ideas to impart—La Mettrie took a problematic moral stance and Rousseau took an unorthodox view of the benefits of culture and the nature of political society. Just as Rousseau was a catalyst for political discussions of the 1770s and 1780s, so La Mettrie functioned as a pivotal thinker in the decade of the 1740s (a period much less well studied than the decades before the Revolution), one who shaped the leading philosophical debates and as his distinctive contribution to the Enlightenment brought to the fore a medical understanding of the philosophical tradition.

But unlike Rousseau, who fits a distinctive niche in Enlightenment historiography, La Mettrie has not been similarly integrated. He left no school and no defenders. The contentions of those who knew him, like Voltaire and Maupertuis, that he was not as depraved as his writings might lead one to believe, are the most vigorous defense he has received. As a result, it has been too easy to take the statements of some philosophes at face value, as though they were valid indications of La Mettrie's importance or, according to standard historiography, his lack of importance to the Enlightenment as a whole. It has also been easy to allow the French Revolution to cast its shadow over historical understanding of the Enlightenment. Because La Mettrie, dead for nearly forty years at the outbreak of the Revolution, had no impact on its concerns and because his writings do not deal primarily with political issues, it has been easy to read him out of the Enlightenment understood as a prelude to the Revolution. Also, perhaps as befits an adept polemicist, La Mettrie has been put to polemical uses in the centuries after his death. Philosophes and antiphilosophes conspired to make his philosophy a caricature of itself; more recently he has been cast as a forerunner of Marx and a source of the evils of the modern world.

The difficulty of integrating La Mettrie into the Enlightenment has been exacerbated by the tardy and halting development of the history of science and medicine. These fields were not well defined until the twentieth century. Because they initially emphasized the heroic figures of science and the most striking scientific innovations, the philosophes have not figured prominently in their accounts. Nor has science been a preeminent concern of historians of the Enlightenment; it has been acknowledged chiefly as a point of departure by historians of the Enlightenment, who have only recently begun to explore the relevant scientific texts and contexts.

But if La Mettrie does not easily fit the traditional Enlightenment historiography and if he cannot easily be used to forecast the coming political crisis, he is nonetheless crucial to the definition of a particular strand of the Enlightenment, a strand that became increasingly important to the Enlightenment itself and to the inheritance the Enlightenment bequeathed to the modern world.[22] As the philosophes began to rely less on God as a source of social structure or the understanding of human beings, La Mettrie's medical conception of nature and human nature became more central. In other words, as the Enlightenment progressively became characterized by increasingly radical or agnostic positions, it became less common to invoke God as a source for understanding the order of the universe, human nature, and human society. Instead, nature, a term loosely defined but widely used, filled the explanatory void. La Mettrie, as has been shown in the preceding chapters, gave a medical cast to fundamental Enlightenment issues; he maintained that all human capabilities, including the ability to acquire knowledge or to behave in a moral fashion, were dependent on physiological processes and physiological constitutions. In general, then, La Mettrie addressed epistemological and metaphysical notions in a pragmatic way, insisting that physiology either provided compelling answers to philosophical dilemmas or at least produced sufficient information to enable one to act. This criticism and reinterpretation of the philosophical tradition was based on an empirical and scientific study of man, deliberately understood not as a metaphysical abstraction or as an uneasy alliance of body and soul but rather as an integral part of the natural order. Man as a physiological creature set a new standard for what was natural, a position that allowed La Mettrie to characterize contemporary moral notions and social conventions as artificial. As a result, La Mettrie's medicalization of both nature in general and human nature in particular as well as his medical reformulation of essential Enlightenment issues became more central to the movement itself.

While La Mettrie's medicalization of the Enlightenment was radical and uncharacteristic of the spirit of the early Enlightenment (so much so that La Mettrie could generally be dismissed by his contemporaries as a pariah), nonetheless, as the Enlightenment developed as a movement, many of the positions he took, which had seemed much too radical to be acceptable in the 1740s, became more mainstream in the 1770s, although they remained unattributed to La Mettrie. However, even if La Mettrie is credited as prescient in defining positions of the later Enlightenment, that is an insufficient recognition of his contributions to the movement.

While La Mettrie's route through the medical tradition to the cause of philosophy is perhaps not the most conventional path to Enlightenment, it was nonetheless particularly productive. La Mettrie understood the mission of Enlightenment in terms of medicine. From his position within the medical profession, he developed a reformist stance and criticized a particular formulation of the corporate order. His familiarity with medical theory and his appreciation of the problematic relationship of medical theory to medical practice led La Mettrie to the epistemological concerns of the philosophes. His exposure to the corruptions of medicine played a crucial role in his own development as a reformer; it transformed him from a concerned physician into a philosophe. Medicine not only provided the model for epistemology and his reformist concern, it also provoked a humanitarian response to the ills of society.

But La Mettrie's development as a philosophe through the medical tradition had a more direct influence on the Enlightenment as a whole. La Mettrie made explicit the radical potential of the French physiological tradition in a way that was to shape the discussion of crucial Enlightenment topics, such as man's role in nature, what that role implied about a distinctly human nature and how morality was to be understood. In other words, La Mettrie brought physiology into the Enlightenment, and the French physiological tradition offered a particularly coherent formulation of radical ideas that La Mettrie forcefully brought to bear on specific Enlightenment issues.

La Mettrie saw the issues of his day through the prism of medicine. As a result his formulation of them is distinctive enough that he could reasonably be considered apart from the Enlightenment and the philosophic movement despite his own attempts to identify with it. For example, on the question of epistemology and methods La Mettrie reflects an Enlightenment perspective skewed by his medicine. He took up the standard of empiricism but adopted such a thoroughgoing epistemological modesty that he was ultimately much more skeptical than any philosophe except Hume. He claimed Lockean sensationalism as the basis of knowledge in the sciences, but unlike most of them he used the biological sciences rather than the physical sciences and very specifically oriented his philosophy around medical issues. La Mettrie can be portrayed as an heir to the heroes of the age, Newton and Locke; his appreciation for Locke was obvious, but his ties to Newton, though more oblique, could be expressed as a commitment to empiricism. But La Mettrie came closer than any of the philosophes to casting aspersions on the usefulness of Newtonianism outside mathematics and physics. And he claimed that Lockean sensationalism was a too-timid materialism. Furthermore, the fact that La Mettrie's appreciation of Newton was muted and of Locke qualified has provided historians with a reason to read him back into the seventeenth century instead of recognizing that his critical stance towards the heroic scientific figures was a way for him to define approaches to Enlightenment that became much more influential after his death.

Perhaps Frederick's remark remains an apt epitaph. He claimed that La Mettrie was not a philosophe. Because La Mettrie's philosophy did not accord well with the conservative beginnings of Enlightenment as characterized by the writings of Voltaire and Montesquieu, only with prescience could Frederick or anyone else writing in the 1740s or early 1750s have recognized the role that La Mettrie would play in defining the radical Enlightenment position on issues such as human nature and morality and in determining the parameters in which they would be discussed. La Mettrie not only espoused eighteenth-century extremes but also exposed the difficulties and inconsistencies of more moderate positions. If, as Frederick points out, La Mettrie was not recognized as a philosophe in the early period of the Enlightenment, nonetheless his "esprit" was philosophically productive. Frederick, like most of his contemporaries, had little respect for La Mettrie's ideas: "He will not give you sane ideas." But Frederick's remark is a fitting assessment of La Mettrie's influence on his fellow philosophes and on subsequent decades: "He will cure you of your old prejudices." The critical appraisal of received ideas was a hallmark of the Enlightenment endeavor in the 1740s. Not content with mere criticism, however, La Mettrie also launched implicit and sometimes explicit challenges to more conventional philosophes. And it would not have endeared La Mettrie to the philosophes to have some of their own approaches, deism for example, exposed as prejudices, ideas without an empirical basis. Ultimately, though there was never any reason to acknowledge them as a debt or an influence, some of La Mettrie's ideas would have been recognized by 1770 as not only sane but also persuasive.

Despite the critical appraisals of his contemporaries, La Mettrie defined one of the most enduring legacies of the eighteenth century to the modern world through his medical approach to philosophical issues. He was the crucial figure in integrating public health issues into the Enlightenment, a concern that became more pronounced in the nineteenth century. And in fact the positions taken by La Mettrie, expunged of their radical and antireligious overtones, cross the chasm of the Revolution to provide a link to the anthropological view of man more common to the physiological foundations of social science in the nineteenth century.[23] The scientists of the nineteenth century presume many of La Mettrie's positions as givens in their own work. But they had no good reason to acknowledge their materialist antecedents. Furthermore, since science, after the Revolution, was under the protection of the state, it was no longer tied to an antireligious stance, and it no longer had a sharp polemical edge. So that, as Vartanian has suggested, even ideologues like Cabanis, who shared many fundamental points of view with La Mettrie, might genuinely have failed to recognize some of their affinities because of the dramatic differences in style.[24]

In the nineteenth century physicians accepted many of La Mettrie's fundamental positions, although they did not acknowledge him. Physicians not only assumed that all ideas were derived from sensations, a perfectly orthodox Lockean position, but also that mental faculties derived from physical organization. They thus subsumed a materialist position under the orthodox rubric of sensationalism because materialism, especially the materialism of La Mettrie, provided a physiological orientation missing from the sensationalism of Condillac. But while physicians and phrenologists believed that mental states were to be explained by the configuration of the brain and that physiological organization was the basis for understanding, they did not acknowledge any debt to La Mettrie or to other materialists, despite the fact that La Mettrie's work was well known in the nineteenth century. (There had, for example, been a new edition of his collected works in 1796.)

Perhaps the most extreme example of an unwillingness to credit La Mettrie was the emendation of the historical record. It became part of the standard accounts of the history of philosophy in the Enlightenment to assert that La Mettrie was influenced in his discussion of Locke by Condillac's *Essai des origines des connaissances humaines*, despite the fact that La Mettrie's *Histoire naturelle de l'âme* had appeared a year earlier. This historical revisionism was a clear attempt to rule La Mettrie out of any significant subsequent development of Enlightenment philosophy; if Condillac preceded La Mettrie, then the philosophes must have absorbed the sensationalist position without the taint of materialism.

Although La Mettrie is sometimes castigated as being retrograde because of his natural and medical science, his less than well-developed political agenda, and his too limited sense of political reform, nonetheless he was avant-garde in his recognition of the role physiology would play in the social sciences. La Mettrie, along with Diderot, who shares so many of his fundamental positions, seems to be the most modern of the philosophes. He was convinced that medicine and science would replace religion as a way to understanding all human behavior, including rationality and morality, and he assumed that physiology was the crucial determinant of all human behavior, including rational and moral behavior. His fundamental premise was that physiology might produce at the least some toleration for deviants and, more optimistically, some real benefits for mankind. His ultimate hope, and one the nineteenth century assiduously sought to fulfill, was that physiology might yield a realistic understanding of human nature.

La Mettrie's approach to moral and social dilemmas resonates in contemporary issues. For example, La Mettrie's medical approach to ethical questions is significant in the insanity defense and arguments about diminished capacity. His attempt to correlate mental states with brain physiology seems to have been substantiated by twentieth-century findings about brain chemistry (for example, as the sources of Alzheimer's disease and schizophrenia). It is also interesting that biomedical and biochemical explanations of human capabilities more strikingly suggest the influence of La Mettrie than the computer analogies sometimes invoked as the derivations of man-machine. Yet although these modern comparisons are intriguing, La Mettrie's most enduring accomplishment was to bring to the fore a medical understanding of the philosophical tradition, to forge that understanding into a weapon for Enlightenment and reform, and finally to bequeath a lasting basis for a medical understanding of human nature.

Notes

Preface

1. For a discussion of seventeenth-century literary influences on La Mettrie, see Ann Thomson, *Materialism and Society in the Mid-eighteenth Century: La Mettrie's "Discours préliminaire"* (Geneva: Librairie Droz, 1981), 69–77; John Falvey, "A Critical Edition of the *Discours sur le bonheur*," in *Studies on Voltaire and the Eighteenth Century* 134 (1975): 40–57; Theo Verbeek, *"Traité de l'âme" de la Mettrie*, edited with commentary, 2 vols. (Utrecht: OMI-Grafisch Bedrijf, 1988), 2:75–117.

2. I agree with Falvey that succeeding editions of *Discours sur le bonheur* show La Mettrie's attempt to ally his moral philosophy to acceptable norms like Montaigne; see "A Critical Edition of the *Discours sur le bonheur*," 50–60. But I see the evolution from *L'Histoire naturelle de l'âme* to *L'Homme machine* as a change of style rather than the fundamental shift of philosophical allegiance that Aram Vartanian suggests; see *La Mettrie's "L'Homme machine": A Study in the Origins of an Idea* (Princeton: Princeton University Press, 1960), 16.

Introduction

1. Paul Hazard, *European Thought in the Eighteenth Century from Montesquieu to Lessing*, trans. J. Lewis May (New Haven: Yale University Press, 1954), 55; Ernst Cassirer, *The Philosophy of the Enlightenment* (Boston: Beacon Press, 1954), 124; Peter Gay, *The Enlightenment: An Interpretation*, 2 vols., vol. 2, *The Science of Freedom* (New York: W. W. Norton, 1969), 3–27.

2. Jacob Leib Talmon, *The Origins of Totalitarian Democracy* (New York: Praeger, 1960).

3. Karl Marx, "Kritische Schlacht gegen den französischen Materialismus," chapter 6 in *Die heilige Familie*, new ed. (Berlin: Dietz, 1965). For a more recent account, see "Notes sur le materialisme au xviiie siècle et ses interpretations marxistes," in Pierre Naville, *D'Holbach et la philosophie scientifique au xviiie siècle*, 2d ed. (Paris: Gallimard, 1967), 404–15.

4. Lester Crocker, *Nature and Culture: Ethical Thought in the French Enlightenment* (Baltimore: Johns Hopkins University Press, 1963); *An Age of Crisis: Man and World in Eighteenth-century French Thought* (Baltimore: Johns Hopkins University Press, 1959).

5. Aram Vartanian, *Diderot and Descartes* (Princeton: Princeton University Press, 1953), 204–14; Vartanian, *La Mettrie's "L'Homme machine,"* 203–49; Falvey, "A Critical Edition of the *Discours sur le bonheur,"* 50–75; Thomson, *Materialism and Society,* 81–133. Verbeek's *"Traité de l'âme" de La Mettrie,* a reprinted Dutch dissertation, was difficult to procure. I was able to see a copy only after I had completed this study. My responses to relevant points are to be found primarily in the notes.

6. This coherence is perhaps explained in part by the rapid literary outpouring and the short period in which these works were produced.

7. Frederick the Great, *Éloges de trois philosophes* (London, 1753).

8. Pierre Lemée, *Julien Offray de La Mettrie, Saint-Malo 1709, Berlin 1751, médecin, philosophe, polémiste, sa vie et son oeuvre* (Mortain: Éditions Mortainais, 1954); Thomson, *Materialism and Society,* 5–20.

9. Some medical historians have suggested that he died of a ruptured appendix.

10. John Falvey, "A Critical Edition of the *Discours sur le bonheur,"* 32–36.

11. Aram Vartanian, "La Mettrie, Diderot, and Sexology in the Enlightenment," in *Essays in the Age of Enlightenment in Honor of Ira O. Wade* (Geneva: Droz, 1977), 347–67.

1   A Source of Medical Enlightenment

1. Peter Gay, *The Enlightenment: An Interpretation,* vol. 2, *The Science of Freedom,* 2.

2. These disconcerting aspects of eighteenth-century medical practice may explain the interest of historians of medicine in the nineteenth century. The reorganization and reform of medical practice and the emergence of the hospital and the clinic make the medicine of that period much more recognizable and perhaps more comfortable terrain for the modern historian. Important studies such as David Vess's work on the innovations in military medicine, *Medical Revolution in France, 1789–1796* (Gainesville, Fla.: University Presses, 1975), and Erwin Ackerknecht's study of the development of the hospital, *Medicine at the Paris Hospital, 1794–1848* (Baltimore: Johns Hopkins University Press, 1967), treat the eighteenth century as a dark prologue to the more enlightened nineteenth century. Matthew Ramsey's recent study, *Professional and Popular Medicine in France, 1770–1830* (Cambridge: Cambridge University Press, 1988), illuminates the slowly changing world of medical practice in its diverse manifestations and the convoluted professional structures of the eighteenth century, but he too is inclined to look ahead to the transformation of

professional organizations in the nineteenth century. And the distance between medical practices in France in the eighteenth century and in the nineteenth has been used by Foucault to argue a radical break in *épistéme* in *The Birth of the Clinic: An Archeology of Medical Perception*, trans. A. M. Sheridan Smith (New York: Vintage Books, 1975).

3. Diderot, "Premier lettre d'un citoyen zélé, qui n'est ni chirurgien, ni médecin . . ." (1748), in *Corréspondence*, 16 vols., ed. Georges Roth (Paris: Minuit, 1955), 1:59–71.

4. Licensed medical practice in France, aptly characterized by Ramsey as "a professional crazy quilt," was divided into three *corps*, physicians, surgeons and apothecaries, each organized as a municipal *corps* exercising a purely local or regional monopoly. This already complex organization was further complicated by the numerous distinctions drawn within each corporation according to certification procedures and specific privileges. Ramsey, *Professional and Popular Medicine*, 18–45.

5. The surgeons of the long robe were constituted as an academic body in 1533 with the creation of the surgical college of Saint Côme, named for St. Cosmus, the twin brother of St. Damien, the patron saint of the doctors.

6. Toby Gelfand, *Professionalizing Modern Medicine: Parisian Surgeons and Medical Science and Institutions in the Eighteenth Century* (Connecticut: Greenwood Press, 1982), 174–88.

7. For a discussion of the connection between Locke and Sydenham see chapter 3.

8. In 1765 the *Encyclopédie* published plates depicting surgical instruments, many of which were reproductions of earlier publications of the Academy of Surgery. Gelfand, *Professionalizing Modern Medicine*, 11.

9. I am indebted to several important sources for this history. There is the contemporary account written by the most famous advocate of the surgeons, François Quesnay, *Recherches critiques et historiques sur les divers états et sur les progrès de la chirurgie en France* (Paris, 1744). Although most physician-historians have considered the pamphlet war to have been a petty squabble, the following works provide a wealth of background information on medical and surgical practice and institutions: Auguste Corlieu, *L'Enseignement au Collège de Chirurgie* (Paris: Bureau de Paris Médical, 1890) and *L'Ancienne Faculté de Paris* (Paris: Adrian Delahaye, 1877); Paul Delaunay, *Le Monde médical parisien au xviii*e *siècle* (Paris: Rousset, 1906) and *La Vie médicale aux xvi*e, *xvii*e, *et xviii*e *siècles* (Paris: Editions Hippocrates, 1935). Important recent sources include Gelfand, *Professionalizing Modern Medicine;* "Empiricism and Eighteenth-Century French Surgery," *Bulletin of the History of Medicine* 44 (Jan.–Feb. 1970), 40–53; "The Paris Manner of Dissection: Student Anatomical Dissection in Early Eighteenth-Century Paris," *Bulletin of the History of Medicine* 51 (Fall 1977), 397–412; Marie-Jose Imbault Huart, *L'École pratique de dissection de Paris de 1750–1822*, thèse, Paris I (1973) (Lille: Reproduction Services, 1975).

10. Despite their limited social and medical status, barber-surgeons, like

Ambrose Paré, Pierre Franco, and Thierry de Hery, made the important surgical advances of the sixteenth century. Gelfand, *Professionalizing Modern Medicine*, 22.

11. Ramsey, in *Professional and Popular Medicine in France*, 21, notes that this kind of union was a pattern characteristic of the seventeenth century.

12. Quesnay, *Recherches critiques et historiques*, 111.

13. Gelfand emphasizes that there was no raison d'être for an academic body of surgeons; they played a limited role in medical practice and had very little support for their profession from the surrounding society. Gelfand also found no evidence that the doctors initiated the union or that surgery declined in the seventeenth century. *Professionalizing Modern Medicine*, 25.

14. Jeanne Rigal, *La Communauté des maîtres-chirurgiens jurés de Paris au xviie et au xviiie siècles* (Paris: Vigot Frères, 1936), 46.

15. Corlieu, *L'Ancienne Faculté de Paris*, 176.

16. Not all barbers actually joined the united surgical company: in 1655 there were approximately 300 barbers and 30 academic surgeons, yet the united company had only 150 members. Although the legislation of 1655 had joined the surgeons and the barber-surgeons into an increasingly uncomfortable union, the course of medical practice throughout the seventeenth century tended to produce a progressive separation of the two groups. Gelfand, *Professionalizing Modern Medicine*, 36.

17. Ibid., 40.

18. Corlieu, *L'Enseignement au Collège de Chirurgie*, 11.

19. Ramsey, *Professional and Popular Medicine in France*, 18–31.

20. Gelfand argues that a population density of surgeons resulting in a ratio in excess of one surgeon per thousand people was a crucial factor in the development of the surgical profession. For discussions of population density and medical practice in France, see Gelfand, "A Monarchical Profession," 151–57; Ramsey, *Professional and Popular Medicine in France*, 58–62; Jean-Pierre Goubert, "The Extent of Medical Practice in France Around 1780," *Journal of Social History* 10 (1976–77): 410–21.

21. Gelfand, *Professionalizing Modern Medicine*, 40.

22. Adrien Helvétius (ca. 1661–1727) was a physician who made his fortune selling powders to combat specific diseases. His remedy in the treatment of dysentery, *ipécacuanha*, was in vogue in Paris in the 1720s. He was the inspector general of military hospitals in Flanders, the first physician to Marie Leczinska, a member of the Academy of Sciences, and a great partisan of the Faculty. Jean-Baptiste Sylva (1682–1742) was a consulting physician to Louis XV, who ennobled him in 1724. He was under the patronage of Pierre Chirac (1650–1732). Chirac seems most deserving of La Mettrie's harsh criticism. Known in his day for his excessive ambition and vanity, he left no notable medical writings.

23. Cited in Gelfand, "A 'Monarchical Profession' in the Old Regime," 159.

24. The few physicians who served in the military were heads of hospitals or high-ranking consultants. Gelfand, *Professionalizing Modern Medicine,* 40.

25. Pierre Huard, *L'Académie Royale de Chirurgie* (Paris: Palais de la Découverte, no. 112, 1966), 21.

26. Louis Gayant and Jean Mery were Parisian surgeons who were members of the Académie des Sciences.

27. Pierre Dionis (1643–1718) was an eminent Parisian surgeon and author of a widely used surgical textbook which went through eight editions, *Cours d'opérations de chirurgie demontrés au Jardin Royal* (Paris, 1707). During the 1670s he taught courses in anatomy and surgery at the Jardin du Roi in which Harvey's medicine was taught in a public setting in France for the first time.

28. Corlieu, *L'Enseignement au Collège de Chirurgie,* 13.

29. First there was the *tentative,* in which the candidate was interrogated by thirteen master surgeons on the subject of physiology. Two months later the candidate had to pass an examination given by nine surgeons on surgical pathology. The most extensive series of examinations still awaited the candidate: the *grand chef d'oeuvre,* four weeks of surgical examinations requiring both theoretical and practical demonstration and covering osteology, anatomy, operations, and medicaments. Corlieu, *L'Enseignement au Collège de Chirurgie,* 57–60.

30. Discussions of French medical education can be found in Paul Delaunay, *La Vie médicale;* Jacques Roger, *Les Sciences de la vie dans la pensée française du xviiiᵉ siècle* (Paris: Armand Colin, 1963), 8–18 and 45–49; René Taton, ed., *L'Organization et diffusion des sciences en France* (Paris: Hermann, 1964), 125–236; C. D. O'Malley, ed., *The History of Medical Education* (Los Angeles: University of California Press, 1970), 121–73; and Georges Gusdorf, *Dieu, la nature, l'homme au siècle des lumières* (Paris: Payot, 1972), 424–38.

31. Roger, *Les Sciences de la vie,* 49.

32. Charles Coury, "The Teaching of Medicine in France from the Beginnings of the Seventeenth Century," in O'Malley ed., *History of Medical Education,* 126.

33. Corlieu, *L'Enseignement au Collège de Chirurgie,* 32.

34. Gelfand, *Professionalizing Modern Medicine,* 57–60.

35. Ibid., 31.

36. Gelfand characterizes this as the difference between the old-style guild of the medical Faculty and the newly formed profession of the reconstituted surgeons of the long robe. See *Professionalizing Modern Medicine,* 31–36.

37. *Mémoire pour l'Université de Paris au projet des patentes du roi, portant l'établissement de cinq démonstrateurs chirurgiens, dans l'amphithéâtre de Saint-Côme* (Signé: Dazoumer, recteur) (Paris, 1725), unpaginated.

38. Ibid.

39. Edouard Christen, *La Chirurgie et les premiers chirurgiens du roi aux xviie et du xviiie siècles* (Versailles: J. M. Mercier, 1930).

40. Gelfand, *Professionalizing Modern Medicine*, 7.

41. *Mémoire pour l'Université de Paris.*

42. Ibid.

43. Ibid.

44. Ibid.

45. Ibid.

46. Delaunay, *Le Monde médical*, 36.

47. See Jacques Roger, *Les Sciences de la vie*, 22–30, for a discussion of the opposition of the Paris Faculty of Medicine to chemistry.

48. *Réponse pour les Chirurgiens de Saint-Côme au Mémoire des Médecins de la Faculté de Paris* (n.p., n.d.), unpaginated.

49. Ibid.

50. *Problèmes philodémiques, si c'est par zèle ou par jalousie que les médecins s'opposent à l'établissement de cinq démonstrateurs chirurgiens dans l'amphithéâtre de Saint-Côme* (n.p., n.d.), 19.

51. *Réponse pour les chirurgiens.*

52. *Problèmes philodémiques.*

53. *Réponse pour les chirurgiens.*

54. *Problèmes philodémiques.*

55. Huard, *L'Académie Royale de Chirurgie*, 7.

56. *Réponse pour les chirurgiens.*

57. *Mémoire pour les chirurgiens de Paris* (Paris, 1730), unpaginated.

58. Keith Baker, "Politics and Public Opinion under the Old Regime," in *Press and Politics in Pre-Revolutionary France*, ed. Jack Censer and Jeremy Popkin (Berkeley: University of California Press, 1987), 202–46.

59. Because venereal disease was discussed in terms of the ulcers or external symptoms it produced, it fell under the domain of surgery.

60. See Gelfand, *Professionalizing Modern Medicine*, 71–73, for a discussion of the venereal disease controversy in the medical profession during the 1730s.

61. *Question de médecine, dans laquelle on examine si c'est aux médecins qu'ils appartient de traiter les maladies vénériennes, et si la sûreté publique exige que ce soient de médecins que se chargent de la cure de ces maladies* (Paris, 1735), unpaginated.

62. Ibid.

63. *Mémoire pour M. Louis de Santeul, docteur régent de la Faculté de Médecine en l'Université de Paris appelant d'une sentence rendue en la chambre criminelle de Châtelet de Paris, le 21 juillet 1721, démandeur et intimes, défendeurs et incidemment appelantes la même sentence* (n.p., n.d.), unpaginated.

64. *Second Mémoire pour les chirurgiens (10 août 1735)* (n.p., n.d.), unpaginated. Haller attributed this particular pamphlet to Petit.

65. In 1728 the surgeons were given a voice in deciding which medicines would be legal, and in 1730 they wrested control over surgical publications

from the Faculty by gaining the right to censor them; see Christen, 18. In 1731 the Royal Academy of Surgery was established to advance the practical knowledge of surgery by publishing observations submitted by surgeons. The Academy also reflected the diversified educational interests of the surgeons, for it considered the practice of surgery to entail a knowledge of anatomy, physiology, pathology, and pharmacy. Gelfand, "Empiricism and Eighteenth-century French Surgery," 40–53. The Academy is often singled out as the crucial factor in raising the educational level of French surgeons, especially in the provinces, and the *mémoires* of the organization are extolled as the accumulated wealth of French surgery. Huard, *L'Académie Royale de Chirurgie*, 12.

66. Ramsey, *Professional and Popular Medicine in France*, 21.

67. Gelfand argues that there was a break in the development of the medical profession in which "ordinary practitioners," i.e., the surgeons, essentially became the medical profession, and thus, to the extent that there was an early modern medical profession, it was represented by the surgical ordinary practitioner. Gelfand identifies several factors as crucial in the transition from surgical practitioner to medical professional, viz., a specified legal status, numerical strength and wide geographical distribution, a low to moderate social origin coupled with an apprenticeship training, strong group identity coupled with versatility of practice, and an egalitarian relationship between practitioner and patient. The pamphlet war seems to offer substantial support for Gelfand's model of professional evolution. Gelfand, "A 'Monarchical Profession,'" 154–59.

68. Gelfand, *Professionalizing Modern Medicine*, 175–76.

2 La Mettrie's Medical Satires

1. Ann Thomson, "Quatre lettres inédités," *Dix-huitième siècle* 7 (1975): 16. Letter to F. W. Van Marshall, 29 June 1751.

2. Raymond Boissier, *La Mettrie: Médecin, pamphlétaire et philosophe* (Paris: Société d'Édition "les Belles Lettres," 1931).

3. On regional corporate control of medical practice, see Ramsey, *Professional and Popular Medicine*, 39–41.

4. La Mettrie, *Ouvrage de Pénélope*, 1:123.

5. La Mettrie, *Ouvrage de Pénélope*, 1:unpaginated preface.

6. Boissier, *La Mettrie*, 121. Jean-Baptiste Senac (ca. 1693–1770) was a renowned anatomist whose most important work, *Traité de la structure du coeur* (Paris, 1749), was the product of twenty years of research on the structure and diseases of the heart. In 1752 he was appointed first physician to Louis XV.

7. La Mettrie, *Ouvrage de Pénélope*, 2, part 5, chap. 14:359–67, entitled "Le caractère d'un grand médecin français," takes Senac as the model of a good physician, specifically because of his work in anatomy.

8. Frederick the Great, *Éloge de La Mettrie*, 7.

9. Jean Astruc (1684–1766) was a mediocre practitioner but a scholar

of note who campaigned vigorously against the surgeons and *variolisateurs*. La Mettrie's character Fum-Ho-Ham in *La Faculté vengée* makes fun of Astruc's incorporation of Chinese characters in his work on venereal disease.

10. Among those who felt the brunt of La Mettrie's satire and who had written either on behalf of the doctors or against the surgeons are Jean-Baptiste Sylva (attributed), *Lettre miraculeuse addressée à M. le Médecin, avocat malgré-lui;* Jean Astruc, *Lettre de M. Astruc, Médecin consultant du Roi, et Professeur roial en médecine, A M. N. Docteur en Médecine de la Faculté de Montpellier, sur un écrit intitulé, Second mémoire pour les Chirurgiens;* J. B. T. Martinenq, *Prétextes frivoles de chirurgiens pour s'arroger l'exercice de la médecine combattus dans leurs principes and dans leurs conséquences;* François Chicoyneau, *Mémoires présentés au Roy par M. Chicoyneau, Conseillier d'Etat ordinaire, Premier Médecin de Sa Majesté;* and Philippe Hecquet, *Le Brigandage de la chirurgie, ou la médecine opprimée par le brigandage de la chirurgie.*

11. La Mettrie, "Lettre à Monsieur Astruc," in *Système de M. Boerhaave sur les maladies vénériennes . . .* (Paris, 1735), 288–301.

12. Jean Astruc, *De Morbis venereis* (Paris, 1736). After La Mettrie's death, Jean Astruc attacked Locke as a supporter of materialism in his *Dissertation sur l'immatérialité et l'immortalité de l'âme* (Paris, 1755). He may have been influenced by La Mettrie's espousal of Locke.

13. La Mettrie, *Système de Hermann Boerhaave sur les maladies vénériennes,* 217.

14. La Mettrie, *Saint Cosme vengé* (Strasbourg, 1744).

15. Dom Augustin Calmet (1672–1757) was an eighteenth-century Benedictine and biblical scholar, who wrote a history of the Old and New Testaments and a biblical dictionary.

16. La Mettrie, *Saint Cosme vengé,* 43.

17. Ibid., 68.

18. In *Julien Offray de La Mettrie,* Lemée dismisses the satires as attacks on Astruc and Haller, 158–60. Boissier, *La Mettrie,* 19, and Vartanian, *La Mettrie's "L'Homme machine,"* 6, consider them to be insignificant.

19. In *La Mettrie,* 70–73, Boissier has attempted to explain La Mettrie's support of the surgeons. However, as a physician writing in 1930, he cannot believe that any doctor would support the barber-surgeons. He therefore concludes that La Mettrie did not "s'engage à fond" in the debate, that he was concerned not with the issues but only with discrediting his colleagues. Boissier has convinced La Mettrie scholars that the satires do not merit consideration.

20. La Mettrie, *Politique du médecin de Machiavel, ou le chemin de la fortune ouverte aux médecins, ouvrage réduit en forme de conseils par le Dr. Fum-Ho-Ham et traduit sur l'original chinois par un nouveau maître-es-arts de S. Cosme. Première partie, qui contient les portraits des plus célèbres médecins de Pekin* (Amsterdam, 1746), v.

21. La Mettrie discusses his position in two chapters, entitled "De la

Prééminence de la médecine ou la chirurgie" and "Des Chirurgiens méde-cins," in *Ouvrage de Pénélope*, 2:217–41.

22. Ibid., 217–19.

23. Ibid., 224, 217, 223.

24. For example, this is the theme of Diderot's pamphlet *Le citoyen zélé*.

25. Gilbert Highet, *The Anatomy of Satire* (Princeton: Princeton University Press, 1962), 4.

26. See especially Diane Guiragossian, *Voltaire's "Facéties"* (Geneva: Librairie Droz, 1963).

27. George Meredith, *An Essay on Comedy and the Uses of the Comic Spirit* (New York: Scribner's, 1918), 82. Cf. David Worcester, *The Art of Satire* (Cambridge, Mass.: Harvard University Press, 1940).

28. Worcester, *The Art of Satire*, 87, 36.

29. La Mettrie, *Politique du médecin de Machiavel*, v.

30. Ibid., 42.

31. Ibid., xxviii–xxix.

32. Professor Donald Lach has pointed out that this name is very close to that of the actual Chinese emperor, Chein-Long.

33. La Mettrie, *Politique du médecin de Machiavel*, xxxviii. La Mettrie developed this idea much more fully in his "Discours préliminaire," in *Oeuvres philosophiques*, 2 vols. (Berlin, 1744), 1:1–54.

34. La Mettrie, *Politique du médecin de Machiavel*, xxxix.

35. Boissier, *La Mettrie*, 118–19.

36. La Mettrie, *Politique du médecin de Machiavel*, xv.

37. Ibid., 25.

38. Pierre Hunauld was a physician from Saint-Malo who studied anatomy under Jacques Winslow. His principal medical work was *Recherches anatomiques sur les os du crâne de l'homme* (Paris, 1730). A friend of Boerhaave's, he was appointed professor of anatomy at the Jardin des Plantes in 1730 and became a member of the Royal Society in 1737.

39. La Mettrie, *Politique du médecin de Machiavel*, 60.

40. Ramsey, *Professional and Popular Medicine*, 42.

41. La Mettrie, *La Faculté vengée, comédie en trois actes par M***, docteur régent de la Faculté de Paris* (Paris, 1747).

42. La Mettrie, *Les Charlatans démasqués, ou Pluton vengeur de la société de médecine, comédie ironique en trois actes en prose* (Paris-Geneva: Aux dépens de la Companie, 1762), iv.

43. Doctor-regents of the Faculty of Paris were at the pinnacle of medical prestige. Outside Paris, doctors were divided into an elite who trained to be doctor regents of medical faculties and were licensed to practice in the urban seat of the faculty and others who were nonresidents of the faculty; these latter pursued a less rigorous medical training and were licensed to practice in smaller cities. See Ramsey, *Professional and Popular Medicine*, 20.

44. La Mettrie, *Les Charlatans démasqués*, 12, 8, 10, 45.

45. Ibid., 51.

46. Ibid., 73.

47. Ibid., 80.

48. In *La Faculté vengée*, 80–82, La Mettrie notes that the theory of the circulation was accepted everywhere else a hundred years before it was taught by the Faculty of Medicine in Paris.

49. La Mettrie, *La Faculté vengée*, 101.

50. Ibid., 120–22, 142.

51. Ibid., 177.

52. Ibid.

53. Guiragossian, *Voltaire's "Facéties,"* 36–40.

54. *La Faculté vengée*, 177–78.

55. Ibid. The devil even allows the unhappily married La Mettrie to leave his wife behind in France.

56. Ibid., 51, 75.

57. *Ouvrage de Pénélope*, 2:223.

58. Aram Vartanian, in "Le Philosophe selon La Mettrie," *Dix-huitième siècle* (Jan. 1969): 161–78, is inclined to take La Mettrie's criticism of Parisian practice as a kind of self-criticism, which he also sees La Mettrie turning against himself as a philosophe in the *Discours préliminaire*. In both cases, I believe this argument neglects La Mettrie's polemical intentions.

59. La Mettrie, *Ouvrage de Pénélope*, 1:unpaginated preface.

60. Hermann Boerhaave, *A Method of Studying Physicis*, trans. Mr. Sanders (London, 1719), 72.

61. La Mettrie, *Ouvrage de Pénélope*, 1:105, 120–21, 136–37.

62. Boerhaave, *A Method of Studying Physicis*, 85.

63. La Mettrie, *Ouvrage de Pénélope*, 1:112, 105, 120.

64. La Mettrie, *Politique du médecin de Machiavel*, 25, 31, 61.

65. La Mettrie, *Ouvrage de Pénélope*, 2, part 4:2.

66. Ibid.

67. Ibid., 90–92.

68. Nina Gelbart, "Medical Journalism and Social Reform in the French Enlightenment," unpublished paper presented at the annual meeting of the Western French Historical Society, November 20, 1986.

69. La Mettrie, *Politique du médecin de Machiavel*, xx.

70. See, for example, Ramsey, *Professional and Popular Medicine*, 65–66.

3   Boerhaave: *The Medical Heritage*

1. In *Ouvrage de Pénélope*, 1:ix, La Mettrie advises his son on how to have a less disgraceful medical career than his father. In *La Vie médicale*, 39, Paul Delaunay cites this as evidence of La Mettrie's debauchery as a medical student.

2. G. A. Lindeboom has worked to establish the authoritative Boerhaave bibliography, edited some of Boerhaave's correspondence, and pro-

duced a thorough biography; see his *Bibliographia Boerhaaviana* (Leiden: E. J. Brill, 1959); *Hermann Boerhaave, the Man and his Work* (London: Methuen, 1968); *Boerhaave's Correspondence*, 3 vols. (Leiden: E. J. Brill, 1962–79); and *Boerhaave and Great Britain* (Leiden: E. J. Brill, 1974).

3. Lindeboom, *Hermann Boerhaave*, 265.

4. For Boerhaave's contribution to botany consult F. W. Gibbs, "Boerhaave and the Botanists," *Annals of Science* 13 (Jan. 1957): 47–61.

5. Hermann Boerhaave, *Institutions de médecine*, trans. Julien Offray de La Mettrie, 2 vols. (Paris, 1740); *Aphorismes sur la connoissance et la cure des maladies*, trans. Julien Offray de La Mettrie (Paris, 1745); *Traité de la matière médicale, pour servira la composition des remèdes indiqués dans Aphorismes par M. Hermann Boerhaave: auquel on a ajouté les opérations chymiques du même auteur*, trans. Julien Offray de La Mettrie (Paris, 1739).

6. Karl Rothschuh, *The History of Physiology*, trans. Guenther Risse (Huntington, N.Y.: Robert Krieger Co., 1973), 115–17; J. D. Cowrie, "Boerhaave and the Early Medical School at Edinburgh," in *Memoralia Hermann Boerhaave Optimi Medici* (Haarlem: De Erven F. Bohn, 1939), 33.

7. Important sources on iatromechanism and iatrochemistry are: Marie Boas, "The Establishment of the Mechanical Philosophy," *Osiris* 10 (1952): 412–541; Robert Le Noble, *Mersenne ou la naissance du mécanisme* (Paris: Vrin, 1943); Robert Schofield, *Mechanism and Materialism: British Natural Philosophy in the Age of Reason* (Princeton: Princeton University Press, 1970); Allen G. Debus, *The Chemical Philosophy: Paracelsian Science and Medicine in the Sixteenth and Seventeenth Centuries*, 2 vols. (New York: Science History Publications, 1977); "The Paracelsians and the Chemists: The Chemical Dilemma in Renaissance Medicine," *Clio Medica* 7 (Sept. 1972): 185–99; "Fire Analysis and the Elements in the Sixteenth and Seventeenth Centuries," *Annals of Science* 23 (Jan. 1967): 127–47; Robert Multhauf, *The Origins of Chemistry* (New York: Watts, 1966).

8. Important sources on Paracelsus are: Walter Pagel, *Paracelsus: An Introduction to Philosophical Medicine in the Era of the Renaissance* (Basel: S. Karger, 1958); Allen G. Debus, *The English Paracelsians* (London: Oldbourne Press, 1965).

9. An important source on van Helmont is Walter Pagel, "The Religious and Philosophical Aspects of van Helmont's Science," *Bulletin of the History of Medicine*, supplement no. 2 (Baltimore: Johns Hopkins University Press, 1944).

10. Friedrich Hoffmann (1660–1742) was predominantly associated with iatromechanism.

11. Discussion in this chapter is based on the fifth and last edition of the work, which was the one translated by La Mettrie. Boerhaave noted that all these editions were necessary because his ideas had continually changed: "Les derniers réflexions qu'on fait sur les ouvrages, sont en effet

toujours les plus sages, and les découverts si fréquentes dans le siècle ou nous vivons, sont souvent apperçues des fonctions inconnus." *Institutions de médecine,* 1:ix.

12. Lester King, "Precursors of Boerhaave's *Institutiones medicae,*" in *Boerhaave and his Time,* ed. G. E. Lindeboom (Leiden: E. J. Brill, 1970), 60.

13. Boerhaave, *Institutions de médecine,* 1:x.

14. Anton Nuck was a celebrated anatomist and the professor of medicine and surgery at the University of Leiden while Boerhaave was a medical student, Jacob Rau was a professor of anatomy there, and Bernard Albinus was appointed by the university in 1702 to teach theoretical and practical medicine. These three professors, as well as Boerhaave himself, helped to make Leiden the outstanding center for medicine in eighteenth-century Europe.

15. Boerhaave, *Institutions de médecine,* no. 28.

16. Ibid.

17. Ibid., no. 24.

18. Ibid.

19. Discussion of Boerhaave's physiology and the injection experiments of the eighteenth century are to be found in F. J. Cole, "The History of Anatomical Injection," in *Studies in the History and Method of Science,* ed. Charles Singer, 2 vols. (Oxford: Clarendon Press, 1921), 2: 285–343; and in Eric T. Carlson and Meribeth M. Simpson, "Models of the Nervous System in Eighteenth-Century Neurophysiology and Medical Psychology," *Bulletin of the History of Medicine* 44 (Sept. 1969): 101–15.

20. Boerhaave, *Institutions de médecine,* no. 224.

21. Ibid., no. 380.

22. Ibid.

23. Ibid., no. 328.

24. Hermann Boerhaave, *Elements of Chemistry,* trans. Timothy Dalhower, 2 vols. (London, 1735), 1:73.

25. Boerhaave, *Institutions de médecine,* no. 328.

26. Ibid., no. 330.

27. Ibid., no. 417.

28. Ibid., no. 571.

29. Ibid., no. 573.

30. Ibid., no. 580.

31. Ibid., no. 570.

32. Hélène Metzger, *Les Doctrines chimiques en France au début du xviie à la fin du xviiie siècle* (Paris: Presses Universitaires de France, 1923).

33. François Duchesneau argues that as a result of Locke's close medical collaborations with Sydenham, Locke's philosophical works were profoundly influenced by Sydenham's medicine. He finds this influence especially strong in Locke's conception of nature, his critique of hypotheses, and his research into the causation and the limits of knowledge. See his *L'Empirisme de Locke* (The Hague: Martinus Nijhoff, 1973), 45–48.

34. Kenneth Dewhurst, *John Locke (1623–1704), Physician and Phi-*

losopher: A Medical Biography (London: Wellcome Historical Medical Library, 1963), 282.

35. More disturbing, this attempt to give Boerhaave some credit by relegating his medical work to a mere reflection of Newton's glory fails to consider the content of Boerhaave's medicine.

36. Boerhaave, Institutions de médecine, no. 330.

37. Boerhaave, A Method of Studying Physicis, trans. Mr. Sanders (London: C. Rivington, 1719), 28. Thomas S. Hall, History of General Physiology (Chicago: University of Chicago Press, 1969), 1:371, presents a more measured view of Boerhaave's relationship to Newton than is usually given: "Newton's emphasis on law—meaning mathematically ordered correlations between phenomena—was praised by Boerhaave but not much applied in his own approach to the organism. Rather, having drawn the foregoing rough comparison of gross structure to various technical artifacts and properly praised Newton's general canons, Boerhaave concentrated in a non-mathematical way on his primary interest in microstructure and microdynamics."

38. Lester King, The Medical World of the Eighteenth Century (Chicago: University of Chicago Press, 1958), 65.

39. Thomas Sydenham, "De Arte Medica," in Dr. Thomas Sydenham, 1624–1689, His Life and Original Writings, ed. Kenneth Dewhurst (London: Wellcome Historical Medical Library, 1966), 81.

40. Ibid., 87.

41. David Riesman, Thomas Sydenham, Clinician (New York: Praeger, 1926), 15.

42. Sydenham, "De Arte Medica," 85.

43. Sydenham, "On Anatomy," in Dr. Thomas Sydenham, 89.

44. Riesman, Thomas Sydenham, Clinician, 45.

45. Lindeboom, ed., Boerhaave's Correspondence, 1:219.

46. Ibid., 2:337.

47. Boerhaave, Aphorismes, nos. 1071–1072, 360–61.

48. Ibid., no. 1075, 360–61.

49. Ibid., no. 570, 163–64.

50. Johann Rudolph Glauber (1604–1670), known as an industrial chemist, developed an extensive chemical laboratory and wrote a pharmacopoeia advocating chemical remedies and a practical chemistry text. For a more extensive discussion, see Kurt F. Gugel, Johann Rudolph Glauber, Leben und Werk (Würzburg: Freunde Mainfränkischen Kunst und Geschichte, 1955).

51. Boerhaave, Aphorismes, no. 879, 278–79.

52. Ibid., no. 1129, 386.

53. Ibid., no. 99, 32.

4 La Mettrie's Practice of Medicine

1. Julien Offray de La Mettrie, Mémoire sur la dyssenterie; Traité de la petite vérole. Verbeek disputes the influence of Boerhaave on La Mettrie

because La Mettrie does not adhere faithfully to Boerhaave's physiology or to Cartesian mechanism, which Verbeek uses to characterize Boerhaave. "Traité de l'âme" de La Mettrie, 2:87–90. But Boerhaave's physiology and practice is more eclectic than Cartesian mechanism. La Mettrie polemicizes Boerhaave, as he does most other thinkers, but this use of Boerhaave does not negate Boerhaave's influence on him.

2. Julien Offray de La Mettrie, Lettres de M.D.L.M., 2.

3. Julien Offray de La Mettrie, "L'Observation de la médecine pratique," Oeuvres de médecine de M. de La Mettrie, 269–325.

4. Those criticisms will be discussed in chapter 5.

5. Boerhaave, Système de M. Hermann Boerhaave sur les maladies vénériennes, 261–65.

6. Jean Astruc, De Morbis venereis (Paris, 1736).

7. La Mettrie, Lettres sur l'art de conserver la santé, 29, 34, 31.

8. La Mettrie, Traité de la petite vérole, 39.

9. La Mettrie, Mémoire sur la dyssenterie, 11.

10. For a discussion of this method of discussing disease, see Lester S. King, Medical Thinking: A Historical Preface (Princeton: Princeton University Press, 1982), 227–44.

11. La Mettrie, Observations de la médecine pratique, 11.

12. Ibid., 128.

13. La Mettrie, "Description d'une catalepsie hystérique," in Mémoire sur la dyssenterie, 278–87.

14. Ibid., 281–85.

15. La Mettrie, Observations de la médecine pratique, 277.

16. Ibid., 284.

17. Ibid., 307.

18. Boerhaave, Système de M. Hermann Boerhaave sur les maladies vénériennes, p. 1 of preface.

19. La Mettrie's abridgment of Boerhaave's Elements of Chemistry appeared in the Observations sur les écrits modernes (1737–38), and his Lettres sur l'art de conserver la santé appeared in the Lettres sur quelques écrits de ce tems (1734).

20. La Mettrie, Mémoire sur la dyssenterie, 87.

21. Ibid., 85.

22. La Mettrie, Traité de la petite vérole, xv.

23. Not all of the philosophes were in favor of inoculation. See d'Alembert's objections in "Réflexions sur l'innoculation," in Oeuvres de d'Alembert, 5 vols. (Paris: A. Berlin, 1821–22), 1:120–84.

24. La Mettrie, Traité de la petite vérole, 5.

25. Ibid., 18.

26. For a recent study of smallpox, see Pierre Darmon, La Longue Traque de la variole, Les Pionniers de la médecine préventative (Paris: Librairie Académique Perrin, 1986).

27. Genevieve Miller, The Adoption of Inoculation for Smallpox in England and France (Philadelphia: University of Pennsylvania Press, 1957), 118–32.

28. King, *Medical Thinking*, 227–44.

29. La Mettrie, *Mémoire sur la dyssenterie*, 66.

30. Ibid., 53.

31. La Mettrie, *Observations de médecine pratique*, (Paris, 1743), 286.

32. After an early career as an English Newtonian who sought to provide mathematical explanations for fever, George Cheyne (1671–1743) wrote popular medical works such as an *Essay of Health and Long Life* (London, 1725) and *The Natural Method of Curing Diseases of the Body and Disorders of the Mind Depending on the Body* (London, 1742). In "Health and Hygiene in the Encyclopedia: A Medical Doctrine for the Bourgeoisie," *Journal of the History of Medicine* 11 (Oct. 1974): 399–421, William Coleman argued that the Hippocratic articles of Arnulfe d'Aumont in the *Encyclopédie* articulated a new bourgeois concern with health. However, this concern was also reflected some thirty years earlier by La Mettrie and seems to have been part of a European-wide Hippocratic revival.

33. La Mettrie, *Lettres sur l'art de conserver la santé*, 2.

34. Ibid., 3–5.

35. Ibid., 20.

36. Ibid., 12.

37. Ibid., 20, 25.

38. La Mettrie, *Traité de la petite vérole*, 66.

39. Ibid.

40. Ibid.

41. Ibid., 49.

42. Ibid., 42.

43. La Mettrie, *Mémoire sur la dyssenterie*, 74.

44. Ibid., 28.

45. La Mettrie, *Traité du vertige avec la description d'une catalepsie hystérique et une lettre à Astruc dans laquelle on répond à la critique qu'il a faite d'une dissertation de l'auteur sur les maladies vénériennes* (Rennes, 1737), 4.

46. Ibid., 9–10.

47. For a discussion of this point, see chapter 6.

48. La Mettrie, *Traité du vertige*, 11.

49. Ibid., 36.

50. Boissier, *La Mettrie*, 41.

51. La Mettrie, *Traité du vertige*, 36, 49–50, 53.

52. Ibid., 21, 26, 27.

53. Ibid., 63.

5 La Mettrie and Boerhaave:
Medical Theory Reappraised

1. *Göttingische Zeitung von Gelehrten Sachen* (June, 1749), 377–78.

2. La Mettrie, *Institutions de médecine*, 2d ed., 8 vols. (Paris, 1743–48), unpaginated preface.

3. Ibid.

4. La Mettrie acknowledged his debt to Boerhaave with these words: "I owe to him this gratitude in light of the immortal works with which he has enriched medicine with the excellent lessons which I attended in 1733 and 4 at Leyden and which I heard with such eagerness and pleasure from his own mouth. It is to his excellent school that I owe the taste that I have for observation and experience. Through it I have acquired understanding of the physiology of the human body without which a physician is only an Empiric. Through it I learned to distinguish sensible medicine from all those miserable conjectures that one gives in the name of medicine; I owe him the little that I am worth." La Mettrie, *Ouvrage de Pénélope*. Verbeek disputes La Mettrie's direct exposure to Boerhaave because during La Mettrie's stay in Leyden, according to the *Ordo Lectionem*, "le texte de ces leçons étaient les *Aphorismes* plûtot que les *Institutions*," 2:14.

5. La Mettrie, *Institutions de médecine*, 1:28.

6. Ibid., 1:24–28.

7. Ibid., 1:10.

8. Ibid., 1:75.

9. Ibid., 1:68.

10. Ibid., 1:75.

11. Ibid., 1:70.

12. Julien Offray de La Mettrie, *Vie de Boerhaave* (Paris, 1740), 46.

13. Ibid., 67.

14. La Mettrie, *Institutions de médecine*, 1:58.

15. Ibid.

16. Ibid., 2:83.

17. Ibid., 2:88–89.

18. Ibid., 2:52. Despite this denunciation, La Mettrie accepted the existence of the chemical elements of water, earth, salt, and oil in the blood and cited the physiological effects produced by too much or too little of any of these substances in the body. *Institutions de médecine*, 2:181.

19. La Mettrie, *Institutions de médecine*, 2:243–44.

20. Ibid., 3:232.

21. Ibid., 2:107.

22. Ibid., 3:136–37.

23. La Mettrie conceded that the chemists, especially van Helmont, had made some important advances in our understanding of the composition of urine. Ibid., 1:309–10.

24. La Mettrie traced the term to Basil Valentine, who used it to describe the faculty whereby living bodies convert other substances into part of themselves. Paracelsus and van Helmont gave this principle a far more active and important role. Ibid., 1:310.

25. La Mettrie, *Traité de l'âme*, in *Oeuvres philosophiques*, 2d ed., 3 vols. (Berlin, 1774), 1:96–98.

26. La Mettrie, *Lettres de M.D.L.M.;* "Observations de la médecine pratique," in *Oeuvres de médecine*, 269–325.

27. La Mettrie, *Institutions de médecine*, 3:248.
28. Ibid., 2:84.
29. Ibid., 2:219.
30. Ibid., 4:63.
31. Ibid., 4:201.
32. Ibid., 2:240–41.
33. Ibid.
34. Ibid.
35. Ibid., 1:89.
36. Ibid., 1:90.
37. Ibid., 3:255.
38. Ibid., 2:258.
39. Boerhaave, *Institutions de médecine*, nos. 24–28.
40. La Mettrie, *Institutions de médecine*, 1:362.
41. Ibid., 2:285.
42. Ibid., 4:142.
43. Ibid., 4:5.
44. La Mettrie, *Politique du médecine*, xx.
45. Kathleen Wellman, "Julien Offray de La Mettrie: Medicine in the Service of Philosophy" (unpublished Ph.D. diss., University of Chicago, 1983), 88–94.
46. La Mettrie, *Institutions de médecine*, 3:232.
47. La Mettrie put Haller's findings on muscular irritability to particularly good use in *L'Homme machine*, in *Oeuvres philosophiques*, 1:333–45.
48. La Mettrie, *L'Homme machine*, 305–10.
49. La Mettrie, *Institutions de médecine*, 2:213.
50. Ibid.
51. La Mettrie, *La Volupté*, in *Oeuvres philosophiques*, 2:219–45; *Discours sur le bonheur*, ibid., 2:83–166.
52. These particular physicians were brought to my attention by Ann Thomson's discussion of them in *Materialism and Society*, 22–30.
53. See Thomas Hankins's discussion of this bifurcation in *Science and the Enlightenment* (Cambridge: Cambridge University Press, 1987), 113–58.
54. The most extensive discussion of this tradition is to be found in Keith Thomas, *Man and the Natural World: A History of the Modern Sensibility* (New York: Pantheon Books, 1983).
55. For a discussion of Aristotelianism in medical education see Paul Delaunay, *Le Monde médicale Parisien au xviiie siècle*, 6–39, and Jacques Roger, *Les Sciences de la vie dans la pensée française au xviiie siècle* (Paris: Armand Colin, 1963), 59–64, 112–27.
56. These physiologists maintained their authority as distinct from religious authority whether or not they argued orthodox positions.
57. The most extensive discussion of the physiology of Lamy is to be found in Roger, *Les Sciences de la vie*, 270–80, 360–64.

58. Guillaume Lamy, *Explications mécaniques et physiques des fonctions de l'âme sensitive* (Paris, 1688), 32.

59. This argument implicitly attacks Descartes's denigration of these faculties and restores them to the traditional Scholastic view of the faculties of memory and imagination. See Dennis L. Sepper, "Descartes and the Eclipse of the Imagination," *Journal of the History of Philosophy* (1989), 379–403. These physiologists then categorized the faculties of the rational soul under the traditional faculties of the sensitive soul which were traditionally located in the organism.

60. Lamy, *Explications mécaniques*, 132.

61. Ibid., 34–35.

62. François Maubec, *Principes physiques de la raison et des passions des hommes* (Paris, 1709), 30.

63. Ibid., 197.

64. Antoine Louis, *Essai sur la nature de l'âme, ou l'on tâche d'expliquer son union avec le corps, et les lois de cette union* (Paris, 1747), v.

65. Ibid., vi.

66. Ibid., 21.

67. Ibid., 30.

68. Ibid., 28.

69. Antoine Le Camus, *Médecine de l'esprit,* 3 vols. (Paris, 1753), viii.

70. Ibid., 11.

71. Ibid., iv.

72. Ibid., 2.

73. Louis Moreau de St. Elier, *Traité de la communication des maladies et des passions* (The Hague, 1738), 99.

74. Ibid., 66.

75. Ibid., 68.

76. Ibid., 59.

77. Ibid.

78. Kathleen Wellman, "La Mettrie's *Institutions de médecine:* A Reinterpretation of the Boerhaavian Legacy," *Janus* 72, no. 4 (1985): 283–304.

79. La Mettrie, *Traité de l'âme,* 1:53–55, 55–68.

80. La Mettrie, *L'Homme machine,* 1:286–90.

81. La Mettrie, *Traité de l'âme,* 1:56–68.

82. Ibid., 1:145–52, 101–5.

83. Ibid., 1:96.

84. La Mettrie, *Discours sur le bonheur,* 2:105.

6 Materialism and Lockeanism:
The Medicalization of Metaphysics

1. That is not to say that the French had no access to Locke's ideas in their native tongue. While he was living in Holland, Locke himself published a hundred-page summary of the *Essay,* which was immediately translated by Jean La Clerc and appeared in 1688 in the *Bibliothèque*

universelle. In 1700, a French translation by Pierre Coste of the entire *Essay* appeared, prepared under Locke's supervision. A discussion of the early dissemination of Locke in France is to be found in Robert G. Weyant's introduction to Condillac's *Essay on the Origin of Human Knowledge* (Gainesville, Fla.: Scholar's Facsimiles and Reprints, 1971), v.

2. For a discussion of the French debate on Locke, see John Yolton, *Locke and French Materialism* (Oxford: Clarendon Press, 1991). In "L'Histoire naturelle de l'âme: The Philosophical Satire of La Mettrie" (Ph.D. diss., New York University, 1973), Lionel Honoré claims that La Mettrie's citation of the Scholastic theologian Antoine Goudin and his use of substantial forms makes *L'Histoire naturelle de l'âme* a philosophical satire of Scholasticism. A revised version of this dissertation appears in a two-part article, "The Philosophical Satire of La Mettrie," in *Studies on Voltaire and the Eighteenth Century,* part 1, 215 (1982): 175–222, and part 2, 216 (1983): 203–28. Honoré assumes that La Mettrie is directly and extensively influenced by the views of the soul of Scholastic and Renaissance thinkers. Verbeek disputes the influence of Locke because the *Abrégé des Systèmes* does not deal directly with the *Essay.* Verbeek sees Locke as an unlikely influence on La Mettrie because, Verbeek contends, Locke was a philosopher primarily concerned with theological issues. He instead sees the clandestine literature which he calls "spinoziste" (a term he uses to mean atheist-materialist) as the crucial influence on La Mettrie. *"Traité de l'âme" de La Mettrie,* 2:86–87, 75–86.

3. La Mettrie, *Institutions de médecine,* 1:1–13; 2:213–25.

4. Although La Mettrie works through many arguments before baldly stating this position, his own fundamental premise is that empirical studies tell us that the soul must be material and mortal. La Mettrie, *Traité de l'âme,* 1:97.

5. Honoré, "The Philosophical Satire," part 1, 196, notes that La Mettrie's reference to Tertullian as a "grand Théologien qui a osé penser" was not only designed to promote hostility among those who revered him as a church father but also to point out that, according to Tertullian, the soul is passed on by the mother and father in the act of generation and is thus both spiritual and material, a position the church did not accept.

6. La Mettrie, *Traité de l'âme,* 1:53.

7. La Mettrie uses Tertullian to make this point, which is crucial to his materialism; *Traité de l'âme,* 1:54.

8. Ibid.

9. Ibid.

10. This argument is more thoroughly developed in La Mettrie's *L'Homme plante,* in *Oeuvres philosophiques,* 2:1–21. See chapter 7 for a more extensive discussion.

11. La Mettrie, *Traité de l'âme,* 1:56.

12. Honoré, "The Philosophical Satire," part 1, 197, suggests that there is "implicit in the metaphor a possible allusion to the biological origin of man as one of the living species of animals" and further concludes that the

mention of a *ver spermatique* puts La Mettrie in the camp of the spermaticists. The first point is possible; the second is not borne out by La Mettrie's physiological works.

13. This point suggests that this text is a philosophical satire against the Scholastics, but Honoré claims that this misrepresentation of Goudin is the result of La Mettrie's haste to gather evidence.

14. One of the things La Mettrie admires about Locke is that he did not become embroiled in religious issues or provoke religious fanaticism; La Mettrie, *Abrégé des systèmes,* in *Oeuvres philosophiques,* 1:212.

15. Honoré, "The Philosophical Satire," part 1, 189, cites this as a defense commonly invoked by Renaissance thinkers such as Cremonini and Pomponazzi. But these same points and thinkers are cited by Pascal, who is a more likely source for La Mettrie's remarks.

16. La Mettrie claims that only faith supports the notion of an immaterial soul. By the standards of truth La Mettrie has argued, i.e., empirical demonstrability and utility, there is no reason to suppose an immortal soul.

17. See chapter 8 for La Mettrie's use of Descartes as spokesman for Christianity.

18. See the dedicatory letter to the Sorbonne attached to "The Meditations," in *The Philosophical Writings of Descartes,* trans. and ed. John Cottingham et al., 2 vols. (Cambridge: Cambridge University Press, 1985), 2:3–6.

19. See, for example, Objection VI to the Meditations in *The Philosophical Writings of Descartes,* 2:278–84.

20. La Mettrie appraises Spinoza, Wolff, Leibniz, and Malebranche in the *Abrégé des systèmes,* 1:194–208, 213–16.

21. La Mettrie, *Traité de l'âme,* 1:57.

22. Ibid., 58.

23. Ibid., 67.

24. Ibid. Honoré, "The Philosophical Satire," part 1, 205, concludes, "My contention that La Mettrie's mockery of Descartes's theory of animals as pure machines is not meant seriously is based on the fact that he is fully aware that the final conclusion of the *Histoire* and of *L'Homme machine* will be that man is also a machine, albeit a machine of feeling." I think this is part of La Mettrie's perfectly serious refutation of Descartes for exactly the same reason: La Mettrie has so redefined the nature of man and machines at variance with Descartes that he can feel free to make fun of him.

25. La Mettrie, *Traité de l'âme,* 1:58.

26. Honoré, "The Philosophical Satire," 203, notes that "Whether sensation is an active quality of matter in its primary state or whether sensation is a quality *in potentia* that is educed or actualized by the organization of the composite is a question La Mettrie is agnostic about at this stage of his treatise."

27. Cf. Honoré, "The Philosophical Satire," part 1, 180. Verbeek sees La Mettrie's use of Aristotle as part of his concern to revive the ancient

position in the ancients vs. moderns debate, see *"Traité de l'âme" de La Mettrie*, 2:123.

28. La Mettrie, *Traité de l'âme*, 1:64.

29. Ibid., 68.

30. Honoré takes this use of Occam's razor as a deliberate irony directed against the medieval tradition. "The Philosophical Satire," part 1, 213.

31. La Mettrie, *Traité de l'âme*, 1:78, 95.

32. Ibid., 96. Verbeek suggests that this text should be understood as a collection of different texts written to further different agendas; see *"Traité de l'âme" de La Mettrie*, 2:114–18.

33. La Mettrie, *Traité de l'âme*, 1:96.

34. This is not to support Vartanian's claim that La Mettrie is dogmatic in *L'Histoire naturelle de l'âme* but not in *L'Homme machine*.

35. La Mettrie, *Traité de l'âme*, 1:96, 97.

36. Vartanian, *La Mettrie's "L'Homme machine,"* 14–18.

37. Ibid., 16.

38. Voltaire praised Locke as "a wise man who modestly recounted its history, unlike earlier writers who wrote romances of the soul . . . Locke has unfolded to man the nature of human reason as a fine anatomist explains the powers of the body." Voltaire, "Letter on Locke," in *Philosophical Letters* (Indianapolis: Bobbs-Merrill, 1961), 53–54.

39. John Yolton, *Thinking Matter: Materialism in Eighteenth-Century Britain* (Minneapolis: University of Minnesota Press, 1983).

40. John Yolton, "French Materialist Disciples of Locke," *Journal of the History of Philosophy* 25, no. 1 (Jan. 1987): 83–104.

41. *L'Âme matérielle*, ed. Alain Niderst (Rouen: Publications de la Faculté de Lettres et Sciences Humaines, 1969).

42. La Mettrie, *Abrégé des systèmes*, 1:212.

43. Ibid., 211–12.

44. Ibid., 212. Verbeek claims that because this account is not an explicit commentary on Locke's *Essay*, Locke was not a direct influence. But I would argue that La Mettrie did not need to discuss in the *Abrégé* issues he had addressed in the text.

45. La Mettrie's consistently serious treatment of Locke undercuts the argument that this text is a philosophical satire.

46. La Mettrie, *Abrégé des systèmes*, 1:210.

47. Condillac, Locke's more orthodox heir, would brook no attempt to relate thought to the body because he claimed that any notion of a body presupposes an aggregate; the body cannot be the subject of thought, because thought is the product of a single indivisible perception. Thus, to seek to connect thought and the body is a misbegotten enterprise. *Essay on the Origin of Human Knowledge*, 15.

48. La Mettrie, *Traité de l'âme*, 1:82–83.

49. La Mettrie applied his knowledge of the physiology of the eye which he had developed in *Traité du vertige*.

50. La Mettrie, *Traité de l'âme*, 1:85.

51. Locke, *An Essay Concerning Human Understanding,* ed. Peter H. Nidditch (Oxford: Oxford University Press, 1975), 139–40.

52. La Mettrie, *Discours sur le bonheur,* in *Oeuvres philosophiques,* 2:83–166.

53. La Mettrie, *Traité de l'âme,* 1:88.

54. Ibid.

55. René Descartes discussed the role of God in the physical universe in "Meditation Three," *The Philosophical Writings,* 2:24–36.

56. La Mettrie, *Traité de l'âme,* 1:78.

57. Ibid., 79.

58. "Thus our ideas do not come from a knowledge of the properties of bodies, but in what the change which affects our organs consists. They form themselves by this change alone. Following its nature and its degrees, ideas arise in our souls which have no connection with their occasional and efficient causes, nor no doubt with the will, despite which take place in the medulla of the brain. Sensations thus do not at all represent things as they are in themselves, since they depend entirely on the corporeal parts which offer them transit." La Mettrie, *Traité de l'âme,* 1:91.

59. Ibid.

60. Locke, *Essay,* 402–5. Condillac gives some quarter to organic qualities but for him they were equally likely to be the result of the soul. *Essay on the Origin of Human Knowledge,* 49.

61. La Mettrie, *Traité de l'âme,* 1:80.

62. There are several striking similarities in the texts. For example, they both point to Pascal's prodigious memory. For Locke, Pascal's ability is comparable to the omniscience of God, but La Mettrie disparagingly notes that a good memory is often in inverse proportion to original thought. Locke, *Essay,* 154; La Mettrie, *Traité de l'âme,* 1:102.

63. Locke, *Essay,* 150–51.

64. La Mettrie, *Traité de l'âme,* 1:99–103.

65. Locke, *Essay,* 229.

66. La Mettrie, *Traité de l'âme,* 1:109.

67. Locke, *Essay,* 231.

68. Ibid., 232.

69. Ibid.

70. La Mettrie, *Traité de l'âme,* 1:111.

71. Locke, *Essay,* 236.

72. La Mettrie, *Traité de l'âme,* 1:110.

73. Ibid., 129.

74. Ibid., 113.

75. La Mettrie's sense of what it means to have an individual constitution is based on Boerhaave's physiology. Lockean "faculties of the soul" have become brain functions. La Mettrie, *Traité de l'âme,* 1:114.

76. This point leads to his moral argument that certain proclivities that would ordinarily meet with disapprobation are simply the result of softness or hardness of the nerves. Ibid., 114.

77. Ibid., 116.

78. Ibid., 117. Verbeek notes that this sense of elasticity derives from inklings of irritability in Haller's *Praelectiones. "Traité de l'âme" de La Mettrie,* 2:28–29.

79. La Mettrie relied on Guillaume-Hyacinthe Bougeant, S.J., *Amusement philosophique sur le langage des bêtes* (Paris, 1739), in his discussion of animal behavior.

80. La Mettrie, *Traité de l'âme,* 1:120.

81. "It is no mistress, able to choose them according to her liking, since they demonstrably depend on causes that are entirely strange to it." Ibid., 129.

82. Ibid., 114.

83. Ibid., 148.

84. Ibid. Condillac too postulates a chain of sensation. But the crucial difference between him and La Mettrie is that for Condillac it is the chain itself that organizes the sensations rather than the organs. *Essay on the Origin of Human Knowledge,* 37–38.

85. La Mettrie, *Traité de l'âme,* 1:153.

86. Ibid., 153, 101.

87. La Mettrie cites Voltaire as the source of this example, but Locke also used it to show that ideas of shape and other qualities are formed by the conjunction of the perceptions of several senses. Locke, *Essay,* 186–87. Condillac, whose theory of perception emphasizes each individual sensation, claimed that sight and touch were not both necessary to perceive the proper shape but that the sight of this blind man was still defective from lack of practice; *Essay on the Origin of Human Knowledge,* 150. See William Paulson, *Enlightenment, Romanticism, and the Blind in France* (Princeton: Princeton University Press, 1987), for an extensive discussion of the role that the notion of the blind restored to sight played in eighteenth- and nineteenth-century French culture.

88. Joseph Conrad Amman (1669–1713), a German physician who practiced medicine in Amsterdam, is best known for his instruction of deaf-mutes. His method of instruction was oral, designed to enable a deaf-mute to articulate different speech sounds after having ascertained, by means of touch and sight, the corresponding disposition of vocal apparatus.

89. La Mettrie used Amman to argue the comparability of man and animals in *L'Homme machine.* Condillac, much more interested than La Mettrie in speech as a vehicle for reform, claimed that with proper and careful use of words "we might reason in metaphysics and in morals with as great exactness as in geometry." *Essay on the Origin of Human Knowledge,* 10. La Mettrie was interested in speech as a purely physiological process which could not negate the comparability between men and animals.

90. In his edition of *L'Homme machine,* 213, Vartanian notes that La Mettrie equated the orangutan with the classical satyr.

91. Condillac also denied the *bête machine* hypothesis, claiming that animals also have a soul but of a much simpler kind. Because he considered

the physical connections to the processes of perception irrelevant, Condillac had no interest in La Mettrie's attempts to connect animals to man and assiduously avoided any possible materialist implications of any of his remarks. *Essay on the Origin of Human Knowledge,* 37.

92. La Mettrie, *Traité de l'âme,* 1:185.

93. Isabel Knight, *The Geometric Spirit: The Abbé de Condillac and the French Enlightenment* (New Haven: Yale University Press, 1968), 34–40.

94. Ibid., 2.

7 La Mettrie's New Philosophy Applied:
The Medicalization of Nature

1. La Mettrie, *Discours préliminaire,* in *Oeuvres philosophiques,* 1:7.

2. This is a broader purpose than is usually given to these three texts. The *Système d'Épicure* is often considered mere musing on Lucretius; see Roger, *Les Sciences de la vie,* 493–94. *L'Homme plante* is usually considered an anachronistic return to the argument from analogy. Even *L'Homme machine,* Vartanian claims, is an attempt to address the failure of metaphysics by clarifying the nature of mind; see *"L'Homme machine" de La Mettrie,* 13.

3. While the opinions of Descartes and Malebranche are discounted at the outset, La Mettrie cites favorably evidence taken from Thomas Willis, Hermann Boerhaave, Joseph Amman, and others.

4. Vartanian moderated the notoriety by placing the work within the context of scientific and philosophical issues of the eighteenth century, and his studies have focused modern interest on La Mettrie. Though this chapter is much indebted to Vartanian's wealth of information on this text, I disagree with him on three issues: the relationship of this work to *L'Histoire naturelle de l'âme;* the relationship of La Mettrie to Descartes; and the degree to which this work can be considered mechanistic.

5. Frederick the Great, *Éloges de trois philosophes* (London, 1753).

6. For some of the uses made of La Mettrie by philosophe and anti-philosophes, see Vartanian's chapter, "L'Homme machine since 1748," in *La Mettrie's "L'Homme machine,"* 114–36, and Ann Thomson, *Materialism and Society,* 169–94.

7. On the development of the man-machine idea, see Heikki Kirkinen, *Les Origines de la conception moderne de l'homme machine* (Helsinki: Academiae Scientarum Fennicae, 1960); and Aram Vartanian, "Man-Machine from the Greeks to the Computer," *Dictionary of the History of Ideas,* 3:131–46.

8. Roger's treatment of La Mettrie's natural philosophy takes this approach in *Les Sciences de la vie,* 487–94. Verbeek argues that La Mettrie's philosophy is an attempt to revive the ancients; see *"Traité de l'âme" de La Mettrie,* 2:45–74.

9. This is a distinction Vartanian makes in *La Mettrie's "L'Homme machine,"* 19.

10. Keith Gunderson, *Mentality and Machines,* 2d ed. (Minneapolis: University of Minnesota Press, 1985), 1–38. Cf. *Oeuvres philosophiques,* 2:29.

11. Descartes, *Traité de l'Homme* (Paris, 1664).

12. "Thus it is evident that La Mettrie was at least in a general way aware of Descartes's argument for making a hard and fast distinction." Gunderson, *Mentality and Machines,* 32.

13. Walter Soffer, *From Science to Subjectivity: An Interpretation of Descartes's Meditations* (New York: Greenwood Press, 1987); Harry G. Frankfurt, *Demons, Dreamers, and Madmen: The Defense of Reason in Descartes's Meditations* (Indianapolis: Bobbs-Merrill, 1970); and Amelia Oksenberg Rorty, ed., *Essays on Descartes's Meditations* (Berkeley: University of California Press, 1987).

14. Vartanian, *Diderot and Descartes,* 182.

15. Many of the examples of a naturalistic or materialistic reading of Descartes were written after La Mettrie made the famous connection in *L'Homme machine.* See Vartanian, *Diderot and Descartes,* 282–90. See, for example, Jacques Gauthier d'Agoty, *Observations sur l'histoire naturelle* (Paris, 1754); Abbé Dufour, *L'Âme ou le sistème des Matérialistes, soumis aux seules lumières de la raison* (Avignon, 1759); Denesle, *Examen du matérialisme* (Paris, 1754); Abbé Gabriel Gauchat, *Lettres critiques, ou analyse et réfutation de divers écrits modernes contre la Religion* (Paris, 1755–63); and Charles François Tiphaigne de la Roche, *Bigarrures philosophiques* (Amsterdam and Leipzig, 1759).

16. La Mettrie, *L'Homme machine* in *Oeuvres philosophiques,* 1:290.

17. Ibid., 316.

18. Ibid., 305.

19. Ibid., 317.

20. Ibid., 315.

21. In *Diderot and Descartes,* 189–90, Vartanian considers innate ideas as a support for the imagination, but that is not the sense in which innate ideas function in Descartes's metaphysics, i.e., as intellection independent of sense impressions, nor is it consistent with Descartes's disparagement of imagination in his later works. Descartes's sense of the imagination is much more favorable in his early works (see Dennis Sepper, "Descartes and the Eclipse of the Imagination," *Journal of the History of Philosophy* [1989], 379–403), but those early writings are not the source of Descartes's reputation in the eighteenth century. Nor does Cartesian rationalism correspond to the way La Mettrie wants to legitimate the imagination. Verbeek discusses La Mettrie's use of the imagination as a confusion of Boerhaave and Haller in *La Mettrie's "Traité de l'âme,"* 2:20–25.

22. While Vartanian's interpretation in *Diderot and Descartes,* 181–200, is by no means so simplistic, he contends that La Mettrie is both a Cartesian and a mechanist. Vartanian's work has been invaluable in pointing to the ways in which the eighteenth century is indebted to Descartes. However, his description of Cartesianism is so all-encompassing that the

term becomes almost meaningless. It embraces any concern with medicine, empiricism, moral reform and even every self-conscious rejection or reinterpretation of Descartes. While it would be ridiculous to suggest that La Mettrie, or any other eighteenth-century thinker, was completely uninfluenced by Descartes, it does not seem legitimate to claim, as Vartanian does, that La Mettrie's fundamental philosophical allegiance was to Descartes.

23. La Mettrie, *L'Homme machine*, 1:289, 295, 355.

24. To claim La Mettrie as a mechanist misconstrues the point of the title and takes it as the thesis of the text. In *La Mettrie's "L'Homme machine,"* Vartanian uses *l'homme machine* as the thesis of the work, exploring the development of the term and arguing persuasively for the subtlety of La Mettrie's argument. But it cannot even be assumed that La Mettrie chose his titles judiciously; he often published a work in different editions with different titles. For example, his *Histoire naturelle de l'âme* became *Traité de l'âme*, and his *Discours sur le bonheur* became *Anti-Sénèque*. In this case of *L'Homme machine* there is no change of title, but La Mettrie does comment satirically on the themes of *L'Homme machine* in *Les Animaux plus que machines,* a text which may illuminate how he wanted his text to be understood.

25. Vartanian, *La Mettrie's "L'Homme machine,"* 17.

26. Ibid., 16.

27. La Mettrie, "Lettre à Mme de Châtelet," in *Histoire naturelle de l'âme,* new ed. (Oxford, 1747), 4. Verbeek argues that La Mettrie attacks Mme. de Châtelet's adherence to Leibniz; see *"Traité de l'âme" de La Mettrie,* 2:59–64.

28. For example, La Mettrie speaks derisively of himself as the author of *L'Homme machine* in *Les Animaux plus que machines.*

29. La Mettrie, *Discours préliminaire,* 2.

30. Vartanian, *La Mettrie's "L'Homme machine,"* 32.

31. Falvey, "Critical Edition of *Discours sur le bonheur,*" 32–36.

32. La Mettrie, *L'Homme machine,* 1:286, 288. Vartanian, *La Mettrie's "L'Homme machine,"* 13, contends that the polemical animus of this treatise is directed primarily against theologians. But his ire seems directed more forcefully against Descartes and Cartesian metaphysics and less directly against the theologians, who are not sufficiently worthy adversaries to merit a full-blown crusade.

33. La Mettrie, *L'Homme machine,* 1:288–89.

34. Ibid., 289.

35. Ibid., 290.

36. Ibid.

37. Ibid., 290.

38. Ibid., 1:290, 292, 295.

39. Ibid., 295.

40. Ibid., 297.

41. Ibid., 297–98.

42. Thomas Willis, *De cerebro anatome* (London, 1673). Secondary sources on Willis are Kenneth Dewhurst, *Thomas Willis as Physician* (Los Angeles: William Andrew Clark Library Publications, 1964); Hans Rudi Isler, *Thomas Willis (1621–78), Doctor and Scientist* (London: Methuen, 1968). La Mettrie concluded about the prospects for reform, "It is the same with the mad; the vices of their brains do not always reveal themselves to our research; but if the causes of imbecility, of madness, etc., are not sensible, where are we to go to look for that which explains all the varieties of spirits?" For the conclusions La Mettrie drew from Willis, see *L'Homme machine*, 1:299–300.

43. Ibid., 304.

44. Ibid., 306.

45. Ibid., 305.

46. Ibid., 333. See Aram Vartanian, "Trembley's Polyp: La Mettrie and Eighteenth-century Materialism," *Journal of the History of Ideas* 11 (Sept. 1950): 259–86, for a discussion of the role of the polyp in the development of eighteenth-century materialism. On the role of Trembley's polyp in eighteenth-century embryology, see Shirley Roe, *Matter, Life, and Generation: Eighteenth-Century Embryology and the Haller-Wolff Debate* (Cambridge: Cambridge University Press, 1981). Roe discusses the religious and metaphysical concerns that influenced the embryology of Haller and Wolff. For a discussion of the concern over irreligious implications of the polyp, see Virginia P. Dawson, *Nature's Enigma: The Problem of the Polyp in the Letters of Bonnet, Trembley, and Reaumur* (Philadelphia: American Philosophical Society, 1987).

47. La Mettrie, *L'Homme machine*, 1:334.

48. Ibid., 337.

49. Ibid., 339.

50. Ibid., 340.

51. Claude Perrault (1623–88), physician and anatomist, was a founding member of the *Académie des sciences* and the author of *Mémoires pour servir à l'histoire naturelle des animaux* (Paris, 1671).

52. La Mettrie, *L'Homme machine*, 1:342.

53. Despite the fact that La Mettrie is given to ironic asides and internal criticism, he nonetheless continues to raise the issues of *L'Histoire naturelle de l'âme* in *L'Homme machine*.

54. La Mettrie, *L'Homme machine*, 1:316.

55. Ibid., 330, 316.

56. Ibid., 317.

57. Ibid., 308.

58. Ibid., 323–24.

59. Denis Diderot, "Pensées philosophiques," in *Oeuvres complètes de Diderot*, ed. J. Assezat and Maurice Tourneux, 20 vols. (Paris: Garnier Frères, 1875–77), 1:125–70.

60. Denis Diderot, "La Rêve d'Alembert," in *Oeuvres complètes*, 2:101–91.

61. La Mettrie, *L'Homme machine*, 1:328.

62. Ibid., 330.

63. Ibid., 331.

64. For a discussion of German opposition, see Vartanian, *La Mettrie's "L'Homme machine,"* 95–102.

65. La Mettrie, *L'Homme plante*, in *Oeuvres philosophiques*, 2:17–18.

66. Arthur O. Lovejoy, *The Great Chain of Being* (Cambridge: Harvard University Press, 1936), 181–242.

67. Blaise Pascal, *Pensées* (Paris: Editions Garnier Frères, 1964), nos. 396–432, pp. 171–74.

68. This notion of a need-fulfilling soul seems to be a deliberate perversion of the Pascalian soul, which becomes stronger in overcoming temptation or in failing to heed needs. La Mettrie, *L'Homme plante*, 2:19.

69. Ibid., 20.

70. La Mettrie argued that sexual responses are natural and good and appropriate to the order and perfection of nature. He develops the moral implications of this view in *Discours sur le bonheur*.

71. La Mettrie, *L'Homme plante*, 2:20.

72. Ibid., 19.

73. La Mettrie, *Traité de la petite vérole*, 39.

74. La Mettrie, *L'Homme plante*, 2:1.

75. "It would not be just that those who live without pleasure, die with pain." Ibid., 11, 19.

76. Vartanian, "Trembley's Polyp," 259–86.

77. Bentley Glass, "Maupertuis, Pioneer of Genetics and Evolution," in *Forerunners of Darwin: 1745–1859,* ed. Bentley Glass, Owsei Temkin, and William L. Straus, Jr. (Baltimore: Johns Hopkins University Press, 1959), 51–83.

78. Vartanian, "Trembley's Polyp," 270.

79. Roger, *Les Sciences de la vie*, 487–93.

80. Crocker, "Diderot's Transformism," in *Forerunners of Darwin*, 125.

81. Diderot, "Pensées sur l'interprétation de la nature," in *Oeuvres complètes*, 2:5–70.

82. La Mettrie, *Le Système d'Épicure*, in *Oeuvres philosophiques*, 2:232–33.

83. Crocker, "Diderot's Transformism," 125.

84. La Mettrie, *Le Système d'Épicure*, 2:233.

85. Benoit de Maillet, *Telliamed, ou Entretiens d'un philosophe indien avec un missionaire français sur la diminution de la mer, la formation de la terre, l'origine de l'homme etc., mis en ordre sur les mémoires de feu de M. de M.****, 2 vols. (Amsterdam: L'Honoré et fils, 1748).

86. *De rerum natura*, book 5, ll. 835–52.

87. Jean-Jacques Rousseau, "Discours sur l'origine et les fondements de l'inegalité parmi les hommes," in *Oeuvres de Jean-Jacques Rousseau, citoyen de Genève*, 5 vols. (Paris: A. Belin, 1817), 3:241–328.

88. La Mettrie, *Le Système d'Épicure*, 2:289.

89. For example, Lester Crocker contends that La Mettrie's statement that men were not always as they are now simply means that when humans were hatching, some of them were hatched with all the organs necessary for life and reproduction, while others were monsters, lacking something essential for life or reproduction. "Diderot's Transformism," 130.

90. La Mettrie, *Le Système d'Épicure*, 2:246.

91. Ibid., 237.

8 Moral Theory in Medical Terms

1. In *Oeuvres complètes de Diderot*, 3:2.

2. Maria Franca Spallanzani's "Lo 'scandalo' di La Mettrie," *Rivista di filosofia* 69, no. 10 (1978): 119–28, is a good recent example of this general treatment of La Mettrie.

3. Lester Crocker, *Nature and Culture: Ethical Thought in the French Enlightenment* (Baltimore: Johns Hopkins University Press, 1959); *An Age of Crisis: Man and World in Eighteenth-Century French Thought* (Baltimore: Johns Hopkins University Press, 1963); and Jacob Leib Talmon, *The Origins of Totalitarian Democracy* (New York: Praeger, 1960).

4. With the recent renewed interest in the publication of the *Encyclopédie*, historians have emphasized the constraints and fears that colored the way the philosophes chose to present some of their ideas. See Jacques Proust, *L'Encyclopédie* (Paris: Armand Colin, 1965); *Diderot et l'Encyclopédie* (Paris: Armand Colin, 1967); John Pappas, *Voltaire and d'Alembert* (Bloomington: Indiana University Press, 1962); D. W. Smith, *Helvétius: A Study in Persecution* (Oxford: Clarendon Press, 1965). Those fears might have led the philosophes to disassociate themselves from the inflammatory statements of La Mettrie, especially since the proponents of conservatism or antiphilosophical sentiments—Palissot, for example— deliberately sought to discredit the philosophic movement by using La Mettrie's most outrageous statements. See Claude Palissot, *Les Philosophes, avec une lettre de l'auteur de la comédie "des Philosophes" au public pour servir de préface à la pièce* (Paris, 1760).

5. La Mettrie's *Discours sur le bonheur*, in *Oeuvres philosophiques*, 2:83–166, is the earliest version of the text. First published in November or December 1748, it appeared in the *Oeuvres philosophiques* in 1751. *Anti-Sénèque*, the first revision of the text, was published by November of 1750. A second revision, also called *Anti-Sénèque*, was probably published by the end of August of 1751. For information on the publication history of this text, see John Falvey's critical edition in *Studies on Voltaire*, 11–22.

6. Angliviel de La Baumelle's *Vie de Maupertuis*, cited in Falvey, 15.

7. Falvey traces a tendency for La Mettrie through the various editions of this text to ally with the forces of moderation, to tone down the radical implications. For this reason (and because it is the rarest of the texts) Falvey has found the latest text to be the most interesting. For the same reasons I

have chosen the least equivocal and most accessible of the texts as the basis of this discussion.

8. See, for example, Diderot, "D'Alembert's Dream" and "Supplement to Bougainville's 'Voyage,'" in *Rameau's Nephew and Other Works*, 89–186.

9. For example, Denis Diderot, "Réfutation de l'ouvrage d'Helvétius intitulé *de L'Homme*," in *Oeuvres complètes de Diderot*, 2:267–456.

10. La Mettrie, *Discours sur le bonheur*, 2:104, 105.

11. Jean-Jacques Rousseau, "Discours sur l'origine et les fondements de l'inegalité," 3:241–328.

12. Thomson, *Materialism and Society*, 19–20.

13. Talmon, *Origins of Totalitarian Democracy* (New York: Praeger, 1960).

14. La Mettrie, *Discours sur le bonheur*, 2:122.

15. François Marie Arouet de Voltaire, "Essai sur les moeurs," in *Oeuvres complètes de Voltaire*, 52 vols. (Paris: Garnier Frères, 1877–1885), vols. 11, 12, 13.

16. Charles Secondat, le Baron de Montesquieu, *The Spirit of the Laws*, trans. Thomas Nugent, ed. Franz Neumann (New York: Hafner Press, 1949), book 1, chap. 1, p. 1.

17. Peter Gay, *The Enlightenment*, 2:174–87.

18. La Mettrie, *Discours sur le bonheur*, 2:108.

19. Ibid., 111.

20. Ibid. Freud also argued that remorse is a holdover from infancy in *Civilization and Its Discontents*, trans. and ed. James Strachey (New York: W. W. Norton, 1961).

21. La Mettrie, *Discours sur le bonheur*, 2:112. This image is taken from Descartes's *Meditations* and used against him.

22. La Mettrie rejected the claim of some moralists that remorse had moral force because it undermined the passions. He claimed that the passions were more in accord with human nature and better served human interests, while "remorse is only an unhappy remembrance, a former way of feeling." *Discours sur le bonheur*, 2:112. This validation of the passions put La Mettrie at odds with some philosophes who predicated their moral systems on controlling the passions. But others, notably Rousseau, considered the passions a source of goodness. Diderot, in early moral works such as his commentary on Shaftesbury, identified the passions as a source of positive moral good; see, for example, "Essai sur le mérite et la vertu," in *Oeuvres complètes*, 10:15.

23. *Discours sur le bonheur*, 2:113. La Mettrie here emends Voltaire's "Autre temps, autre moeurs" to draw more radical conclusions.

24. Ibid., 115.

25. Ibid.

26. Ibid., 85.

27. Ibid., 85, 90. La Mettrie's medical practice furnished him with case studies to support his argument. "Illness produces every day, before the

eyes of the physician, the most surprising metamorphoses, it reduces the man of intelligence to an idiot who will never recover and raises the idiot to the level of an immortal genius." Other evidence of the physical nature of happiness is the sense of well-being produced by drugs like opiates, "which have no other origin than the smooth equalizing of the circulation and a soft relaxation of solid fibers." *Discours sur le bonheur,* 2:90.

28. Ibid., 87.

29. Diderot, *Rameau's Nephew and Other Works,* 72.

30. La Mettrie, *Discours sur le bonheur,* 2:87.

31. Ibid., 122.

32. Ibid.

33. Ibid., 121.

34. Ibid., 122.

35. Ibid., 123.

36. Helvétius, "De l'homme," in *Oeuvres complètes,* 5 vols. (Paris, 1795), 4:1–320.

37. La Mettrie, *Discours sur le bonheur,* 2:119.

38. Ibid., 135.

39. Ibid., 127.

40. This is admittedly not a well-developed theory of politics, but it ought to rescue La Mettrie from the charge of simply catering to established regimes; see Thomson, *Materialism and Society,* 19–20.

41. La Mettrie, *Discours sur le bonheur,* 2:127, 131.

42. Ibid., 102.

43. Ibid., 101.

44. Descartes, "Discourse on Method," in *The Philosophical Writings of Descartes,* 1:122.

45. John Falvey suggests that La Mettrie's rather perfunctory treatment of Descartes is also directed against seventeenth-century moral notions, since Descartes's *Lettres sur la morale* emphasized a code similar to that of Seneca, based on self-control through will-power; "A Critical Edition," 55–60.

46. La Mettrie, *Discours sur le bonheur,* 2:98.

47. Voltaire's letter of 27 January 1752, cited in Falvey, "A Critical Edition," 16.

48. La Mettrie, *Discours sur le bonheur,* 2:84.

49. Ibid., 103.

50. Diderot, "Essai sur les règnes de Claude et Néron," *Oeuvres complètes,* 3:2.

51. "Stoicism, so very much disparaged, nonetheless brings us the weapons of victory; it offers us a harbor where we can repair our ship which has been battered by the storm. What better compass!" La Mettrie, *Discours sur le bonheur,* 2:124.

52. Ibid., 127, 100.

53. Ibid., 132–33.

54. Ibid., 133.

55. Ibid., 141.

56. Ibid., 83.

57. Ibid., 147.

58. This work was, however, meant either to cause discomfiture or to proclaim his affiliation with the philosophe camp. La Mettrie dedicated the work to la Marquise de *** as his source of information. The Marquise is usually assumed to be Mme. de Châtelet, and the dedication broadly suggests that the inspiration was of a personal nature. He also held up Voltaire as an example of the *voluptueux,* saying that he was too great a poet not to enjoy the pleasures of *volupté* and too tasteful to be debauched. La Mettrie, *La Volupté,* in *Oeuvres philosophiques,* 2:219. This work was also published as *L'École de la volupté* (Cologne: Pr. Marteaux, 1747) and later reprinted as *L'Art de jouir* (Paris, 1800).

59. La Mettrie, *La Volupté,* 2:220.

60. Donatien Alphonse François, Comte [called Marquis de] Sade, *Histoire de Juliette, ou les propertés du vice,* 6 vols. (Paris: Sceaux, 1954). For comparisons between La Mettrie and de Sade, consult Crocker, *Nature and Culture,* 327–429, and Robert Mauzi, *L'Idée du bonheur au dix-huitième siècle* (Paris: Armand Colin, 1960), 249–52.

61. A standard source on the *libertin* tradition is Antoine Adam, *Les Libertins au xviiᵉ siècle* (Paris: Buchet-Chastel, 1964).

62. La Mettrie cited the effects of the imagination in sexual stimulation as an example of the physiological connections between the imagination and the body. Honoré cites the denunciation; see "The Philosophical Satire," 216.

63. La Mettrie, *La Volupté,* 2:222.

64. La Mettrie, *Discours sur le bonheur,* 2:151.

65. Ibid., 152, 154.

66. Ibid., 156. Dr. Bordeu of "D'Alembert's Dream," sometimes said to have been modeled on La Mettrie, offers a similar self-exoneration: "whatever judgment you may form of my ideas, I hope, for my part you will not come to any conclusions against the honesty of my mind." Diderot, "D'Alembert's Dream," in *Rameau's Nephew and Other Works,* 97.

67. Paul Henri Dietrich Holbach, baron d', *The System of Nature,* 3 vols. (London, 1820; reprinted, New York: Garland, 1984), 2:69.

68. Ibid., 3:85–117.

69. Ibid., 1:325.

70. Ibid., 2:65.

71. Diderot, "Réfutation *de l'Homme,*" 330–31, 310–11, 380–81.

9   From Philosopher to Philosophe:
The Role of the Médecin-Philosophe

1. La Mettrie, *Discours préliminaire,* in *Oeuvres philosophiques,* 1:1.

2. Ann Thomson claimed that the *Discours préliminaire* was "the culminating point of La Mettrie's materialism and a synthesis of his materialism, of its aims, and its significance for the author." *Materialism and*

Society, 1. While I agree that this text is significant, I disagree with her definition of La Mettrie's materialism as the application of a particularly grim interpretation of the *Discours sur le bonheur*. For a more extensive discussion, see my review in the *Journal of Modern History* (Mar. 1985): 301–3.

3. See in particular Crocker, *Nature and Culture* and *An Age of Crisis*.

4. Thomson, *Materialism and Society*, 19–20.

5. Thomson discusses La Mettrie's links to the *libertin* tradition in *Materialism and Society*, 69–77.

6. Ibid., 90–93.

7. The final paragraph of La Mettrie's text extols Frederick as a model of the way rulers should treat philosophes, but it must be recognized that La Mettrie needed to protect his place of refuge. Given the context of the remarks—he has just raised the question of the danger of relying on *les grands*—the possible irony of this argument should not be overlooked.

8. Critics were quick to point out the radical nature of this supposedly conciliatory text; see Thomson, 90–93.

9. La Mettrie, *Discours préliminaire*, x.

10. Thomson raises the question of audience but concludes that since this treatise is obviously a defense and since so much of the criticism La Mettrie provoked came from the German periodical press, La Mettrie intended to defend himself against his most proximate and vociferous critics. But this treatise would in no way have effectively responded to those critics or allayed their fears about his philosophy. Thomson acknowledges La Mettrie's appeal to the philosophes in the second part of the treatise, but she does not see it as relevant to the rest of his philosophy and therefore discounts it.

11. La Mettrie, *Discours préliminaire*, 1:10.

12. Ibid., 12.

13. Ibid., 141.

14. Ibid., 12.

15. This distinction is developed in Cassirer, *The Philosophy of the Enlightenment*, 3–37.

16. Thomson, *Materialism and Society*, 69–73.

17. La Mettrie's atheism is at odds with the deism of the *libertins*. See Adam, *Les Libertins*.

18. Thomson mentions La Mettrie's dismissal of Fontenelle as a mere "bel esprit," but she does not see this as significant for La Mettrie's attitude toward *libertinage*. *Materialism and Society*, 75–76. Verbeek argues that La Mettrie objects to Fontenelle as a modern; see *"Traité de l'âme" de La Mettrie*, 2:26–56.

19. Thomson argues that La Mettrie's use of Epicurus indicates his fundamentally retrograde and aristocratic outlook rather than the "embourgeoisement," characteristic of eighteenth-century epicureanism, the thesis advanced by Jean Ehrard in *Le xviiie siècle: Littérature française*, vol. 1, 1720–1750 (Paris: Arthaud, 1974), 50.

20. Thomson, *Materialism and Society*, 19–23.

21. For example, La Mettrie concluded that philosophy would certainly destroy the groundless belief in the soul: "I would dare to say that all the rays which flow from the breast of nature, fortified and as if reflected by the precious mirror of philosophy, destroy and turn to dust a dogma which is only founded on some pretended moral utility." *Discours préliminaire*, 1:5.

22. These two references were pointed out by the religious apologist Picot, in his *Mémoires pour servir à l'histoire ecclésiastique* (1853), 3:120. Cf. Thomson, *Materialism and Society*, 177.

23. Voltaire, "Letter on Locke," 59.

24. Ibid., 56.

25. La Mettrie, *Discours préliminaire*, 1:5.

26. See Alan Kors for an extensive discussion of Bayle's role in the debate on atheism, *Atheism in France, 1650–1729, Volume I: The Orthodox Sources of Disbelief* (Princeton: Princeton University Press, 1990).

27. Elisabeth Labrousse, *Pierre Bayle*, 2 vols. (The Hague: Martinus Nijhoff, 1963–64).

28. La Mettrie, *Discours préliminaire*, 1:26, 27.

29. Ibid., 111–15.

30. Ibid., 17.

31. Cf. Thomson, *Materialism and Society*, 96. One of the charges La Mettrie made against Haller was that he was a sexual profligate.

32. La Mettrie, *Discours préliminaire*, 1:11.

33. Immanuel Kant, *Foundation of the Metaphysics of Morals. What is Enlightenment? And a Passage from the Metaphysics of Morals*, trans. and ed. Lewis White Beck (Chicago: University of Chicago Press, 1950).

34. Denis Diderot, "Les Sages," in *Oeuvres philosophiques de Diderot*, 354.

35. La Mettrie, *Discours préliminaire*, 1:23.

36. Ibid., 19, 20.

37. Voltaire, *Correspondence*, ed. Theodore Bestermann, 135 vols. (Geneva: Institute Voltaire, 1953–77). Each letter is identified by number and hereinafter is cited as Best., with its number. Best. 7200.

38. Voltaire, "Letter on Locke," 58.

39. La Mettrie, *Discours préliminaire*, 19–20.

40. In *The Philosophes and the People* (New Haven: Yale University Press, 1976), Harry C. Payne discusses the evolution of the philosophes' attitude toward the people over the course of the eighteenth century.

41. *Encyclopédie* 12:509, cf. Payne, *The Philosophes and the People*, 20.

42. Voltaire, "Notebooks," in *The Complete Works of Voltaire*, ed. Theodore Bestermann et al., 115 vols. (Geneva: Society for Voltaire Studies, 1968), 81:534, 82:60.

43. Claude Adrien Helvétius, "De l'Homme," in *Oeuvres complètes*, 4:11.

44. Thomson, *Materialism and Society*, 90–92.

45. Thomson sees a radical dichotomy in the style of the first and second

parts of this work (the first more rational and clear-cut, the second more impassioned). That distinction does not persuade me, as it does Thomson, that the first part is to be taken more seriously. Instead, the first part seems stilted, an attempt to use the justifications of others; the second part seems more in keeping with the style of La Mettrie's other medical and philosophical works. Furthermore, it does not make sense to see the first part as genuine when the motivation is safety and then argue that the second, with its glorification of the broad powers of the philosophe, is disingenuous and a mere rhetorical flourish, when the incautious rhetoric would have completely undermined the security supposedly sought by the first part. Thomson, *Materialism and Society,* 87–88.

46. La Mettrie, *Discours préliminaire,* 1:34.

47. Ibid., 36, 38.

48. Ibid., 38.

49. Ibid.

50. Ibid.

51. Ibid., 40.

52. La Mettrie, *Discours sur le bonheur,* 1:110–15.

53. Ibid., 44.

54. Discussion of the political positions taken by the philosophes in the 1750s are to be found in Peter Gay, *Voltaire's Politics: The Poet as Realist* (Princeton: Princeton University Press, 1959); John Pappas, *Voltaire and d'Alembert;* and Anthony Strugnell, *Diderot's Politics: A Study of the Evolution of Diderot's Political Thought after the Encyclopédie* (The Hague: Martinus Nijhoff, 1973).

55. Helvétius, "De l'Homme," vii, preface.

56. d'Alembert, "Essai sur les gens des lettres et des grands," in *Mélanges de littérature, d'histoire, et de philosophie,* new ed., 5 vols. (Amsterdam, 1759–68), 1:321–412.

57. La Mettrie, *Discours préliminaire,* 1:50.

58. Ibid., 49.

59. Herbert Deickmann, *Le Philosophe: Texts and Interpretation* (St. Louis, Mo.: Washington University Press, 1948).

60. Ibid., 30, 36, 56.

61. In large part, the philosophic self-definition developed in response to the criticisms of their enemies; see Keith M. Baker, *Condorcet: From Natural Philosophy to Social Science* (Chicago: University of Chicago Press, 1975), 16–23.

Conclusion: *The Legacy of a Medical Enlightenment*

1. Frederick the Great, *Éloge de La Mettrie,* 1.

2. The German criticism of La Mettrie is thoroughly discussed in Vartanian, *La Mettrie's "L'Homme machine,"* 95, 99–101, 103–5.

3. d'Alembert, *The Preliminary Discourse to the Encyclopedia* (Indianapolis: Bobbs-Merrill, 1963), 144–45.

4. For a discussion of the historical and literary uses of materialism in the nineteenth century, see Olivier Bloch, ed., *Images au xixe siècle du matérialisme du xviiie siècle* (Paris: Declée, 1979).

5. Ernst Bergmann, in *Die Satiren des Herrn Maschine* (Leipzig: E. Wiegandt, 1913), sought to rehabilitate La Mettrie from eighteenth-century German critics as part of the German Enlightenment because La Mettrie spent time at the court of Frederick. But François Picavet, in *La Mettrie et la critique allemande* (Paris: Félix Alcan, 1913), argued that Bergmann's interest was provoked by German chauvinism and that La Mettrie was an insignificant thinker.

6. Thomson claims that for d'Holbach nature and society are fundamentally in harmony in a way that they are not for La Mettrie; see *Materialism and Society*, 182–85.

7. Vartanian, *La Mettrie's "L'Homme machine,"* 19.

8. Baker, *Condorcet*, 18–23.

9. See John Pappas, "Berthier's *Journal de Trévoux* and the Philosophes," *Voltaire Studies* 3 (1957): 1–240 for an extensive exposition of the similarities between the ideas of the philosophes and those of one of their sharpest critics, the Jesuit Berthier. Expressions of unphilosophic sentiments by philosophes are noted by Peter Gay in *The Party of Humanity: Essays in the French Enlightenment* (New York: Alfred A. Knopf, 1964), 115–18.

10. John Pappas, *Voltaire and d'Alembert,* discusses differing strategies for the philosophes and the concern over materialism among leaders of the philosophical party.

11. Peter Gay, *The Enlightenment*, 1:3–27.

12. In *La Faculté vengée* the play on the names of doctors is obvious. When a second edition was published, La Mettrie provided a frontispiece which identified each of the figures.

13. Voltaire's correspondence demonstrates a consistent concern to mobilize the movement, especially from 1758 to 1770. For example, Voltaire wanted to be informed of all charges against the philosophes, especially those which appeared in the *Journal de Trévoux,* and attempted to galvanize the philosophes against the Jesuits, Best. 7415. He pointed out that all philosophes were susceptible to persecution and that the time to fight rather than flee had come, Best. 7908, 7955. John Pappas, in *Voltaire and d'Alembert,* 41, details d'Alembert's efforts to keep Voltaire apprised of the threats to the philosophes. Voltaire eagerly took on the role d'Alembert urged on him as principal defender and advocate for the philosophes; see Best. 8155, 8114, 8196, 8206.

14. Voltaire campaigned for Diderot's election to the French academy; see Lucien Brunel, *Les Philosophes et l'Académie Française au dix-huitième siècle* (Paris: Librairie Hachette, 1884), 92. For Voltaire's account of his effort to make Diderot acceptable to the academic establishment see Best. 8381, 8378, 8375.

15. Cited in Arthur M. Wilson, *Diderot, The Testing Years, 1713–1759* (New York: Oxford University Press, 1957), 310.

16. Best. 7137, 7231.

17. Wilson, *Diderot*, 335.

18. Claude Joseph Boncerf, *Le vrai Philosophe, ou l'usage de la philosophie* (Paris, 1762).

19. John Pappas, "Voltaire et la guerre civile des philosophes," *Revue d'histoire littéraire de la France* 61 (Oct.–Dec., 1961): 525–49.

20. Cf. Pappas, "Voltaire et la guerre civile," 527.

21. Denise Leduc Lafayette, "Le 'cas' La Mettrie," in Bloch, ed., *Images*, 111.

22. As materialism has become less of an anathema, historians have become more inclined to acknowledge its influence even on more conservative thinkers. For example, Michel Paty notes that d'Alembert's notion of nature seems influenced by a "matérialisme dynamique"; see "La Position de d'Alembert par rapport au matérialisme," *Revue philosophique* 171, no. 1 (1981): 49–66.

23. See Jan Goldstein, *Console and Classify: The French Psychiatric Profession in the Nineteenth Century* (Cambridge: Cambridge University Press, 1987), 49–63. For an extensive discussion of medical philosophy at the turn of the century, see Martin Staum, *Cabanis: Enlightenment and Medical Philosophy in the French Revolution* (Princeton: Princeton University Press, 1980).

24. Aram Vartanian, "Cabanis and La Mettrie," *Studies on Voltaire and the Eighteenth Century* 145 (1976): 2149–166.

Bibliography

Primary Sources

d'Alembert, Jean. "Réflexions sur l'innoculation." In *Oeuvres de d'Alembert,* 1:120–84. 5 vols. Paris: A. Belin, 1821–22.

———. *The Preliminary Discourse to the Encyclopedia.* Indianapolis: Bobbs-Merrill, 1963.

———. "Essai sur les gens des lettres et des grands." In *Mélanges de littérature, d'histoire, et de philosophie,* new ed., 1:321–412. 5 vols. Amsterdam, 1759–68.

Astruc, Jean. *De Morbis venereis.* Paris, 1736.

———. *Dissertation sur l'immaterialité el l'immortalité de l'âme.* Paris, 1755.

———. *Lettre de M. Astruc, Médecin consultant du Roi, et Professeur roial en médecine, A. M. N., Docteur en Médecine de la Faculté de Montpellier, sur un écrit intitulé, Second mémoire pour les Chirurgiens.* N.p., n.d.

Boerhaave, Hermann. *Aphorismes sur la connoissance et la cure des maladies.* Translated by Julien Offray de La Mettrie. Paris, 1745.

———. *Elements of Chemistry.* Translated by Timothy Dalhower. 2 vols. London, 1735.

———. *Institutiones medicae.* Leyden, 1708.

———. *Institutions de médecine.* Translated by Julien Offray de La Mettrie. 2 vols. Paris, 1740.

———. *A Method of Studying Physicis.* Translated by Mr. Sanders. London, 1719.

———. *Traité de la matière médicale pour servira la composition des remèdes indiqués dans les Aphorismes par M. Hermann Boerhaave; auquel on a ajouté les opérations chymiques du même auteur.* Translated by Julien Offray de La Mettrie. Paris, 1739.

Bougeant, Guillaume-Hyacinthe, S.J. *Amusement philosophique sur le langage des bêtes.* Paris, 1739.

Cheyne, George. *Essay of Health and Long Life.* London, 1725.

————. *The Natural Method of Curing Diseases of the Body and Disorders of the Mind Depending on the Body.* London, 1742.

Chicoyneau, François. *Mémoires présentés au Roy par M. Chicoyneau, Conseillier d'Etat ordinaire, Premier Médecin de Sa Majesté.* Paris, 1736.

Condillac, Etienne Bonnet de. *Essay on the Origin of Human Knowledge.* Edited by Robert G. Weyant. Gainesville, Fla.: Scholar's Facsimilies and Reprints, 1971.

Descartes, René. *The Philosophical Writings of Descartes.* Translated and edited by John Cottingham et al. 2 vols. Cambridge: Cambridge University Press, 1984–85.

Diderot, Denis. *Corréspondence.* Edited by Georges Roth. 16 vols. Paris: Minuit, 1955–70.

————. *Oeuvres complètes de Diderot.* Edited by J. Assezat and Maurice Tourneux. 20 vols. Paris: Garnier Frères, 1875–77.

————. *Rameau's Nephew and Other Works.* Translated by Jacques Barzun. Edited and with an introduction by Ralph H. Brown. Indianapolis: Bobbs-Merrill, 1964.

Dionis, Pierre. *Cours d'opérations de chirurgies demontrés au Jardin Royal.* Paris, 1707.

Frederick the Great. *Éloges de trois philosophes.* London, 1753.

Haller, Albrecht von. *Mémoires sur la nature sensible et irritable des parties du corps animal.* Lausanne, 1756.

Hecquet, Philippe. *Le Brigandage de la chirurgie.* Utrecht, 1738.

Helvétius, Claude Adrien. "De l'homme de ses facultés intellectuelles et de son éducation." In *Oeuvres complètes,* 4:1–320. 5 vols. Paris, 1795.

Hunauld, Pierre. *Recherches anatomiques sur les os du crâne de l'homme.* Paris, 1730.

La Mettrie, Julien Offray de. *Histoire naturelle de l'âme.* New ed. Oxford, 1747.

————. *Institutions de médecine de M. Hermann Boerhaave traduites du Latin en française par M. de La Mettrie et avec une commentaire par M. de La Mettrie.* 2d ed. 8 vols. Paris, 1743–50.

————. *La Faculté vengée, comédie en trois actes par M***, docteur régent de la Faculté de Paris.* Paris, 1747.

————. *Les charlatans démasqués, ou Pluton vengeur de la société de médecine, comédie ironique en trois actes en prose.* Paris-Geneva: Aux dépens de la Companie, 1762.

————. *Lettres de M.D.L.M., docteur en médecine sur l'art de conserver la santé et prolonger la vie.* Paris, 1738.

————. *Mémoire sur la dyssenterie.* Leyden, 1750.

————. *Observations de médecine pratique.* Paris, 1743.

————. *Oeuvres de médecine de M. de La Mettrie.* Berlin, 1750.

————. *Oeuvres philosophiques.* 3 vols. Berlin, 1774.

————. *Ouvrage de Pénélope, ou Machiavel en médecine.* 3 vols. Berlin, 1748–50.

———. *Politique du médecin de Machiavel, ou le chemin de la fortune ouvert aux médecins, ouvrage réduit en forme de conseils par le Dr. Fum-Ho-Ham et traduit sur l'original chinois par un nouveau maître-es-arts de S. Cosme. Première partie, qui contient les portraits des plus célèbres médecins de Pekin.* Amsterdam, 1746.

———. *Saint Cosme vengé.* Strasbourg, 1744.

———. *Système de Hermann Boerhaave sur les maladies vénériennes, traduit en français par M. de La M. Avec des notes et un dissertation du traducteur sur l'origine, la nature, et la cure de ces maladies.* Paris, 1735.

———. *Traité de la petite vérole avec la manière de guérir de cette maladie.* Paris, 1740.

———. *Traité du vertige avec la description d'une catalepsie hystérique et une lettre à Astruc dans laquelle on répond à la critique qu'il a faite d'une dissertation de l'auteur sur les maladies vénériennes.* Rennes, 1737.

———. *Vie de Boerhaave.* Paris, 1740.

Lamy, Guillaume. *Explications mécaniques et physiques des fonctions de l'âme sensitive.* Paris, 1688.

Locke, John. *An Essay Concerning Human Understanding.* Edited by Peter H. Nidditch. Oxford: Oxford University Press, 1975.

Louis, Antoine. *Essai sur la nature de l'âme, ou l'on tâche d'expliquer son union avec le corps, et les lois de cette union.* Paris, 1747.

Lucretius. *De rerum natura.* Cambridge, Mass.: Harvard University Press, 1937.

Maillet, Benoit de. *Telliamed, ou Entretiens d'un philosophe indien avec un missionaire français sur la diminution de la mer, la formation de la terre, l'origine de l'homme, etc., mis en ordre sur les mémoires de feu de M. de M***.* 2 vols. Amsterdam: L'Honoré et fils, 1748.

Martinenq, J. B. T. *Prétextes frivoles de chirurgiens pour s'arroger l'exercice de la médecine combattus dans leur principes and dans leurs conséquences.* Paris, n.d.

Maubec, François. *Principes physiques de la raison et des passions des hommes.* Paris, 1709.

Mémoire pour les chirurgiens. Paris, 1730.

Mémoire pour M. Louis de Santeul, docteur régent de la Faculté de Médecine en l'Université de Paris appelant d'une sentence rendue en la chambre criminelle de Châtelet de Paris, le 21 juillet 1721, démandeur et intimes, défendeurs et incidemment appelantes la même sentence. N.p., n.d.

Mémoire pour l'Université de Paris au projet des patentes du roi, portant l'établissement de cinq démonstrateurs chirurgiens dans l'amphithéâtre de Saint-Côme. Signé: Dazoumer, recteur. Paris, 1725.

Montesquieu, Charles Secondat, Baron de. *The Spirit of the Laws.* Translated by Thomas Nugent. Edited by Franz Neumann. New York: Hafner Press, 1949.

Moravia, Sergio, ed. *Opere filosofiche: Julien Offray de La Mettrie*. Rome: Editori Laterza, 1978.

Moreau de St. Elier, Louis. *Traité de la communication des maladies et des passions*. The Hague, 1738.

Palissot, Claude. *Les Philosophes, avec une lettre de l'auteur de la comédie "des Philosophes" au public pour servir de préface à la pièce*. Paris, 1760.

Pascal, Blaise. *Pensées*. Paris: Editions Garnier Frères, 1964.

Problèmes philodémiques si c'est par zèle ou par jalousie que les médecins s'opposent à l'établissement de cinq démonstrateurs chirurgiens dans l'amphithéâtre de Saint-Côme. N.p., n.d.

Quesnay, François. *Recherches critiques et historiques sur les divers états et sur les progrès de la chirurgie en France*. Paris, 1744.

Question de médecine, dans laquelle on examine si c'est aux médecins qu'il appartient de traiter les maladies vénériennes, et si la sûreté publique exige que ce soient de médecins qui se chargent de la cure de ces maladies. Paris, 1735.

Réponse pour les chirurgiens de Saint-Côme au mémoire des médecins de la Faculté. N.p., n.d.

Représentations pour le Sr. de la Martinière, premier chirurgien du Roi, et les prévots et collège des maîtres en chirurgie de Paris, sur la confirmation de leurs droits et privilèges, etc. Pour servir de reponse aux représentations de M. Chicoyneau, premier médecin du roi et des médecins de Paris. Paris, 1748.

Rousseau, Jean-Jacques. "Discours sur l'origine et les fondements de l'inegalité parmi les hommes." In *Oeuvres de Jean-Jacques Rousseau, citoyen de Genève*, 3:241–328. 5 vols. Paris: A. Belin, 1817.

Sade, Donatien Alphonse François, Comte [called Marquis de]. *Histoire de Juliette, ou les propertés du vice*. 6 vols. Paris: Sceaux, 1954.

Second Mémoire pour les chirurgiens (10 août 1735). N.p., n.d.

Senac, Jean. *Traité de la structure du coeur*. Paris, 1749.

Sydenham, Thomas. *The Works of Thomas Sydenham*. Translated by R. G. Latham. 2 vols. London: The Sydenham Society, 1848–50.

Sylva, Jean-Baptiste (attributed). *Lettre miraculeuse addressée à M. le Médecin, avocat malgré-lui*. N.p., n.d.

Voltaire, François Marie Arouet de. *The Complete Works of Voltaire*. Edited by Theodore Bestermann. 115 vols. Geneva: Society for Voltaire Studies, 1963–70.

———. *Correspondence*. Edited by Theodore Bestermann. 135 vols. Geneva: Institute Voltaire, 1953–77.

———. *Philosophical Letters*. Indianapolis: Bobbs-Merrill, 1961.

Willis, Thomas. *De cerebro anatome*. London, 1673.

Secondary Sources

Ackerknecht, Erwin R. *Medicine at the Paris Hospital, 1794–1848*. Baltimore: Johns Hopkins University Press, 1967.

Adam, Antoine. *Les Libertins au xviie siècle*. Paris: Buchet-Chastel, 1964.
Baker, Keith M. *Condorcet: From Natural Philosophy to Social Matheme-tics*. Chicago: University of Chicago Press, 1975.
———. "Politics and Public Opinion under the Old Regime." In *Press and Politics in Pre-Revolutionary France*, edited by Jack Censer and Jeremy Popkin, 204–46. Berkeley: University of California Press, 1978.
Bariety, Maurice, and Charles Coury. *L'Histoire de la médecine*. Paris: Librairie Fayard, 1963.
Becker, Carl. *The Heavenly City of the Eighteenth-Century Philosophers*. New Haven: Yale University Press, 1932.
Bergmann, Ernst. *Die Satiren des Herrn Maschine*. Leipzig: E. Wiegandt, 1913.
Bloch, Olivier, ed. *Images au xixe siècle du matérialisme du xviiie siècle*. Paris: Declée, 1985.
Boas, Marie. "The Establishment of the Mechanical Philosophy." *Osiris* 10 (1952): 412–541.
Boissier, Raymond. *La Mettrie: médecin, pamphlétaire et philosophe (1710–51)*. Paris: Société d'Édition "les Belles Lettres," 1931.
Bowler, Peter J. "Evolutionism in the Enlightenment." *History of Science* 12 (Sept. 1974): 159–83.
Brunel, Lucien. *Les Philosophes et l'Académie Française au dix-huitième siècle*. Paris: Librairie Hachette, 1884.
Brunet, Pierre. *Les Physiciens hollandais et la méthode experimentale en France*. Paris: Librairie Scientifique Albert Blanchard, 1926.
Campbell, Blair. "La Mettrie: The Robot and the Automaton." *Journal of the History of Ideas* 31 (1970): 555–72.
Canguilhem, Georges. *La Formation de concept de reflexe aux xviie et xviiie siècles*. Paris: Presses Universitaires de France, 1955.
Carlson, Eric T., and Meribeth N. Simpson. "Models of the Nervous System in Eighteenth-Century Neurophysiology and Medical Psychol-ogy." *Bulletin of the History of Medicine* 44 (1969): 101–15.
Cassirer, Ernst. *The Philosophy of the Enlightenment*. Boston: Beacon Press, 1954.
Christen, Edouard. *La Chirurgie et les premiers chirurgiens du roi aux xviie et xviiie siècles*. Versailles: J. M. Mercier, 1930.
Cole, F. J. "The History of Anatomical Injection." In *Studies in the History and Method of Science*, edited by Charles Singer. 2 vols. Oxford: Clar-endon Press, 1921.
Coleman, William. "Health and Hygiene in the Encyclopedia: A Medical Doctrine for the Bourgeoisie." *Journal of the History of Medicine* 11 (1974): 399–421.
Corlieu, Auguste. *L'Ancienne Faculté de Paris*. Paris: Adrian Delahaye, 1877.
———. *L'Enseignement au Collège de Chirurgie*. Paris: Bureau de Paris Médical, 1890.
Coury, Charles. "The Teaching of Medicine in France from the Beginning of the Seventeenth Century." In *The History of Medical Education*,

edited by C. D. O'Malley, 121–73. Los Angeles: University of California Press, 1970.

Cowrie, J. D. "Boerhaave and the Early Medical School at Edinburgh." In *Memorialia Hermann Boerhaave Optimi Medici, 27–43*. Haarlem: De Erven F. Bohn, 1939.

Crocker, Lester. *An Age of Crisis: Man and the World in Eighteenth-Century French Thought.* Baltimore: Johns Hopkins University Press, 1959.

———. *Nature and Culture: Ethical Thought in the French Enlightenment.* Baltimore: Johns Hopkins University Press, 1963.

———. "Diderot's Transformism." In *Forerunners of Darwin: 1745–1859,* edited by B. Glass, O. Temkin, and W. Strauss. Baltimore: Johns Hopkins University Press, 1959.

Dagan, Jean. *L'Histoire de l'esprit humain dans la pensée française de Fontenelle à Condorcet.* Paris: Librairie Klincksieck, 1972.

Darembourg, Charles. *Histoire des sciences médicales.* 2 vols. Paris: J. B. Bailliere, 1870.

Darmon, Pierre. *La Longue Traque de la variole, Les Pionniers de le médecine préventative.* Paris: Librairie Académique Perrin, 1986.

Davis, Audrey. *Circulation Physiology and Medical Chemistry in England (1650–1680).* Lawrence, Kans.: Coronado Press, 1973.

Dawson, Virginia. *Nature's Enigma: The Problem of the Polyp in the Letters of Bonnet, Trembley, and Reaumur.* Philadelphia: American Philosophical Society, 1987.

Debus, Allen G. *The Chemical Philosophy: Paracelsian Science and Medicine in the Sixteenth and Seventeenth Centuries.* 2 vols. New York: Science History Publications, 1977.

———. *The English Paracelsians.* London: Oldbourne Press, 1965.

———. "Fire Analysis and the Elements in the Sixteenth and Seventeenth Centuries." *Annals of Science* 23 (Jan. 1967): 127–47.

———. "The Paracelsians and the Chemists: The Chemical Dilemma in Renaissance Medicine." *Clio Medica* 7 (Sept. 1972): 185–99.

Delaunay, Paul. *Le Monde médical parisien au xviiiᵉ siècle.* Paris: Rousset, 1906.

———. *La Vie médicale au xviᵉ, xviiᵉ, et xviiiᵉ siècles.* Paris: Editions Hippocrates, 1935.

Dewhurst, Kenneth, editor. *Dr. Thomas Sydenham, 1624–1689, His Life and Original Writings.* London: Wellcome Historical Library, 1966.

———. *John Locke (1632–1704), Physician and Philosopher: A Medical Biography.* London: Wellcome Historical Medical Library, 1963.

Duchesneau, François. *La Physiologie des Lumières: Empirisme, modèles et théories.* The Hague: Martinus Nijhoff, 1982.

———. *L'Empirisime de Locke.* The Hague: Martinus Nijhoff, 1973.

———. "Vitalism in Late Eighteenth Century Physiology: The Cases of Barthez, Blumenbach and John Hunter." In *William Hunter and the Medical World of the Eighteenth Century,* edited by William Bynum and Roy Porter. Cambridge: Cambridge University Press, 1988.

Ehrard, Jean. *L'Idée de la nature en France à l'aube des lumières*. Paris: Flammarion, 1970.

Falvey, John. "The Aesthetics of La Mettrie." *Studies on Voltaire and the Eighteenth Century* 87 (1972): 397–472.

———. "A Critical Edition of the *Discours sur le bonheur*." *Studies on Voltaire and the Eighteenth Century* 134 (1975): 1–140.

———. "The Individualism of La Mettrie." *Nottingham French Studies* 4 (May 1965): 15–27.

Foucault, Michel. *The Birth of the Clinic: An Archeology of Medical Perception*. Translated by A. M. Sheridan-Smith. New York: Vintage Books, 1975.

———. *The Order of Things: The Archeology of the Human Sciences*. Translated by A. M. Sheridan-Smith. New York: Vintage Books, 1975.

Frankfurt, Harry G. *Demons, Dreamers, and Madmen: The Defense of Reason in Descartes's Meditations*. Indianapolis: Bobbs-Merrill, 1970.

Gay, Peter. *The Enlightenment: An Interpretation*. 2 vols. New York: W. W. Norton, 1969.

———. *Voltaire's Politics: The Poet as Realist*. Princeton: Princeton University Press, 1959.

Gelbart, Nina. "Medical Journalism and Social Reform in the French Enlightenment." Unpublished paper presented at the annual meeting of the Western French Historical Society, November 21, 1986.

Gelfand, Toby. "Empiricism and Eighteenth-Century French Surgery." *Bulletin of the History of Medicine* 44 (Jan.–Feb. 1970): 40–53.

———. "A 'Monarchical Profession' in the Old Regime: Surgeons, Ordinary Practitioners, and Medical Professionalization in Eighteenth-Century France." In *Professions and the French State, 1700–1900*, edited by Gerald L. Geison, 149–80. Philadelphia: University of Pennsylvania Press, 1984.

———. "The Paris Manner of Dissection: Student Anatomical Dissection in the Early Eighteenth-century Paris." *Bulletin of the History of Medicine* 51 (Fall 1977): 397–412.

———. *Professionalizing Modern Medicine*. Westport, Conn.: Greenwood Press, 1982.

Gibbs, F. W. "Boerhaave and the Botanists." *Annals of Science* 13 (Jan. 1957): 47–61.

Gillispie, Charles Coulston. *Science and Polity in France at the End of the Old Regime*. Princeton: Princeton University Press, 1980.

Glass, Bentley, "Maupertuis, Pioneer of Genetics and Evolution." In *Forerunners of Darwin: 1745–1859*. Edited by Bentley Glass, Owsei Temkin, and William L. Straus, Jr. Baltimore: Johns Hopkins University Press, 1959.

Goldstein, Jan. *Console and Classify: The French Psychiatric Profession in the Nineteenth Century*. Cambridge: Cambridge University Press, 1987.

Goubert, Jean-Pierre. "The Extent of Medical Practice in France Around 1780." *Journal of Social History* 10 (1976–77): 410–21.

————. *Malades et médecins en Bretagne, 1770–1790*. Paris: Klincksieck, 1974.

Greenbaum, Louis S. "Scientists and Politicians: Hospital Reform in Paris on the Eve of the French Revolution." In *The Consortium on Revolutionary Europe, 1740–1850*, edited by Harold Parker, 168–91. Gainesville, Fla.: University Presses, 1975.

Greenwood, E. "Attributes of a Profession." *Social Work* 2 (July 1957): 44–55.

Gugel, Kurt F. *Johann Rudolph Glauber, Leben und Werk*. Würzburg: Freunde Mainfränkischen Kunst und Geschichte, 1955.

Gunderson, Keith. *Mentality and Machines*. 2d ed. Minneapolis: University of Minnesota Press, 1985.

Guiragossian, Diana. *Voltaire's "Facéties."* Geneva: Librairie Droz, 1963.

Gusdorf, Georges. *Dieu, la nature, l'homme au siècle des lumières*. Paris: Payot, 1972.

Hahn, Roger. *The Anatomy of a Scientific Institution: The Paris Academy of Sciences 1666–1803*. Berkeley: University of California Press, 1971.

Hall, Thomas S. *History of General Physiology*. 2 vols. Chicago: University of Chicago Press, 1969.

Hankins, Thomas L. *Jean d'Alembert. Science and the Enlightenment*. Oxford: Oxford University Press, 1970.

————. *Science and the Enlightenment*. Cambridge: Cambridge University Press, 1987.

Hannaway, Caroline. "Public Welfare and the State in 18th-Century France: The Société Royale de Médecine of Paris (1776–1783)." Ph.D. diss., Johns Hopkins University, 1974.

————. "The Société Royale de Médecine and Epidemics in the Ancien Régime." *Bulletin of the History of Medicine* 46 (May–June 1972): 257–73.

Hazard, Paul. *European Thought in the Eighteenth Century, from Montesquieu to Lessing*. Translated by J. Lewis May. New Haven: Yale University Press, 1954.

Highet, Gilbert. *The Anatomy of Satire*. Princeton: Princeton University Press, 1962.

Honoré, Lionel. "L'Histoire naturelle de l'âme: The Philosophical Satire of La Mettrie." Ph.D. diss., New York University, 1973.

————. "The Philosophical Satire of La Mettrie." *Studies on Voltaire and the Eighteenth Century*. 215 (1982): 175–222; and 216 (1983): 203–28.

Huard, Pierre. *L'Académie Royale de Chirurgie*. Paris: Palais de la Découverte, no. 112, 1966.

Huard, Pierre, and Mirko Grmek. *La Chirurgie moderne, ses débuts en occident au xvie, xviie, et xviiie siècles*. Paris: Edition Roger Dacosta, 1968.

Huart, Marie-Jose Imbault. *L'École pratique de dissection de Paris de 1750–1822*. Thèse, Sorbonne, Paris I, 1973. Lille: Reproduction Services, 1975.

Isler, Hans Rudi. *Thomas Willis (1621–1678), Doctor and Scientist*. London: Methuen, 1968.

Johnson, Terence J. *Professions and Power*. London: Macmillan, 1972.

Keel, Othmar. "The Politics of Health." In *William Hunter and the Medical World of the Eighteenth Century*, edited by William Bynum and Roy Porter. Cambridge: Cambridge University Press, 1988.

Kerker, Milton. "Hermann Boerhaave and the Development of Pneumatic Chemistry." *Isis* 46 (Jan. 1955): 35–49.

King, Lester S. "Medical Theory and Practice at the Beginning of the Eighteenth Century." *Bulletin of the History of Medicine* 46 (Jan.–Feb. 1972): 1–15.

———. *Medical Thinking: A Historical Preface*. Princeton: Princeton University Press, 1982.

———. *The Medical World of the Eighteenth Century*. Chicago: University of Chicago Press, 1958.

———. *The Philosophy of Medicine: The Early Eighteenth Century*. Cambridge: Harvard University Press, 1978.

———. "Precursors of Boerhaave's *Institutiones mediciae*." In *Boerhaave and his Time*, edited by G. E. Lindeboom. Leiden: E. J. Brill, 1970.

———. *The Road to Medical Enlightenment, 1650–1695*. New York: American Elsevier, 1970.

Kirkinen, Heikki. *Les Orgines de la conception moderne de l'homme machine*. Helsinki: Academiae Scientiarum Fennicae, 1960.

Knight, Isabel. *The Geometric Spirit: The Abbé de Condillac and the French Enlightenment*. New Haven: Yale University Press, 1968.

Kors, Alan C. *Atheism in France, 1650–1729, Volume I: The Orthodox Sources of Disbelief*. Princeton: Princeton University Press, 1990.

Kuhn, Thomas S. *The Copernican Revolution: Planetary Astronomy in the Development of Western Thought*. Cambridge: Harvard University Press, 1957.

Labrousse, Elisabeth. *Pierre Bayle*. 2 vols. The Hague: Martinus Nijhoff, 1963–64.

Larson, Magali Sarfatti. *The Rise of Professionalism: A Sociological Analysis*. Berkeley and London: University of California Press, 1977.

Le Brun, François. *Les Hommes et la mort en Anjou aux xviie et xviiie siècles*. Paris: Mouton, 1971.

Le Houx, Françoise. *Le Cadre de vie des médecins parisiens aux xvie et xviie siècles*. Paris: Picard, 1976.

Lemée, Pierre. *Julien Offray de La Mettrie, Saint-Malo–1709, Berlin–1751, médecin, philosophe, polémiste, sa vie et son oeuvre*. Mortain: Éditions Mortainais, 1954.

Le Noble, Robert. *Mersenne ou la naissance du mécanisme*. Paris: Vrin, 1943.

Lindeboom, G[errit] A. *Bibliographia Boerhaaviana*. Leiden: E. J. Brill, 1959.

———. *Boerhaave and Great Britain*. Leiden: E. J. Brill, 1974.

———. *Boerhaave's Correspondence*. 3 vols. Leiden: E. J. Brill, 1962–79.
———. *Hermann Boerhaave, the Man and his Work*. London: Methuen & Co., 1968.
Lovejoy, Arthur O. *The Great Chain of Being*. Cambridge: Harvard University Press, 1936.
Marx, Karl. *Die heilige Familie*. New ed. Berlin: Dietz, 1965.
Mauzi, Robert. *L'Idée du bonheur aux dix-huitième siècle*. Paris: Armand Colin, 1960.
Maza, Sarah. "Le Tribunal de la nation: Les mémoires judiciares et l'opinion publique à la fin de l'ancien régime," *Annales: ESC* 42, no. 1 (1987): 73–90.
Metzger, Hélène. *Les Doctrines chimiques en France au début du xviie à la fin du xviiie siècle*. Paris: Presses Universitaires de France, 1923.
———. *Newton, Stahl, Boerhaave et la doctrine chimique*. Paris: Librairie Felix Alcan, 1930.
Meyer, Jean. "L'Enquête de l'Académie de médecine sur les epidémies, 1774–94." *Annales: ESC* 21, no. 4 (1966): 729–49.
Miller, Genevieve. *The Adoption of Inoculation for Smallpox in England and France*. Philadelphia: University of Pennsylvania Press, 1957.
Multhauf, Robert. *The Origins of Chemistry*. New York: Watts, 1966.
Naville, Pierre. *D'Holbach et la philosophie scientifique au xviiie siècle*. 2d ed. Paris: Gallimard, 1967.
O'Malley, C. D., ed. *The History of Medical Education*. Los Angeles: University of California Press, 1970.
Pagel, Walter. *Paracelsus: An Introduction to Philosophical Medicine in the Era of the Renaissance*. Basel: S. Karger, 1958.
———. "The Religious and Philosophical Aspects of van Helmont's Science." *Bulletin of the History of Medicine*. Supplement no. 2. Baltimore: Johns Hopkins University Press, 1944.
Pappas, John. "Berthier's *Journal de Trévoux* and the Philosophes." *Voltaire Studies* 3 (1957): 1–240.
———. *Voltaire and d'Alembert*. Bloomington: Indiana University Press, 1962.
———. "Voltaire et la guerre civile des philosophes." *Revue d'histoire litteraire de la France* 61 (Oct.–Dec. 1961): 525–49.
Paulson, Ronald. *The Fictions of Satire*. Baltimore: Johns Hopkins University Press, 1967.
Paulson, William. *Enlightenment, Romanticism, and the Blind in France*. Princeton: Princeton University Press, 1987.
Picavet, François. *La Mettrie et la critique allemande*. Paris: Félix Alcan, 1889.
Poritzky, Julien E. *Julien Offray de La Mettrie, sein Leben und seine Werke*. Berlin: Ferd. Dummlers Verlagsbuchhandlung, 1900.
Proust, Jacques. *Diderot et l'Encyclopédie*. Paris: Armand Colin, 1967.
———. *L'Encyclopédie*. Paris: Armand Colin, 1965.
Ramsey, Matthew. *Professional and Popular Medicine in France, 1770–1830: The Social World of Medical Practice*. Cambridge: Cambridge University Press, 1988.

Rather, Leland J. *Mind and Body in Eighteenth-Century Medicine. A Study Based on Jerome Gaub's "de regimine mentis."* London: Wellcome Historical Medical Library, 1965.

Riesman, David. *Thomas Sydenham, Clinician.* New York: Praeger, 1926.

Rigal, Jeanne. *La Communauté des maîtres-chirurgiens jurés de Paris au xviie et au xviiie siècles.* Paris: Vigot Frères, 1936.

Risse, Guenther. *Hospital Life in Enlightenment Scotland.* Cambridge: Cambridge University Press, 1986.

Ritterbush, Philip. *Overtures to Biology: The Speculations of Eighteenth-Century Naturists.* New Haven: Yale University Press, 1964.

Roe, Shirley. *Matter, Life, and Generation: Eighteenth-Century Embryology and the Haller-Wolff Debate.* Cambridge: Cambridge University Press, 1981.

Roger, Jacques. *Les Sciences de la vie dans la pensée française du xviiie siècle.* Paris: Armand Colin, 1963.

Roggerone, Giuseppe A. *Controilluminismo: Saggio su La Mettrie ed Helvetius.* 2 vols. Lecce: Edizioni Milella, 1975.

Rorty, Amelia Oksenberg, ed. *Essays on Descartes's Meditations.* Berkeley: University of California Press, 1987.

Rosenfield, Leonore Cohen. *From Beast Machine to Man-Machine: Animal Soul in French Letters from Descartes to La Mettrie.* New Haven: Yale University Press, 1968.

Rothschuh, Karl. *The History of Physiology.* Translated by Guenther Risse. Huntington, N.Y.: Robert Krieger Co., 1973.

Schofield, Robert. *Mechanism and Materialism: British Natural Philosophy in an Age of Reason.* Princeton: Princeton University Press, 1970.

Seidel, Michael. *Satiric Inheritance: Rabelais to Sterne.* Princeton: Princeton University Press, 1979.

Smith, D. W. *Helvétius: A Study in Persecution.* Oxford: Clarendon Press, 1965.

Soffer, Walter. *From Science to Subjectivity: An Interpretation of Descartes's Meditations.* New York: Greenwood Press, 1987.

Spallanzani, Maria Franca. "Lo 'scandalo' di La Mettrie." *Rivista di filosofia* 69, no. 10 (1978): 119–28.

Spink, John S. *French Free Thought from Gassendi to Voltaire.* London: Athlone Press, 1960.

Staum, Martin. *Cabanis: Enlightenment and Medical Philosophy in the French Revolution.* Princeton: Princeton University Press, 1980.

Strugnell, Anthony. *Diderot's Politics: A Study of the Evolution of Diderot's Political Thought after the Encyclopédie.* The Hague: Martinus Nijhoff, 1973.

Talmon, Jacob Leib. *The Origins of Totalitarian Democracy.* New York: Praeger, 1960.

Taton, René, ed. *L'Organization et diffusion des sciences en France.* Paris: Hermann, 1964.

Temkin, Oswei. "The Classical Roots of Glisson's Doctrine of Irritation," *Bulletin of the History of Medicine* 38 (July–Aug. 1964): 297–328.

Thomas, Keith. *Man and the Natural World: A History of the Modern Sensibility.* New York: Pantheon, 1983.

Thomson, Ann. *Materialism and Society in the Mid-Eighteenth Century: La Mettrie's "Discours préliminaire."* Geneva: Librairie Droz, 1981.

———. "Quatre lettres inédits," *Dix-huitième siècle* 7 (1975): 12–18.

Van Kley, Dale. *The Damiens Affair and the Unraveling of the Ancien Régime.* Princeton: Princeton University Press, 1984.

Vartanian, Aram. *Diderot and Descartes.* Princeton: Princeton University Press, 1953.

———. "La Mettrie, Diderot, and Sexology in the Enlightenment." In *Essays in the Age of Enlightenment in Honor of Ira O. Wade,* edited by Jean Macray, 347–67. Geneva: Droz, 1977.

———. *La Mettrie's "L'Homme machine": A Study in the Origins of an Idea.* Princeton: Princeton University Press, 1960.

———. "Le Philosophe selon La Mettrie." *Dix-huitième siècle* (Jan. 1969): 161–78.

———. "Man-Machine from the Greeks to the Computer." *Dictionary of the History of Ideas.* 5 vols. Edited by Philip Weiner. New York: Scribner's, 1973–74.

———. "Trembley's Polyp: La Mettrie and Eighteenth-Century French Materialism." *Journal of the History of Ideas* 11 (Sept. 1950): 259–86.

Verbeek, Theo. *"Traité de l'âme" de La Mettrie.* Edited with commentary. 2 vols. Utrecht: OMI-Grafisch Bedrijf, 1988.

Vess, David. *Medical Revolution in France, 1789–1796.* Gainesville, Fla.: University Presses, 1975.

Wade, Ira O. *The Clandestine Organization and Diffusion of Philosophic Ideas in France from 1700 to 1750.* Princeton: Princeton University Press, 1938.

Wellman, Kathleen. "La Mettrie's *Institutions de médecine:* A Reinterpretation of the Boerhaavian Legacy." *Janus* 72, no. 4 (1985): 283–304.

Wilson, Arthur. *Diderot, The Testing Years, 1713–1759.* New York: Oxford University Press, 1957.

Wolfe, David E. "Sydenham and Locke on the Limits of Anatomy." *Bulletin of the History of Medicine* 35 (May–June 1961): 200–218.

Worcester, David. *The Art of Satire.* Cambridge, Mass.: Harvard University Press, 1940.

Yolton, John. "French Materialist Disciples of Locke." *Journal of the History of Philosophy* 25, no. 1 (Jan. 1987): 83–104.

———. *Locke and French Materialism.* Oxford: Clarendon Press, 1991.

———. *Thinking Matter: Materialism in Eighteenth-Century Britain.* Minneapolis: University of Minnesota Press, 1983.

Index

Newton, Isaac, 61, 73, 126, 175, 243, 282
Newtonianism, 72, 282; Boerhaave and, 72–73
Nuck, Anton, 65

Ordinance of 1724, 18, 20, 22, 24, 29
Ordinance of 1743, 30

Palissot, Claude, 277
Pamphlet war between doctors and surgeons, 10–13, 20–33; La Mettrie's involvement in, 40–41, 57. *See also* Doctors; Surgeons
Paracelsians, 112
Paracelsus, Theophrastus, 63, 81, 112, 186
Pascal, Blaise, 151, 200–201, 314 n.68
Passions, 157–58
Patin, Guy, 51, 113
People, the: La Mettrie and, 257–59; the philosophes and, 257–59
Perrault, Claude, 195
Philip, Duke of Orleans, 19
"Le Philosophe," 258, 270
Philosophes: the Church and, 253; La Mettrie allies with, 248, 251; La Mettrie's definition of, 249, 262–66, 269–70; La Mettrie differs from, 259–61; La Mettrie uses arguments of, 254–60; response to La Mettrie, 213, 239, 275–76; on society, 226
Philosophy: La Mettrie praises, 249, 254; medicine and, 250
Physicians: authority, 211–12; moral role, 199–200, 224. *See also* Doctors; *Médecin-philosophe*
Physiology: eighteenth-century French, 126–32; La Mettrie and, 132–34
Pitcairn, Archibald, 63, 111
Plato, 139, 146
Pliny, 164
Premier chirurgien, 19
Premier médecin, 17–18, 19
Privilege: La Mettrie's attack on, 52–53, 59

Procope, Michel, 46
Public health: La Mettrie's concern with, 52, 57, 86, 89–98, 111

Quesnay, François, 14

Ramsey, Matthew, 288 n.2, 289 n.4, 290 n.11, 295 n.43
Rau, Jacob, 65
Réaumur, René Antoine Ferchault de, 203
Remorse, 197, 220–22, 238; La Mettrie refutes Descartes's theory of, 197–98; philosophes and, 220
Roger, Jacques, 204
Rousseau, Jean-Jacques, 1, 208, 236, 242; comparison with La Mettrie, 216–17, 279

Sade, Donatien Alphonse François, Comte (called Marquis) de, 4, 237
Saint-Cyr, Guy de, 277
Sainte-Beuve, Charles Augustin, 273
Sapere aude, 146
Satire, 43; La Mettrie's medical satires, 34, 36, 38–39, 47, 51
Saunderson, Nicholas, 164
Scholastics, 33, 148, 182, 229
Senac, Jean, 37
Seneca, 214, 230, 232, 233, 235
Sensorium commune, 145, 153, 159
Skepticism: La Mettrie and, 205, 206
Smallpox, 85, 92–95, 98–99; Sydenham's treatment of, 77–78
Society: La Mettrie's notion of, 216–20, 226, 228, 264–66; the philosophes' theory of, 218–20, 267
Soul: and eighteenth-century physiology, 127, 128, 129, 131, 230–31; La Mettrie and, 139, 141, 146, 186; La Mettrie's critique of Descartes's view of, 178–79; physical nature of, 189, 190, 192, 195, 202
Spinoza, Baruch, 61
Stahl, Georg Ernst, 116, 159, 194
Stenon, Nicolaus, 192
Stoicism, 232–33
Stoics, 232–33

Surgeons: arguments in the pamphlet war, 23–27, 28–29; education of, 18, 31; Enlightenment and, 13, 25, 29, 30, 32–33; history of, 13–20; La Mettrie's support for, 7, 35–36, 40, 42, 43; social status and role, 16–20, 26, 30
Surgeons of the long robe, 13
Surgeons of the short robe, 13. *See also* Barber-surgeons
Swieten, Gerard van, 63, 84
Sydenham, Thomas, 13, 72, 86, 98, 103; Boerhaave and, 75–77; chemistry and, 113; La Mettrie's critique of, 87–89, 90; Locke and, 79, 298 n.33; opposition to the medical establishment, 77–78
Sylva, Jean-Baptiste, 16, 45, 46
Sylvius de la Boë, François, 63, 69, 113, 116

Tabula rasa, 162
Talmon, Jacob L., 4, 247
Theologian, 141; La Mettrie's attack on the authority of, 186, 212, 252–53
Thomson, Ann, 4, 5, 251, 252, 318 n.2, 319 n.10, 319 n.18, 319 n.19, 320 n.45
Transformism, 204–11
Two-book theory of knowledge, 186

Variolation, 93–94. *See also* Inoculation
Vartanian, Aram, 4, 183, 185, 204, 273, 287 n.2, 296 n.58, 310 n.4, 311 n.21, 311 n.22, 312 n.24, 312 n.32; interpretation of La Mettrie and Descartes, 172, 175–77
Vascular injection experiments, 66
Venereal disease, 27–29, 40–41, 85, 86, 91
Verbeek, Theo, 4, 288 n.5, 299 n.1, 305 n.2, 306 n.27, 307 n.44, 309 n.78, 312 n.7
Vertigo, 85, 99–105
Vita contemplativa, 234
Vitalism, 159
Voltaire, François Marie Arouet de, 1, 43, 51, 135, 231, 240–42, 253, 257–58, 307 n.38, 322 n.13, 322 n.14; *Essai sur les moeurs*, 219; "Letter on Locke," 150, 253, 282; role as philosophe, 274–78
Volupté, 224, 225, 235–37
Volupté d'esprit, 233

Will, 158–59, 179
Willis, Thomas, 114, 121, 191, 195

Yolton, John, 150, 305 n.2

About the Author

Kathleen Wellman is Assistant Professor of History
at Southern Methodist University.